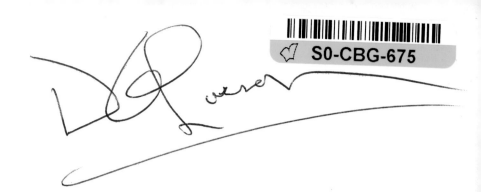

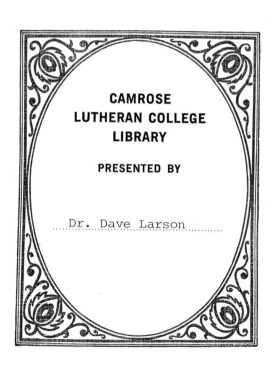

All About Allergy

Also by M. Coleman Harris, M.D., and
Norman Shure, M.D.

PRACTICAL ALLERGY

SENSITIVITY CHEST DISEASES (EDITORS)

All About Allergy

•

M. Coleman Harris, M. D.
and
Norman Shure, M. D.

•

Prentice-Hall, Inc., Englewood Cliffs, N.J.

ALL ABOUT ALLERGY, by M. Coleman Harris, M. D. and Norman Shure, M. D.

© 1969 by M. Coleman Harris and Norman Shure

13-022186-4

Library of Congress Catalog Card Number: 69-13718

Printed in the United States of America • *T*

Prentice-Hall International, Inc., London
Prentice-Hall of Australia, Pty. Ltd., Sydney
Prentice-Hall of Canada, Ltd., Toronto
Prentice-Hall of India Private Ltd., New Delhi
Prentice-Hall of Japan, Inc., Tokyo

Second printing...... December, 1969

Acknowledgment is made for permission to reprint material from
the following works:

Practical Allergy by M. Coleman Harris and Norman Shure. Reprinted
by permission of the publisher, F. A. Davis Company.

Sensitivity Chest Diseases, M. Coleman Harris and Norman Shure, editors.

Reprinted by permission of the publisher, F. A. Davis Company.

To our patients
whose perceptive inquiries
have stimulated and encouraged us to write
this book

Foreword

Why another book on allergy? Over the past thirty years several books have been written as well as innumerable pamphlets by, among others, the American Medical Association, agencies of the Federal Government, life insurance companies, pharmaceutical firms, and the Allergy Foundation of America. Yet in our combined medical practices of more than fifty-five years, we have been asked repeatedly about general problems in allergy and have spent thousands of hours explaining them to patients. People are now more generally knowledgeable and are no longer satisfied with elementary texts. Allergy, moreover, is no longer confined merely to hay fever, asthma, hives, and eczema. In becoming a broader subject it is involving the lives of larger numbers of our population.

Written for the intelligent layman, *All About Allergy* is an explicit and scientific probing of subjects previously not covered or inadequately described. With explanations of the newer theories we hope to provide an understanding of what allergy is, how it develops, and what can be done about it. We discuss the diseases that are currently attributed either to allergy alone or to allergy in combination with other causes. We also examine such pioneering research subjects as the problem of the body's "rejection" mechanism in transplantation of vital organs.

We have included the practical facets of allergy disease, such as those dealing with hay fever, hives, eczema, and asthma. These readily observable diseases of allergy will be discussed in all their important aspects: diagnosis, treatment, prevention, and cure. Thus is included what the doctor can do for the patient, and what the patient can do for himself. The information discussed encompasses the geographical location and the identification of plants producing allergy symptoms, the source of hidden constituents in foods, and the nature of the common inhalant substances that are likely to be allergenic. Sample diets to detect

vii

food allergy are presented. The composition of antihistamines, creams, lotions, ointments, compounds, and nose drops that are widely advertised and readily purchased at a drugstore without a doctor's prescription are tabulated and compared with those requiring a doctor's prescription.

The current technical explosion has brought into existence many new chemicals and materials to which people are allergic. Some of these have been determined; others are suspect; but for all of them is needed clarification of the symptoms they produce and the measures that can be taken to eliminate their reactivity and to relieve the afflicted individual.

Numerous prescription drugs have been developed for use by doctors within the last decade or so, and among them are the antihistamines and the cortisone products. Knowledge of how these drugs act—their value, as well as the side effects or bad reactions which may occur if the drugs are taken in improper dosage or for too long a time—is a matter of concern to every patient using them. Those drugs which are prone to cause adverse side effects are listed, and the common reactions they produce are described.

In addition, emotional problems can be a major factor in allergy diseases, and a clear understanding of their influence requires unbiased discussion

We also describe the newer forms of injection treatment and measure them by the time-honored multiple-injection form.

Unusual allergy diseases, like the dire effects that follow the bite of stinging insects in individuals who are sensitive to them, will be presented, along with information for the reader on how to cope with them.

However, we do not necessarily advocate or recommend the use of any of the treatments or drugs mentioned in this book. Our purpose is only to report what is being used.

We acknowledge our indebtedness to F. A. Davis Company, medical publishers, who have given us permission to use photos, tables and other material from our other text books.

M. Coleman Harris, M.D.
Norman Shure, M.D.

Contents

Chapter One	A Short History of Allergy............	1
Chapter Two	Fundamentals of the Allergic Reaction....	8
Chapter Three	The Initial Consultation..............	19
Chapter Four	Diagnostic Allergy Tests..............	30
Chapter Five	Pollen in Allergy...................	43
Chapter Six	Inhalant Causes of Allergy Other Than Pollen................	61
Chapter Seven	The Injection Treatment of Allergy Diseases	80
Chapter Eight	Food Allergy......................	94
Chapter Nine	Drug Reactions....................	120
Chapter Ten	Reactions to Biting and Stinging Insects...	139
Chapter Eleven	Hay Fever—Seasonal and Perennial......	149
Chapter Twelve	Bronchial Asthma..................	173
Chapter Thirteen	Allergy of the Skin.................	207
Chapter Fourteen	Physical Allergy...................	225
Chapter Fifteen	Less Frequent Manifestations of Allergy...	233
Chapter Sixteen	Occupational Allergy................	261
Chapter Seventeen	Newer Aspects of Allergy.............	285
Chapter Eighteen	The Emotional Factor in Allergy........	299
Chapter Nineteen	What To Do About Your Allergy........	307
Chapter Twenty	Unconventional Treatment of Allergy Diseases..................	322
	Glossary of Allergy Terms.............	341
	Index...........................	361

All About Allergy

Chapter One

A Short History of Allergy
2641 B.C. — A.D. 1920

EARLY DESCRIPTIONS

Contrary to popular opinion, allergy was recognized and mentioned in antiquity, although not in the same terms in which it is understood today. Deciphered Egyptian hieroglyphic tablets traced to the year 2641 B.C. indicate that King Menes died from the bite of a hornet. The vivid description of his symptoms correspond with our present-day knowledge of the effects of stinging insect bites on susceptible or allergic persons.

The Roman poet and philosopher Lucretius, who lived in the first century before the birth of Christ, seemed to describe allergy in his aphorism, "What is one man's meat is another man's poison." Although now a cliché, the statement suggests that an individual allergic to milk, for example, may become violently ill after drinking it, while others may drink the same liquid with impunity.

Migraine, characteristically described as a one-sided headache accompanied by nausea and vomiting and commonly referred to as a "sick headache," may be due to allergy. In the writings of Aretaeus of Cappadocia, dated A.D. 110, can be found an excellent description of this headache with the characteristic symptoms of a slow onset, a premonitory phase with lightning flashes before the eyes, followed by headache and upset stomach. Aretaeus also gave a detailed report of attacks of shortness of breath, coughing, and wheezing — obviously asthma. Botallus in 1565, writing on the duty of a doctor to his patient, confirmed the observation of the famed Greek physician Galen that some people sneeze in the presence of certain flowers. "I know men," Botallus wrote, "who, at the smell of roses, were seized with a loathing, as to be subject to headaches, or a sneezing fit, or a running of the nostrils, so that for two days it could not be stopped. ... I know, likewise, of a woman who at the smell of must, would fall over, collapse, ... be forced to vomit, or have a severe headache ... therefore doctors should refrain

1

from using this perfume, or any other that may affect the patient." His admonition is as pertinent today as it was four centuries ago.

Even the specific treatment of allergy disease was discussed in early literature. The Father of Medicine, Hippocrates, who lived from 460 B.C. to 357 B.C., wrote in his 64th Aphorism, "It is a bad thing to give milk to persons having sick headaches." This has been interpreted as indicating milk allergy as a cause of migraine.

In the Babylonian Talmud is a description of a method to build up the tolerance of individuals who suffer from stomach and intestinal distress after eating eggs. The procedure described is essentially the same as the one recommended today for desensitizing, or building a tolerance, to egg allergy. This, very simply, is the concept of eating a very small amount of egg and then at regular and specified intervals increasing the quantity eaten. Such a procedure is currently used for many foods, especially those that cannot be eliminated from one's diet or are difficult to avoid.

MODERN HISTORY

In 1819 the London physician John Bostock, a victim of severe hay fever and asthma, wrote and published a meticulous account of his symptoms in a treatise aptly titled, "Case of Periodic Affection of the Eyes and Chest." Nine years later he wrote another treatise, "Of Catarrhus Aestivus or Summer Catarrh." In that publication he used the term "hay fever," adopting the term applied to the disease because it occurred during the haying season. The term, of course, is a misnomer because symptoms do not include fever, and contact with hay is not the cause. Although in the nineteenth century the term "fever" indicated any indisposition or illness, we continue to use the name "hay fever," wrong as it may be. While Dr. Bostock recognized that his symptoms occurred during the summer months, he did not connect them with summer plants. Instead, he concentrated on temperature changes, particularly the effect of heat, and wrote at great length about the direct rays of the sun.

It remained for Dr. W. R. Kirkman in 1852 to demonstrate the true cause of hay fever by performing an experiment on himself. A day or two before Christmas he collected some pollen of sweet vernal grass in his hothouse, rubbed it on his hands, and sniffed it. A severe hay fever attack resulted, and for an hour he suffered paroxysms of sneezing. It is strange that despite Dr. Kirkman's published *Case of Hay Fever,* physicians years later were still inclined to regard hay fever as caused by vegetable matter in the atmosphere, "bright, hot, dusty sunshine," and "heat."

Dr. Charles Harrison Blackley of Manchester, England, also a hay fever sufferer, began experimenting on himself in 1859 and wrote a scholarly book on his findings to reconcile most of the earlier theories with the one he proposed and which, incidentally, is still accepted. Blackley's great contribution was the description of a pollen test he had performed on himself in a rather crude fashion, but a test roughly similar to the type of allergy skin tests performed today. He reported the appearance of the typical hive that developed at the site of the test (with which allergic patients who have undergone such skin testing are very familiar):

> Whilst I was suffering from my usual attack of hay fever during the summer of 1865, as much pollen as could be obtained from two anthers of *Lolium italicum* was applied to the center of the anterior surface of one forearm after the skin had been abraded as in the ordinary method of vaccinating. ... The center of the other forearm was treated in exactly the same way except that no pollen was applied to it. The scratching with the lancet raised a wheal such as seen in urticaria or in stinging with nettles. In a few minutes after the pollen had been applied the abraded spot began to itch intensely; the part immediately around the abrasion began to swell.... The arm to which no pollen had been applied did not exhibit any sign of swelling or irritation.

Just as Dr. Blackley proved that the cause of his summer hay fever was Italian ryegrass, Dr. Morril Wyman of Cambridge, Massachusetts, identified ragweed as the cause of the characteristic August to October hay fever, the plague of most hay fever sufferers in the United States.

MODERN THEORY

Although the symptoms and causes of allergy disease had now been described in detail, there still was no hint of the underlying mechanisms involved. Why should the body react in a disturbed manner to certain substances? Why did only some people have the symptoms while others did not, even though they all encountered the same substance? Why were the symptoms so similar, although the "cause," or contact, was different?

When Dr. Clemens von Pirquet suggested the term "allergy" in 1906, it was in the midst of an important era in medical history. Bacteria had been found and isolated as the cause of infectious disease. In 1893 von Behring had introduced diphtheria antitoxin, a substance which, it seemed, almost magically neutralized the effects of the lethal products of diphtheria organisms. Not long after, a similar antitoxin was found for tetanus, another disease which almost invariably had been fatal. Attention now became focused on preventive as well as curative measures.

But there were confusing results from the experiments being performed. First, the antitoxins, although intended to protect the patient from the diseases for which they were administered, often produced symptoms totally different from those of the diseases, and at times even more severe. Furthermore, attempts to prevent a disease by the use of serums occasionally produced a similar peculiar reaction or chain of symptoms.

The decreased sensitivity (immunity) to a disease produced by the injected serum would often render the patient more sensitive (hypersensitive) to some component in the material used. But interestingly, the symptoms usually had their onset only after the second injection of the serum. There had been recorded indications of such reactions with reference to smallpox vaccine as far back as 1798. We now term this an "accelerated reaction" to the vaccination. In 1839 Francois Magendie had also observed that rabbits who several times were given injections of the liquid portion of dog's blood (serum) eventually showed strange and unusual reactions. Similar observations were being recorded all over the world but without adequate explanation.

The precise explanation must be credited to Dr. Charles Robert Richet in the years between 1898 and 1902. He and his associates were cruising on the Indian Ocean with the Prince of Monaco, studying the cause of the hives produced by the Portuguese man-of-war, a species of nettlefish, or jellyfish. After returning to Paris, Richet studied the sea anemone, another variety of stinging nettle, on the assumption that there was a poisonous (toxic) substance present in the nettlefish family which produced the hives, as is true of the *urtica,* or nettle plant.

Upon administering the toxin to dogs, he found that the initial injection was completely harmless. Subsequent injections, however, in many cases produced severe and sometimes fatal symptoms. This was what others had vaguely noted but had not pursued in further studies. Richet continued his experiments and was impressed with the fact that they could almost be reproduced at will. He concluded, first, that the initial injection of a foreign substance into an animal is usually harmless, but second, that when the same material is reinjected into the same animal in similar or even smaller doses, severe or even fatal symptoms can occur, and, finally, that an interval of several days must elapse between the first and subsequent injections for the reaction to take place. To this reaction or series of events, Richet gave the term *anaphylaxis* to indicate lack of protection as opposed to *prophylaxis,* the increase of protection.

For the standardization of diphtheria antitoxin it was customary at that time to inject both the diphtheria toxin and the diphtheria antitoxin into guinea pigs. Dr. von Pirquet observed that the guinea pigs developed the same symptoms that had been described by Richet in his original experiments with the sea anemone. It was a stroke of ingenuity for him to associate these symptoms in animals with the peculiar symptoms evidenced by humans following the use of protective serums, and thus explain the origins and anticipate or predict additional alterations in bodily functions.

Antitoxin was then manufactured, as it is now, by injecting the actual toxin into a horse, because the defense mechanism of a horse is capable of producing large amounts of antitoxin. The protecting material, therefore, contained elements of horse serum protein, and it was determined that the horse protein produced the symptoms in guinea pigs and in humans. The paradoxically increased sensitivity with unusual and peculiar symptoms was not caused, therefore, by hypersensitivity to the disease but by an induced sensitivity to horse serum, a foreign substance.

Von Pirquet objected to Richet's limited term *anaphylaxis* and consequently proposed in 1906 the more general term *allergy* to indicate deviation from the original state.

> I propose the term, Allergy: Allos implies deviation from
> the original state, from the behavior of normal individuals. . . .
> A foreign substance which by one or more applications

> stimulates the organism of a change in reaction is an Allergen.
> . . . Among the allergens should be included the poison of
> mosquito and bees . . . the pollen producing hay fever . . . the
> urticaria-producing substance of strawberries and crabs.

Not long after, the knowledge of this phenomenon, allergy, was
applied. In 1905, W. P. Dunbar of Hamburg, Germany, had attempted
to manufacture an antitoxin to pollen which would counteract the
symptoms of hay fever, then thought to be due to some poison contained
in the plant. Dunbar's procedure was to inject pollen into horses to
produce an antitoxin, just as diphtheria was injected into horses to
produce a diphtheria antitoxin. His recommendation was to use this
"pollen antitoxin" locally in the nose. W. Weichardt in 1906 had
attempted a similar production of pollen antitoxin by feeding large
amounts of the plant that was suspected of causing trouble to cattle. But
as von Pirquet disclosed later, these methods of prophylaxis were based
upon an entirely wrong premise. The correct method does not involve an
intermediate animal; it consists of administering the foreign material
directly to the patient, in small but increasing doses, at frequent and
regular intervals.

Drs. Leonard Noon and John Freeman of London must be credited
with the development of the allergy injection treatment as we now know
it. They began their work in 1911, and — except for refinements in
technique and in the production of allergy extracts, developed mostly by
American clinicians — their treatment is still important. Among the
American physicians who participated in the improvement of this form
of therapy were Drs. Robert A. Cooke and Albert Vander Veer, Jr., of
New York. In 1916 they also were the first to suggest that the tendency
to become sensitized is inherited in accordance with the Mendelian law,
as a dominent characteristic.

Current and experimental developments in allergy are discussed in
subsequent chapters.

SUMMARY

Clinical allergy as we know it has existed and has been recorded from
antiquity. The description of the death of King Menes in 2641 B.C. after
he was bitten by a hornet corresponds with our present knowledge of the

effects of stinging insect bites on susceptible or allergic persons. Lucretius' aphorism, "What is one man's meat is another man's poison," is often quoted as descriptive of allergy. In the Babylonian Talmud there is even advice on building up tolerance to egg for those who react to it with stomach or intestinal distress.

Hay fever and asthma were accurately described by John Bostock of England in 1819. Although he recognized that his symptoms occurred only in the summer, he had no idea of their cause. It was not until Dr. Blackley in 1859 performed a crude allergy skin test with Italian rye-grass that the connection with vegetation was noted and proved.

Despite many earlier observations on the causes of allergy symptoms, it was in 1902 or thereabouts that several French scientists, studying the cause of hives produced by certain fish, provided the essentials necessary for a more thorough understanding of sensitivity diseases. This was at about the time that diphtheria and tetanus antitoxins were being used and were causing incomprehensible reactions.

Treatment of hay fever and asthma due to pollen was begun by Drs. Noon and Freeman of London in 1911, and except for modifications and refinements, their method constitutes our present-day "desensitization treatment."

Chapter Two

Fundamentals of the Allergic Reaction

When the average person humorously uses the word "allergic" to indicate a feeling of antipathy or repugnance, it may be considered in poor taste, but it accurately portrays the general characteristic of allergic reactions and symptoms. Translating this emotional reaction into organic reactions or symptoms, one might simply infer that allergy is an unusual sensitivity to certain substances. But this is not entirely true. For medical purposes the definition must be clarified; otherwise, many changes in the body would be included which are not true evidences of allergy.

DEFINITION OF ALLERGY

Webster defines allergy as "the altered degree of susceptibility caused by a primary inoculation or treatment, as with a specific germ or foreign substance, and manifested in reaction to a subsequent inoculation or treatment with the same thing. . . ." This long definition is accurate but is best reduced to this less complex statement: Allergy is an acquired, specific, altered capability to react, based on an antigen-antibody reaction.

Acquired indicates that allergy symptoms do not under ordinary circumstances occur with the initial use of the substance which subsequently can produce the symptoms. For example, a very common allergy is poison ivy dermatitis or rash, caused by contact with the oil from the plant of a particular species of ivy. Similar reactions occur after brushing against poison oak or poison sumac varieties. This is acquired. Previous contact or some exposure must have taken place; perhaps unknowingly, as is often the case.

Another common example is that of the late-summer hay fever

sufferer who moves from the eastern portion of the United States to an area west of the Rocky Mountains. He will likely be free of symptoms after the move because of the different plants that grow in the new location. In the course of time, however, he is likely to acquire a sensitivity to the plants of his new surroundings and will eventually develop symptoms of allergy.

The term *specific* is necessary in the definition of allergy because the symptoms, although variable—depending upon the person and the part of the body involved in the allergic reaction—are the result of a definitive, special, or "specific" contact. If a person should develop hives from eating strawberries, he will not necessarily get hives from eating grapes, chocolate, or any other particular food; specifically the consumption of strawberries is required for the development of hives. The same principle applies to inhaled substances. If a patient develops hay fever from inhaling pollen of the ragweed plant, he will not have symptoms from inhaling house dust unless, of course, he is also allergic to house dust. Although the symptoms may vary from hay fever to hives or to asthma, the cause must be the same or "specific."

Altered which refers to the inherent constitutional difference in people, indicates the changed reaction which the researcher von Pirquet noted and described sixty years ago when he was injecting for the second time his protective serum to prevent disease in some people. Just as in von Pirquet's experiments all people did not react peculiarly to the second dose of the serums he administered, neither do all people develop the symptoms of an allergy disease from repeated contact with substances which the average person ordinarily encounters daily. Most of us breathe house dust, plant pollen, animal hair, and similar substances without any harmful effects; most of us can eat foods with impunity. Yet a certain number, perhaps 10 percent of the population or more, display unusual, unexpected, or "altered" reactions.

The term *capability to react*, rather than the simpler term "reaction," is used in the definition to indicate that this capability must be present before an allergic response can take place, even though no symptoms have ever occurred. For the common allergies the "capability to react" is in many instances a nonspecific inheritance. One's parents may have been allergic to cat hair, but the offspring may be allergic to foods and develop eczema. What is inherited is the *tendency* to be allergic and the underlying capability to react under given circumstances. Or the tendency may not be inherited at all.

Then there is the group of sympton-free allergic persons who may be so because, among other reasons, they may never come in contact with the particular substance which might initiate the allergic reaction; or they may maintain good resistance; or they may not come in contact with sufficient amounts of allergen for a sufficiently long time. Although this is not the entire answer, it accounts for some people not developing "allergy" until late in life. However, they were always "capable."

ANTIGENS

The *antigen-antibody reaction* is the key to the underlying mechanism of the entire allergic reaction. *Antigens* are substances that enter the body and start off the chain of circumstances which results in the allergic reaction and subsequent allergy symptoms. Pollen, foods, house dust, molds, and chicken, duck, and goose feathers are common antigens. There are many, many more. The term "allergen" is sometimes used as a synonym for antigen.

Antigens are large molecular substances, usually proteins, although starch and oily material can be antigenic as well. These substances may be introduced into the body in a variety of ways: by ingestion, inhalation, injection, or by absorption through contact with the skin. Antigens are usually considered complete or incomplete. A complete antigen is one which can produce antibodies *and* unite with them to produce an observable reaction. Incomplete antigens cannot fulfill both these requirements.

ANTIBODIES

Antibodies are a part of a protein substance in the blood produced in response to antigen stimulation. Subsequently, when the antigen, on reintroduction to the body, joins with the antibody, a series of events occurs which results in allergy symptoms. These *antibodies* are specific for the *antigen*. There are some for pollen, some for certain foods, others for anything one can be allergic to. They therefore explain the *specificity* aspect of the concept. Were these antibodies to remain in the bloodstream, little or no harm might be done, but they are released and tend to attach themselves to certain body tissue cells such as the nose and bronchial tubes. When the identical antigen which produced the specific antibody enters the body again, it unites with this antibody and joins in an antigen-antibody reaction. (This mechanism is accepted by most allergists although it is not always demonstrable by laboratory means.) As a result of this reaction or union, several chemicals such as histamine and similar substances are liberated at the spot where the antigen and antibody united. These chemicals produce such allergy symptoms as hay fever and asthma.

HAPTENS (INCOMPLETE ANTIGENS)

There are some small molecular substances which in their natural form cannot be considered complete antigens, yet they are known to be involved in causing allergy symptoms. This class of substances is known as *incomplete antigens,* or *haptens.* Simple chemicals and drugs are examples. By themselves they are not capable of manufacturing antibodies and leading to an allergic reaction, but when a hapten hooks on to a protein within the body, a chemical bond is formed which is capable of provoking antibodies. It has now become a complete antigen and then may enter into antigen-antibody relationship, resulting in allergy symptoms. The interesting point about this union is that the antibody produced is specific for the hapten rather than for the protein portion to which the hapten became attached to make a complete antigen. Once the antibody is produced, the antigen which must enter the body subsequently to produce allergy symptoms must contain the simple chemical, the hapten. The hapten may be compared to a hitchhiker and the person who gives him a ride is really not important except as a means of transportation.

SHOCK TISSUE

The shock tissue, part of the shock organ, is the place where the antigen-antibody reaction takes place. When this shock tissue happens to be the lining of the inside of the nose, hay fever or its equivalent results. If the shock tissue is the bronchial tubes, symptoms of bronchial asthma will result. If the skin is the shock tissue, hives, eczema, or a rash of some sort may develop. Abdominal cramps, eye trouble, heart irregularities, and numerous other less common manifestations of allergy may develop, depending upon the shock organ or tissue involved.

SENSITIZATION

The production of the capacity to react, that is, the capability of the patient to have allergy symptoms, is *sensitization*. An Eskimo, for example, who has lived in an area devoid of poison ivy, but at some point in his life moves south, becomes sensitized by coming in contact with the poison ivy plant. A hay fever victim who moves west of the Rocky Mountains becomes sensitized to an entirely different plant. Sensitization indicates the production of specific antibodies as a result of contact with a new antigen.

ATOPY

Atopy designates allergy in the human, considered in most cases to be hereditary. Underlying the concept of *atopy* is the supposition that people with allergy symptoms have inherent defects in their immunologic reactions and respond abnormally to ordinarily harmless substances. *Anaphylaxis* is the term which is used for artificially induced allergic reactions in the lower animals. Anaphylaxis has a connotation of severity, and its counterpart in the human has been designated as *anaphylactoid reaction*. Many physicians prefer to use the term anaphylaxis to indicate a very severe allergic reaction in either the laboratory animal or the human.

HYPERSENSITIVITY

Hypersensitivity can be considered synonymous with allergy, since the antigen-antibody reaction almost invariably results in allergy symptoms. *Immunity* from disease is also due to an antigen-antibody reaction, but the result is freedom from symptoms of the disease rather than the onset of illness. Both are antigen-antibody reactions, yet one produces symptoms while the other prevents them. The common explanation given for the difference is that in allergy the antibody is of a special kind, usually called a *reagin*. When the antibody (reagin) joins with the antigen, the result of the union is typical allergy symptoms.

On the other hand, if the antigen unites with the usual protective antibody, the result is protection from the disease. A common example is the injection of humans with a serum used for diphtheria. The serum introduced into humans stimulates the formation of antibodies *against* diphtheria, counteracting the disease.

IDIOSYNCRASY: INTOLERANCE

These terms are often erroneously used as synonyms of allergy. It is not true that all apparent allergic reactions are caused by allergy. This is valid only when the antigen-antibody mechanism is involved. Fear of the dark is not an allergy, nor necessarily is intolerance or an idiosyncratic reaction to drugs or medicines—as in the instances of alcohol or quinine, quantities of which may be relatively well or poorly tolerated by different individuals. These variations are usually based on differences in *tolerance* or *idiosyncrasy* rather than on allergy.

SUMMARY OF THE STEPS IN THE ALLERGIC REACTION

The following sequence of events is a resumé of what must occur for the symptoms of allergy to appear:

1. Primary contact with the antigen. This may be by ingestion, inhalation, injection, absorption, or any other means by which antigen can enter the body.

2. Formation of antibodies (reagins) in the bloodstream in response to the entrance of the antigen.

3. The release of antibodies from the bloodstream.

4. Attachment of antibodies to the cells of the shock tissues. (At this point sensitization has taken place.)

5. Reexposure to the specific antigen.

6. Union of the antigen and antibody (antigen-antibody reaction) in the shock tissue.

7. Release of certain chemicals, such as histamine, as a result of the union.

8. Allergy symptoms as a result of the action of the released chemicals on the tissues at the site of the antigen-antibody reaction (the shock tissue).

There are several obvious questions which occur at this point. One is how and why symptoms occur as a result of the antigen-antibody union. The best current explanation is that histamine or other chemicals are released. Their effect on the blood vessels of the skin, on the bronchial muscle, and on the lining of the nasal passages and the bronchial tubes can explain practically all of the allergy symptoms encountered. The efficacy of the antihistamines which people use for certain allergy symptoms attests to the importance of histamine in particular.

THEORY OF EXPLAINING ALLERGY

A specific antigen causes the body of an allergic person to produce an antibody which will react with it and with no other one when it is reintroduced. Since a person is usually not allergic to one thing only, the body manufactures a separate antibody for each antigen. Inasmuch as there are thousands and thousands of substances to which one may be allergic, the body must have a store of all those available so as to be ready to enter into an antigen-antibody reaction when the proper antigen comes along. There are two main theories which suggest how this is accomplished.

It has been amply proved that the antibody is part of a protein fraction found in the body and often measurable in the bloodstream; more specifically it is the gamma globulin fraction. By complex electrical methods it has been shown which fractions of the gamma globulin protein found in the body are primarily involved. The antigen is the largest molecule, most often protein in nature, although it may be starch or fat as well, which enters the body from the outside and combines with this globulin antibody to produce the antigen-antibody (allergic) reaction.

The antigen must exactly interlock with the antibody in order to join with the proper one. This is a unique process and may be understood more easily if one thinks of an antigen as an irregularly shaped three-dimensional object, much like a piece of a jigsaw puzzle. It must fit its counterpart, the complementary piece to which it conforms. Antigens have been described as having "molecular warts" on their surface. Therefore the antibodies must have large holes on the surfaces into which the "warts" can fit. Each antigen to which the person is allergic may be assumed to have a different shape: the animal dander, the weed pollen, egg white, grass pollen, house dust, or the thousands of other possible allergenic materials. Each of these must seek and fit its mate to produce the symptoms of a given allergy. Some allergic individuals may have only the antibodies of a grass or a weed; others may have those of certain foods. Most persons who are allergic harbor specific antibodies of many different substances.

The existence of these antibodies, or reagins, can be demonstrated graphically through *passive transfer* followed by allergy skin tests specific to the antigen. The serum portion of the blood of an allergic individual will contain these antibodies, which are called skin-sensitizing antibodies because they can be transferred to the skin. (For description of technique of passive transfer see Chapter 4.)

THEORIES OF ANTIBODY FORMATION

The two major theories of specific antibody formation relate to whether the antibody has existed as specifically predetermined-shaped globulin particles, each specific to an antigen or, another possibility, whether all the globulin in the body acts like a piece of soft wax or putty, on which each individual antigen makes its exclusive imprint and like a pattern or template leaves a permanent configuration. This is like cutting cookie dough with a specially shaped cutter. The first theory is known as the *clonal selection theory;* the second as the *template theory.*

A *clone* is a family of cells derived from a common ancestor. The clonal selection theory suggests that there are a large number of clones which by inheritance have a predetermined ability to produce specific antibodies. These cells, which become antibodies, achieve their specificity during fetal life, perhaps by mutations (an alteration from one generation to another). Thus, each group of cells having the same specific antibody-producing ability is descended from a cell which underwent a given mutation. The clone has developed the potential for manufacturing antibodies specific to the antigen which joins it. All the antigen needs to do is to meet the clone with the appropriate configuration to fit or to complement it and the proper union is accomplished. The predetermined antibody cell merely waits for a "knock on the door" by the antigen.

In the template theory it is assumed that all of the material within a certain spectrum of globulin is capable of being changed to specific antibodies. There is no hereditary mutation necessary as in the clonal selection theory, merely the presence of the proper specific antigen to "instruct" it, to impress it, or to mold it into the proper configuration.

THE INHERITANCE FACTOR THEORY

Allergists generally agree that there is a strong hereditary factor present in the transmission of allergy disease. However, the exact type and degree is in controversy. Statistics vary according to the investigator but all agree that there is a much greater chance for the child with both parents who are allergic to develop an allergy than there is for the child with only one allergic parent. Similarly the child with bilateral antecedent allergy will develop symptoms earlier in life than the child with one allergic parent. It is interesting to note that allergy has been reported in one identical twin but not in the other so that the hereditary factor in allergy is sometimes confusing.

Of course many individuals do not know their family history of previous illnesses and are likely to give erroneous or misinterpreted information. Also, years ago, many cases of allergy disease were not recognized as such; others may have been termed allergic but the diagnosis not substantiated by proper laboratory tests. Likewise in children it is not uncommon to find evidence of an allergic disease before one has developed in either parent. For these reasons obtaining evidence of a familial history of allergy is often unreliable.

But certain facts are clear. *Direct* transmission of allergy from the mother to her unborn child cannot take place; that is, specific skin-sensitizing antibodies do not pass through the placenta to the fetus. However, an antigen can be passed through the placenta from mother to child during intrauterine life. At birth, an infant is unable to produce its own antibodies. But since the capacity to do so is inherited, when the

antibody-producing mechanism becomes active, symptoms may develop.

There is another concept that heredity is determined by a single pair of genes and is transmitted (by both homozygous and some heterozygous subjects). Still another concept is that more than one pair of genes is involved. The role of the genetic material, DNA (deoxyribonucleic acid), an important part of the cell, is not of special interest to the nontechnical reader. Of much more practical importance is the question of whether allergic individuals should marry and have children. Many young people fear that their offspring will by inheritance most certainly be allergic and perhaps develop bronchial asthma or some other form of allergy disease which might be equally distressing. Our advice to these young people is not to let the fact that either one or both are allergic deter them. Many such couples have perfectly normal children. However, we do advise that when pregnancy occurs, the obstetrician be informed of the family history of allergy. This information is useful also to the pediatrician when the baby arrives, so that he may take proper precautions to prevent as far as possible the allergy tendency from developing into an allergy disease.

SUMMARY

Allergy is best defined as an acquired, specific, altered capability to react to certain substances. This response is due to a definite cellular and chemical reaction within the body known as the *antigen-antibody reaction*. There are specific reasons for the need of the qualifying adjectives in the definition. The reason for the inclusion of the "antigen-antibody reaction" is to differentiate the allergic response from other types of reactions such as those due to certain medicines, which are merely *idiosyncrasies* or an *intolerance*.

There are two theories for the production of antibodies in the body. One, known as the template theory, presupposes that the antibody-producing protein in the body is not predetermined but that the antigen impresses itself on it like a pattern (template) to make it a specific antibody. The clonal, or selective, hypothesis states that the mass of antibody-producing protein is predetermined and that the function of the antigen is merely to select the proper one. Both theories explain many facets of the fundamental allergic reaction; neither explains the reaction completely.

It is generally believed that the *tendency* to be allergic is inherited rather than allergy diseases themselves. Heredity in allergy does not always and exactly fulfill the criteria of the Mendelian law, such as can be demonstrated in the heredity of blond hair and blue eyes. Evidences of allergy disease among young people should not deter them from having children. No assurance can be given to them that their offspring will or will not develop an allergy disease. Knowing that the tendency exists, precautions can always be taken to help prevent the occurrence of allergy.

Chapter Three

The Initial Consultation

The initial consultation between doctor and patient serves more than one purpose. Although purportedly it is a record of the chronological events of the patient's illness, it is also an introduction, a meeting, a reciprocal appraisal of personalities, and an opening for a relationship which usually extends far beyond the limited confines of mere discussion of clinical symptoms. It is the beginning of the necessarily intimate doctor-patient relationship.

The patient is asked to recall certain aspects of his illness which he may have temporarily forgotten but which may be significant to the physician either in making a proper diagnosis or in determining the cause, and sometimes in both. An annotated history sheet may remind the doctor to ask certain questions, thus preventing omissions.

In general medicine a formula like the following one is frequently used: 1) The present complaint. The symptoms are usually listed numerically in order of their importance. 2) History of the present complaint. This is a chronological sequence of the onset and course of the illness in the patient's words. 3) Inquiry regarding possibly related symptoms. These are questions in connection with organs or systems of the body other than that of which the patient complains. 4) Past illnesses, including operations and accidents. These may have a bearing on the illness of which the patient complains. 5) Family history (some diseases are hereditary). 6) Personal history. This relates principally to occupation, home surroundings, eating and sleeping habits, smoking, drinking, and related data.

In allergy the purpose of this history, or anamnesis ("recalling to mind"), is slightly different from the usual diagnostic history. The doctor who treats allergy diseases is especially interested in the cause of the illness and so the causative, or etiological, factors are particularly stressed.

19

Most patients entering the doctor's office for the first time are nervous and apprehensive. This is a natural reaction, so some doctors have prepared medical history questionnaires to supplement oral interviews. They ask their patients to fill these out at home. But fortunately, most patients soon feel at ease with their doctor, and if they are unable to answer all questions at the first visit, they are able to do so on subsequent visits.

CHIEF COMPLAINT

An allergy medical history usually begins with questions by the doctor relative to the chief complaint. Is it bouts of sneezing, or difficulty in breathing; is it a cough, a rash, headaches, or what? Sometimes it is difficult to secure an exact complaint from a person regarding the chief complaint. The patient may respond to the question, "What do you complain of?" with a reply such as, "I have an allergy." Clearly this means little to the consulting physician.

Another way in which some people answer the simple question of what is bothering them is by reciting a series of events that began in childhood. These may have a bearing on the present illness, but the doctor wishes to know at the start of the consultation what the patient complains of, so that he can list the complaints on his history sheet and bear them in mind according to their importance.

CHRONOLOGICAL HISTORY OF PRESENT ILLNESS

After the chief complaints have been listed, the doctor usually desires some information about previous similar attacks, and particularly about the very first time the person was troubled the same way. What were the circumstances surrounding the attacks? At what age did it occur? What was the individual doing when the attack took place? What was the time of day, the season of the year? In fact, all the circumstances surrounding the first attack are of importance. So also are the events which attended subsequent attacks and especially the most recent one, for which the physician is being consulted.

Allergy illnesses are ubiquitous and involve every aspect of one's life and environment. Inquiry into habits, employment, living conditions, and emotional state may be just as important as questions relative to onset, course, and severity of symptoms. The allergy patient, therefore, must come to the first consultation prepared to answer a battery of questions, many of which may seem at the moment to be irrelevant and not at all connected to his illness.

For example, if an attack of sneezing occurs only in the fall when a certain weed is pollinating, the diagnosis of hay fever is obvious and the etiology of the hay fever is likewise clear—namely, the weeds that are in the general area of the individual. To take another example, if the chief symptom in a child is difficulty in breathing, and the first attack occurred when a cat was adopted in the home; and if the attack always recurs when playing with the pet, asthma is the probable diagnosis and the cat hair or dander is the likely cause.

Naturally all cases are not this simple and in any case no doctor ever makes a diagnosis by history alone; it is made only after a careful physical examination and correlation of all the facts he has gathered. Many times laboratory data are also required.

PREVIOUS TREATMENT

It is of great help to a doctor to know what an allergy patient has been taking for the relief of his condition and whether or not it has been beneficial. Today many doctors direct the pharmacist to type the name of the drug if it is a single drug r the trade name, if it is a manufactured compound, on the outside of the vial or package. This is a good practice. The doctor is much concerned about a patient's reaction to certain medicines. Such information stops him from prescribing drugs which have already proved ineffectual for this patient or to which the patient has reacted badly.

Knowledge of previous consultations with some other doctor and what laboratory or allergy tests he performed may prevent duplication. Upon proper written request by the doctor, signed by the patient, the prior consultant will always send a summary of the prior care. This is in the best interest of the patient.

Any medicine may affect allergic response. The doctor finds it important to ask a patient if he takes any drugs or medication *routinely*, including pain-killers and sleeping pills. Unfortunately, the latter are often taken regularly and without any qualms. Formerly these were different types of barbiturates or a form of bromide, but nowadays many antihistamines are marketed as sleep aids. Years ago, people thought it dreadful to take a sleeping pill; they were afraid of addiction. This is not true today. Sleeping pills of all kinds can be found in the medicine cabinets of many homes and people take them regularly if they have the least bit of difficulty in falling asleep.

Antihistamines are frequently of great benefit to hay fever sufferers, and may induce sleep, but for some people they may be harmful and have disturbing side effects.

It would be difficult to find a person who at some time or other has not taken vitamins; many feel that these "pep them up" or "ward off disease." They are fed to children to "increase their appetite" or "put on weight." Seldom are they necessary unless prescribed by the doctor. Cathartics are sold over the counter at drugstores under many names, and people who take them do not consider them drugs. Most cathartics are innocuous except for their purgative action, but some contain phenolphthalein which may produce rashes in certain people.

ENVIRONMENTAL FACTORS

Where a person lives is important to the doctor, particularly information relative to the vegetation in the vicinity: whether there are trees, a lawn in the front or back yard, a flower garden. The doctor should be told of any changes in the home or other environment.

If an allergic person has entered a new business or occupation, he should bring to the doctor a list of the new chemicals, goods, or material with which he may be working.

Sometimes it may be necessary for the attending physician to visit the home personally to secure more information than he is able to obtain by mere questioning. A plant or living-room sofa of innocent appearance may harbor the cause of the illness. Surrounding the home of an allergic patient there may be many trees, grasses, or weeds to which he may be allergic. A nearby farm with rusts and smuts (molds), or with chickens and other animals, may be the reason for increased symptomatology. But remote sources of pollen can be almost as important as those of local origin. Small bits of allergens, such as pollen and molds, flaxseed (used as stock feed for chickens) and dust, can be carried in the air miles from their source.

Pets, especially dogs and cats, are well-known causes of allergy symptoms. The hair and dander are potent allergens. But it is exceedingly difficult for a doctor to persuade a pet owner to give up the pet who has invariably become "like one of the family." The argument is often given that the pet is kept outside and is allowed in the house only on special occasions. This may lessen the contact, it is true, but the animal's hair may be found in the home nevertheless. It can be brought in on wearing apparel, and once hair gets into carpets or settles on the fabrics of furniture it is difficult to remove. Fleas which an animal may harbor are not infrequently a cause of urticaria (hives) or other allergies.

HABITS

The doctor may find it imperative to inquire deeply into the habits of an allergy patient with particular reference to hours of work, rest, and play. Some people literally "work themselves to death." They do not get sufficient rest and have never learned to play. Others, on the other hand, tend to be lazy and do not exercise sufficiently. They become fat, their muscles flabby, and their circulation may become impaired. A well-regulated life with plenty of rest but also some amount of regulated exercise, in accordance with one's age, is essential to everyone's well-being. It is appalling how eating habits have changed in recent years. Sitting at a lunch counter and rushing through a meal is a common practice among workers, particularly the white-collar workers. Seldom is the meal a balanced one. Factory workers are often required to bring their lunches with them.

Just as allergies are aggravated by nonspecific factors, such as infections and emotional problems, so they are also influenced by the general well-being and health of an individual. An active, robust person is less likely to suffer from an allergy disease than one who is undernourished and indolent. On the other hand, a very severe asthmatic cannot exercise, and the history of lassitude and laziness may indicate severe illness with insufficient oxygen in his blood, caused by chronic persistent respiratory difficulty. In either instance, a knowledge of habits is important to the doctor.

ADDITIONAL SYMPTOMS OF ALLERGY

It is not at all unusual for allergy sufferers to present more than one allergy disease at the same time. Bronchial asthma, for example, is not infrequently associated with allergic rhinitis, either the seasonal type (hay fever) or the perennial type, which, as its name implies, lasts all year. Headaches frequently occur along with gastrointestinal allergy disease. The doctor should be told of any coexisting allergy disease; for while he is relieving the symptoms of one he can be treating the other as well.

PAST HISTORY

Some patients do not understand why the doctor should be interested in their past illnesses; they would seem to be inconsequential. In some cases, however, they denote a pattern. It is not unusual, for example, for a person with asthma to relate a history of eczema in infancy, hay fever in young adult life, and bronchial asthma later on—one allergy disease following the other. The significance of such a recital of illnesses may cause the doctor to suspect that the present illness, bronchial asthma, may be due to a combination of pollen and foods that may also have been instigators of the infant's rash. Upper respiratory infections, repeated sinus infection, recurrent bronchitis attacks, make an allergic person more susceptible to allergens than he would otherwise be. Chronic disturbance of the gastrointestinal tract may designate it as the site for an allergic reaction. Previous operations for nasal polyps suggest that nasal allergy and lung infections have paved the way for asthma.

Overindulgence in specific foods by a mother during her pregnancy may result in the offspring becoming allergic to them. In a breast-fed baby, nearly any food or drug which the mother takes can pass through the mother's milk to the infant, making the question of whether the allergic child was a breast-fed baby pertinent. If the baby was not breast-fed, any feeding problems with various formulas must be ascertained. Infants who have difficulty of this sort and who have or have had recurrent attacks of vomiting, diarrhea, or colic are usually allergic babies. If a child has experienced reactions to previously administered antibiotics or to another drug, this should be reported on the first visit to the doctor.

Immunizing injections against most of the childhood diseases have proved so successful that they are required by law in many states before a child may start school. If the attending doctor did not give them himself, he should be told when they were given and whether any untoward reactions followed their administration. The usual immunizations are for diphtheria, whooping cough, tetanus, smallpox (vaccination) and poliomyelitis (either in the form of live virus by mouth or the dead virus by injection). Special immunizations, such as for rabies, following a dog bite, should also be told to the doctor.

Inquiry about past infections may throw some light on the sudden appearance of an allergy disease. Infection has an important effect, if not by sensitization to the bacteria or its toxins, extension, or reabsorption, then by lowering the allergy threshold and disturbing the normal allergy equilibrium. The history of a past infection of the teeth, tonsils, or nasal sinuses may point to a focus of infection. Some doctors feel that this is significant in the production of an allergy disease, particularly in children.

FAMILY HISTORY

When the diagnosis of a disease as allergic is in doubt, a strong family history may sway the doctor. But frequently, the patient is unaware of a family history; perhaps, too, the allergy had been unrecognized, was diagnosed as something else, or has appeared in the patient prior to its appearance in a parent or other relative. Formerly, it was thought that allergy appears early in the life of those whose parents were allergic and later in life in those who had only one allergic parent. Recent studies appear to disprove this belief and the view has been expressed that the time of onset of symptoms depends primarily upon the extent of exposure to the allergen. The subject of heredity and transmission of the allergy state is discussed in Chapter 2.

PSYCHOLOGICAL ASSOCIATION

Although the doctor may ask the allergy patient questions relative to emotional disturbances accompanying the allergy disease during the first consultation, these are usually not exhaustive and sometimes not explored at all. It is often adequate for the physician to observe his patient and obtain a satisfactory estimate of the person's behavior. People vary greatly when they visit a new doctor. They may be apprehensive and fearful; some are authoritative, while others such as children are reluctant visitors having been brought by a father or mother "for their own good." Their hostility is obvious. Then, of course, there are those patients who are too ill to discuss any emotional problems.

Despite the paucity of evidence, it is a common experience to have the patient or the person with him ask, "Isn't this all emotional, anyway, Doctor?" So often is this asked of a doctor at the first interview that he frequently must explain briefly the relationship of psychological problems to allergy symptoms.

If time permits, the physician will ask such questions relating to the following and on subsequent visits will follow them up if he thinks it is necessary:

In infancy: Bed-wetting. Thumb-sucking. Nightmares. Relation of infant to parents. Brothers. Sisters.

In childhood: Social adjustment with other children and teachers. Influence of older people. Play, recreation, likes, dislikes, and hostilities.

In adolescence: School or college problems with grades, teacher, or fellow students. Sports, competitive or otherwise. Occupational assignments during school or summer vacations. Military training. Sexual development.

In adult life: Sexual activity. Marriage, work, recreation. Military service. Children.

Other questions may be asked with profit in determining a person's psychological reaction to life's experiences. For example, some people may have had trouble with the law and this may influence allergy symptoms. Others may have developed religious philosophies which influence their reaction to allergy discomfiture. Foremost, perhaps, is the person's behavioral pattern and attitude to current life stresses.

SYSTEMATIC REVIEW OF SYMPTOMS

To be certain that nothing is omitted some physicians review the symptoms systematically; that is, they start with the eyes, ears, nose, and throat and proceed to the respiratory tract, the heart, gastrointestinal tract, and finally the genitourinary tract, asking questions relative to each. This constitutes a thorough medical history. Yet it must be emphasized that every patient is unique and many of the questions implied in our outline may not be necessary in a given case. If a person has an obvious case of hay fever, he need not be asked whether he wet his bed when a child. A doctor's good sense determines which questions are pertinent and which are not. Despite the importance of the history in reaching a diagnosis, no physician makes a diagnosis in any patient without a physical examination.

PHYSICAL EXAMINATION

Usually the doctor examines the patient at the time of the first consultation. If there is insufficient time, he may examine only the organs involved in the illness complained of. Each doctor has his own procedure which he uses in conducting his physical examination. Most start with examination of the eyes, ears, nose, and throat, and continue from there to an examination of the chest, abdomen and extremities, the skin, and reflexes of the nervous system (when indicated). Vaginal and rectal examinations are infrequently required in an allergist's office, since few allergy diseases involve these portions of the body. The decision is a matter of the physician's discretion.

Occasionally a doctor will perform some simple laboratory examination such as a blood count, urine examination, or nasal smear at the first consultation, but more often these and other laboratory tests which may be required are left for another time. The blood count may be done to determine if there is any anemia, evidence of infection, or the existence of a large number of eosinophiles. Eosinophiles are a form of white blood cell which are often found in excess in allergy diseases. The urine may be examined for sugar and for albumin. The specific gravity of the urine determines its concentration. Rarely is a microscopic examination of the urine performed, since this is done to ascertain the presence of urinary tract infection or kidney disease. A nasal smear is done to discover the presence or number of eosinophiles relative to polymorphonuclear leukocytes (white blood cells with nuclei of many varying forms). Just as a preponderance of eosinophiles in the nasal smear indicates allergy, a large number of polymorphonuclear leukocytes signifies infection.

SUMMARY

At the first consultation between a doctor and his allergy patient many questions must be asked, since the doctor is concerned not only with making a diagnosis, but also with obtaining as many clues as he can relating to the cause of the illness. An allergy patient may be expected to be asked questions as indicated in the following table, which essentially is the type of outline most physicians treating allergy diseases follow:

Chief Complaint: Sneezing, itching of eyes, difficulty in breathing, cough, rash, headaches, etc.

Chronological History of Present Illness: Previous attacks: date of first attack, mode of onset, circumstances, duration; date of last attack, mode of onset, circumstances, duration.

Environmental Factors: Neighborhood: trees, lawn, flowers, weeds, insecticides; carpeting, rug and padding; bedroom: mattress, pillows, bed covers; heating system; cleaning methods; pets.

Previous Treatments: Laboratory tests: results; allergy tests: when, where, results; injection therapy: results.

Precipitating Factors: Season; time of day; location: home, outdoors; at work, rest, play; exertion; excitement; history of infections; menses; smoking; dust; soaps; cosmetics; odors; gardening, flowers; insects; food idiosyncrasies.

Usual Activities: Sports, sleep, hobbies, work, etc.

Additional Symptoms of Allergy: Hay fever, asthma, eczema, headaches, gastrointestinal symptoms.

Past History: Previous illnesses (especially respiratory), accidents, operations (especially nose and throat).

Family History:	Hay fever, asthma, eczema, headaches, gastrointestinal, cardiac symptoms, etc.
Psychological Association:	Bed-wetting, social adjustment, school record, sports, military training, marital problems.
Systematic Review of Symptoms:	Eyes: irritation, watering, burning, swelling, etc.
	Ears: itching, fullness.
	Nose: itching, sneezing, congestion.
	Throat: sore throat, postnasal drip.
	Respiratory: difficulty in breathing, cough, expectoration (amount, color).
	Cardiac: palpitation, pain, radiation, at rest or upon exertion.
	Gastrointestinal: appetite, pain after eating, heartburn, bowels, straining at stool.
	Genitourinary: frequency, blood, tenesmus (straining at stool or in urination).
	Skin: rashes, itching, swelling.
	Bones and joints: pain, swelling, stiffness.

After the medical history a physical examination is performed and occasionally a certain number of laboratory tests, although the latter are often postponed until a later visit.

Chapter Four

Diagnostic Allergy Tests

When a patient enters a hospital, often before he is visited by his physician or a nurse, a laboratory assistant obtains a blood sample and a urine specimen for examination in the laboratory. The allergist, like the internist, the cardiologist, and other medical specialists, looks to the laboratory for helpful information. In addition to routine laboratory examinations, the allergist usually performs a series of tests known as diagnostic allergy tests. Since they are for the most part performed on the skin, they are frequently spoken of as allergy skin tests. They are used to corroborate the diagnosis of the allergy disease and more often performed to confirm or determine the cause (etiology) of the illness which the doctor suspects from his medical history. In many instances these tests disclose etiological factors which might otherwise go unnoticed; in some cases they help to indicate the type of treatment that should be pursued.

Diagnostic allergy tests are usually performed in the doctor's office. They are neither difficult to perform nor painful. Since the testing extracts have been carefully standardized with their strength and potency well known, they seldom cause any unpleasant or untoward physical disturbance. Usually the tests are performed and interpreted by the doctor himself; otherwise the tests are administered by a trained assistant and the doctor interprets them.

Currently, there are several methods of skin testing, two of which are in common use. The scratch method consists of scarifying (scratching) the skin through the outer layer and depositing the material to be tested (antigen) in the area of scarification. The second type of testing is known as the intradermal or intracutaneous method because the antigen in solution is injected within the layers of the skin.

A control test, consisting of a similar test with the diluent used in

30

preparing the antigen extract (but without the active allergen), is essential in each type of testing. Positive reactions from tests with the antigen extracts are compared with the appearance at the control site to verify that they are true positive allergic skin reactions and not merely a nonallergic or irritating reaction to the diluent, or perhaps the result of injury to the tissues in performing the tests.

In both types of testing a positive reaction consists of the formation of a hive or a wheal (more or less round elevation of the skin, white in the center) surrounded by a zone of redness (erythema) of variable size. This ordinarily disappears within an hour or less and leaves no scar or other aftereffect. The allergy skin test is an allergy reaction in miniature. Since the dose of antigen is known and carefully measured by the physician, then injected into a chosen site, the reaction is completely under control. Nevertheless, the hive produced in a positive reaction is a reproduction of the antigen-antibody reaction that occurs in an allergy reaction elsewhere in the body and is testimony of an allergy disease.

THE SCRATCH TEST

Simple to perform and practically painless, the scratch (or cutaneous) test is chosen by most doctors as a preliminary screening test and for testing infants and young children. Essentially, it consists of a series of scarifications or scratches on the skin into which soluble or powdered antigens in solution are gently rubbed. With proper technique, no blood is drawn and there is no need for skin sterilization with alcohol or any other agent, as required with other tests. Sometimes, when small children are to be "scratch tested" it is necessary to cleanse the area to be used. Soap-and-water washing followed by careful drying is adequate for this.

For infants and young children the area on the back between the shoulder blades (interscapular region) is the site commonly chosen for scratch testing. The child can be placed on his stomach or cradled in his mother's arms while the tests are performed. The interscapular area is excellent because its large area permits many tests to be performed at one time if required.

In older children and in adults the common site for scratch tests is the inner (flexor) surface of the forearm. The interscapular area is considered slightly more sensitive than the flexor surface of the forearm, however, and some allergists prefer this. When they do not secure anticipated reactions on the forearm, they repeat the tests on the back. Many doctors select the forearm as the site in children to permit the patients to see what is going on, eliminating the mystery.

Every physician who does the scratch allergy skin tests has his special technique; all are generally similar. To produce the scratches one doctor may prefer a specially manufactured scarifying instrument; another may choose the blunt edge of a knife such as that used for cataract eye operations; still other doctors adhere to the familiar (and traditional) darning needle. The object is to make a small horizontal scratch about an eighth of an inch long on which to place the antigen. These scratches must be separated from each other by at least a full inch so that if a positive reaction should result at the site of two nearby scratches, they do not run into each other and confuse interpretation.

In order to determine what antigens have been placed in the different scratches, the doctor numbers the scratches with ink or skin-writing pencil conforming with numbers already on the antigen vials and on his skin test reaction sheet. The usual procedure is to make twenty scratches on the skin of the back or the forearm in two vertical rows of ten each.

Many antigens today are available in solution and are equipped with droppers. If this is the case, all that the technician has to do is to place a drop of the antigen extract on the scratch and gently rub it in. If the antigen is not in solution but is in powdered form, as many of the older ones were and some still are, it is necessary to put it into a solution, commonly one of sodium hydroxide. A drop is placed upon the scratch; then the powdered antigen is mixed in it and rubbed into the scratch with a toothpick, which is discarded after use.

A variation in the technique is for the technician to place the liquid antigen on the skin first, and then scarify the skin through the solution. If the same scarifier or needle is used for all tests, one test extract may be carried over to another. This can be prevented if a different scarifier or needle is used for each test. If the same scarifier is used, it is washed with alcohol and dried before application to each new area.

Each test site represents the test of a separate and distinct antigen. As many as twenty different antigen tests may be done at one time. If no positive reactions occur, twenty more may be applied. Rarely are more than forty tests performed at one sitting unless the interscapular area is used. There, as many as sixty or more may be done if there are no marked positive reactions.

Scratch test reactions are read in fifteen to thirty minutes after scarification and application of the antigen. During the interval the doctor or technician examines the test area frequently. If a very large positive reaction is developing at a test site—a conclusive result— the antigen is wiped off with alcohol immediately to prevent the hive from becoming any bigger and to avoid additional absorption of the antigen. Some is absorbed anyway, and if a person is extremely sensitive, absorption of too much of the antigen may cause an unpleasant reaction.

Doctors grade reactions differently. One item of great significance is the reactivity of a person's skin. The skin of some people is highly reactive. The slightest pressure makes a mark on it and causes a local swelling (dermographia). In such a person a hive at the site of the scratch is of little importance; a reaction to be considered positive has to consist of a large hive or wheal with the formation of small protrusions or extensions from the hive (pseudopodia), surrounded by a zone of redness (erythema).

Grading of positive reactions is usually made as follows: A one-plus reaction is a small hive or wheal running along the sides of the scratch and surrounded by a slight amount of pale erythema. A two-plus reaction is a wheal that extends above and below the borders of the scratch and is surrounded by a larger area of erythema. A three-plus reaction is a wheal with pseudopodia surrounded by an intense and irregular erythematous area. A four-plus reaction is a further aggravation of a three-plus reaction in which there are several pseudopodia and a large expansive area of erythema. While this is the common method of grading reactions, some allergists prefer to record them as mild (one- or two-plus reactions), moderate (a three-plus reaction), and marked (a four-plus reaction).

Although the size of a positive reaction probably indicates the degree or sensitivity of the person being tested, it does not always parallel the severity of symptoms. Sometimes a positive skin reaction represents a potential sensitivity and has nothing whatsoever to do with the symptoms for which the doctor was consulted. At other times positive reactions only indicate past or insignificant sensitivities. Allergists always attempt to correlate positive skin tests with the symptoms and the clinical history of the patient.

THE PUNCTURE OR PRICK TEST

The puncture (or prick) test is a modification of the scratch (or cutaneous) test. It is less time-consuming, and many allergists consider it more informative. It may be performed with a stainless steel surgical darning or embroidery needle with a large eye which has been cut evenly across and blunted. With the needle point inserted into the cork stopper of the vial containing the antigen in solution, the blunted cut eye of the needle will remain in the extract when the bottle is closed. Upon removal of the cork, the cut blunt eye will carry with it a small amount of the extract. When this is pressed to the skin of the person to be tested and twisted slightly at the same time, it produces a slight puncture, comparable to a scratch, depositing the antigen in it. A modification of this technique utilizes a small glass medicine dropper which is usually supplied with vials of antigens. By breaking off the end and filing it to remove any excessively jagged edges of glass, it becomes an efficient scarifier as well as an applicator of the antigen. The appearance of a needle is likely to frighten youngsters; a rubber-capped glass dropper will not. Puncture tests are as painless as scratch tests. No blood is drawn, and positive tests are graded similarly.

THE INTRADERMAL OR INTRACUTANEOUS TEST

"Intradermal" and "intracutaneous" are synonymous: both mean "within the substance of the skin." This test is more sensitive and more difficult to perform than the scratch or puncture test, and many allergists utilize it only for scratch tests which have proved negative. The tuberculin syringe and hypodermic needles that are used may arouse suspicion that it is a painful procedure, but actually, it is not more uncomfortable than the scratch tests, partly because very sharp needles are used which only partially penetrate the skin. Nevertheless, children are notoriously afraid of "needles," and unless a child has complete confidence in the doctor or technician, he may squirm and make the testing more difficult. Many physicians who are not allergists and do not perform diagnostic allergy tests frequently do not use this method of testing which also requires more complex equipment and facilities.

The technique of intradermal or intracutaneous testing consists of introducing a small amount of the antigen in solution between the layers of the skin without piercing any of the superficial blood vessels. The outer surface of the upper arm is the usual chosen site, although the interscapular region can be selected. In contrast to the scratch tests, sterilization of the testing area is essential; alcohol is ordinarily used for this purpose. The tiniest amount of antigen in solution necessary to produce a visible wheal or hive is injected. A distance of about an inch is left between each test site, and each test is customarily performed below the other in a vertical line in two rows of five each (plus one which is the control). As in scratch testing, some method of designating which tests are being done on the skin must be kept, either by marking the skin of the subject at the site of each injection with a number corresponding with the number on each antigen vial and syringe or by other methods devised by the individual doctor.

The tests are read in about ten to fifteen minutes after application and are generally considered to be more rapidly reactive than the scratch tests. Because of this, and because the antigen can be absorbed very quickly possibly producing a disagreeable reaction, the testing strengths of antigen extracts for intradermal testing are frequently as much as one hundred times more dilute than those employed in scratch testing. Some doctors do not approve of intradermal testing, arguing that this method of testing produces many false positive reactions sometimes by mere introduction of the needles, the irritation of the extracts, or faulty introduction of air when making the tests. All allergists realize these factors, however, and take them into consideration when evaluating the result; very few allergists rely entirely upon the results of the skin tests. They must be correlated with the symptoms and clinical medical history.

STRENGTH OF TESTING SOLUTIONS

It has been mentioned that there is a difference in strength between extracts used for scratch and intradermal testing. There is also a difference of strength employed in the solutions of the various antigens. Some produce positive reactions more readily than others and in more dilute strengths; others may foster the production of generalized or constitutional reactions. To guard against this possibility, carefully standardized extracts are used and only in those testing strengths that have been proved to be safe. Some of the antigens used in weak solutions because of their pronounced reactivity are pollen, cottonseed, kapok, flaxseed, animal hairs, fish glue, and silk. The foods which are considered most reactive are mustard, navy beans, nuts, shellfish, and seafood in general.

All doctors who perform diagnostic allergy tests and particularly intradermal tests keep on hand such drugs as adrenalin and soluble cortisone derivatives, as well as others for immediate treatment of generalized or constitutional reactions. Similar reactions described in Chapter 7 may result from improper dosage of a pollen extract in the treatment of hay fever.

THE PASSIVE TRANSFER (PRAUSNITZ-KÜSTNER TEST)

Although this has been considered the most reliable of all diagnostic allergy tests, since it demonstrates skin sensitizing antibodies or reagins, it is used today only in certain circumstances. Its primary applications are for infants or children, adults who cannot make repeated visits to the doctor's office, for youngsters who are difficult to test in any other way, for those whose skin is highly reactive to any kind of pressure, and for patients whose skin is so covered with lesions that skin testing is impossible. A number of people who have had a long siege of eczema or other skin disease may have skin too tough and leathery for the introduction of allergy tests.

The basis of the passive transfer test is the transference of the skin sensitizing antibody from the bloodstream of the allergic person and its deposition in the skin of a subject who is not allergic, thus rendering each injected site temporarily allergic to the same substances as the donor. This necessitates withdrawal of blood (serum) from the allergic person. The serum is injected within the layers of the skin of the subject utilizing those sites employed for routine intradermal tests.

The recipient subject must not himself be allergic nor have a family history of allergy and so he cannot be any member of the ill person's immediate family. If possible, the subject should undergo a complete series of intracutaneous tests to prove conclusively that he has no allergy predisposition or sensitivities. It has been suggested that on the day of the tests, he should not eat any of the following foods: eggs, fish, bananas, mustard, or chicken. These may interfere with the accuracy of the passive transfer tests. Another requirement is that the recipient not eat any food to which a positive reaction may be anticipated from the history of the allergic person, as this, too, would hamper the practicability of employing passive transfer tests. A firm indication should be present.

Although either the outer surface of the upper arm or the intrascapular regions may be used for passive transfer, the back is commonly chosen because the larger area allows a greater number of tests to be done at one sitting. The allergist numbers the sites in order to recognize where the various antigens have been placed. Most not only perform the intradermal pollen and food tests on the prepared sites, but repeat them in a series alongside on the nonsensitized skin as a control and for comparison. If a positive reaction appears on the sensitized site but not on the nonsensitized site, he knows immediately that the reaction is valid. If a positive reaction appears on both sites, it indicates a false reaction.

This method of skin testing permits a large number of tests to be done at one time. Only the area to be tested and the cooperation of the subject limit the number. There is no danger of any reaction since the subject is a nonallergic person. The tests are read and graded in a manner similar to the intradermal tests done directly on the allergic patient. The recipient's skin has been known to remain sensitive for as long as four to six weeks. However, it is best for the tests to be performed as soon as possible after the initial redness, where the serum has been injected, has subsided, usually within twenty-four to seventy-two hours.

Ultimately, however, the sites do lose their sensitivity. There is no danger of transference of any of the sensitivities of the allergic person to the subject since the response is temporary and local. All in all, it is a harmless procedure. Only the many difficulties involved in performing this type of test have interfered with making it as popular as it probably deserves to be.

THE CONJUNCTIVAL TEST

When cutaneous and intradermal tests are negative but a pollen or some other inhalant sensitivity is suspected from the medical history, it is sometimes necessary to resort to conjunctival (lining of the eye) testing. The theory of this test is that specific antibodies present in the conjunctiva of the eye more readily unite with the antigen at this site than in the skin, producing a positive reaction. In the performance of the conjunctival test, various strengths of sterile dilutions in series, of the suspected antigen or the powdered antigen, are used. When a solution of the antigen is employed, the first tests are done with a very weak dilution. This is followed if necessary by drops of a stronger dilution.

The technique is as follows: A single drop of a very dilute antigen extract is placed in the eye with an eyedropper. If, after five minutes, no reaction is apparent, a drop of a dilution ten times stronger is used. This procedure is repeated until a final concentrated dilution is introduced. If no reaction has been obtained, the powdered or full strength antigen may now be used.

As much of the powdered antigen necessary to cover the end of a toothpick is placed on the inner surface of the lower lid, and the patient being treated is asked to close his eye. After two or three minutes, the powdered antigen which has collected on the conjunctiva is removed with a small cotton swab, and the eye is washed out with salt solution. Ordinarily, any injury or irritation to the eye by a foreign substance will produce some amount of conjunctival redness, irritation, or inflammation. This is to be expected, but if this inflammation or redness persists for more than five minutes after the application of the antigen in solution, or after the powdered antigen has been removed, the persistence is considered a positive reaction.

Doctors grade positive reactions numerically as in skin tests. These ordinary gradings are subject to the individual doctor's interpretation in accordance with his experience. To prevent the reaction from developing further and to clear it up quickly, a few drops of epinephrine or some form of a soothing eyedrop is placed in the eye. The eye is then washed out well with boric acid solution.

Many, if not most, allergists believe that this method of testing gives more accurate information with respect to a person's sensitivity to inhalant substances, but it is not employed in the average allergy case. Most people, anticipating a possible inflammatory reaction, do not enjoy having materials placed in their eyes, and the inflammation, although quickly disposed of, is uncomfortable. Moreover, once a positive reaction is obtained, the eye cannot be used again as a testing site for some time. Fortunately, skin tests will usually give the required information.

THE NASAL INHALATION TEST ("SNIFF TEST")

This diagnostic allergy test is not employed in the United States with any degree of frequency, primarily because of the severe reaction it can induce. The test is never performed without epinephrine and other drugs readily available in case of the not uncommon severe reaction.

As the name implies, it is performed by simply inhaling or sniffing up some of the suspected substance to be tested. In addition to the nasal or general reaction which is apt to occur, it is impractical because only a few tests can be performed at one sitting. Yet a positive reaction consisting of paroxysms of sneezing or wheezing and difficulty in breathing is bona fide evidence of the veracity of the reaction.

THE NASAL INSTILLATION TEST

In this test, which is similar to the nasal inhalation test, drops of an antigen in solution are instilled into the nose. A positive reaction consists of the nasal and bronchial symptoms indicated above, and this method of testing is characterized by all the problems of the nasal inhalation test.

Although both nasal inhalation tests and nasal instillation tests are used principally for determining pollen sensitivity, other inhalants can be tested in the same manner. Orris root, which has been used as a basic ingredient of perfumed and scented cosmetics, and house dust are some of the other substances which have been tested by these methods.

THE BRONCHIAL INHALATION TEST

It is clear that when an antigen to which a person is sensitive is inhaled, the bronchial tubes will react, producing asthmatic symptoms. This has led some doctors to use bronchial inhalation of a suspected substance as a provocative test procedure.

Either powdered antigen or antigen in solution is used. A powdered antigen is blown directly into the bronchial tract by a blowing device, while a liquid antigen is placed in a nebulizer and inhaled as a fine mist. The machine used for inducing intermittent positive pressure breathing for the relief of bronchial asthma has been made into a testing instrument for the bronchial inhalation test by replacing the medicinal liquid in the chamber with liquid antigen and forcing it into the bronchial tract. There are only a few instances when doctors resort to this method of testing; the possibility of an unpleasant or constitutional reaction is too great.

THE PATCH TEST

The patch test is reserved for cases in which a given material is suspected of producing skin symptoms. In general, there are two methods of performing a patch test, the covered and the uncovered, or open, patch test. In both instances, the suspected substance is placed in direct contact with the skin. The inner surface of the forearm is the usual site for the patch tests, although the back can also be used. The purpose is to reproduce the skin rash in miniature.

In the covered patch test, the test material is kept covered for the duration of the test. The technique consists of placing a very small amount, no more than required to cover a quarter of an inch of space, on the skin and covering it with a one-inch square of four-ply gauze, oiled silk, cellophane, glazed paper, or other type of impermeable material. This square is then sealed to the skin with a larger square of adhesive tape. The patch is left on for twenty-four, forty-eight, or seventy-two hours. If it becomes disturbing, if the skin becomes hot or inflamed, it should be removed immediately, the area quickly washed off, and a soothing cream applied.

The uncovered or open patch test is used when the material to be tested is either an adhesive liquid such as fingernail polish, or a volatile substance such as gases or fumes with which a person may come in contact at work. Commercial products such as hair dyes often include an extra vial of material for such tests.

The strength of the solution to be employed is often a perplexing problem for the allergist as reactions to various strengths vary widely in different patients. Published tables accessible to the doctor provide a rough guide.

The results of both the covered and open patch tests are graded as negative when no reaction is observed at the test site at any time (either immediately or twenty-four to forty-eight hours later). Then the reaction is graded from a small papule (a red elevated area on the skin varying from the size of a pinhead to that of a pea), which is termed a one-plus reaction, to a four-plus reaction, in which there is scaling of the skin (desquamation), some oozing of fluid, and actual destruction of the skin at the site of the test (necrosis).

Diagnostic allergy tests are also used in many diseases, including tuberculosis and pertussis (whooping cough), other than those usually considered to be allergy diseases. Most of these tests are performed just as one does the intradermal allergy test. Some have proved valuable in clinical medicine; others have doubtful significance. However, in the recognizable allergy diseases they are invaluable.

Other tests have been in vogue. A test which introduces the antigen into the skin by a weak electrical current is known as the iontophoresis test. Placing the suspected substance, usually a food, under the tongue for absorption and subsequent reaction is known as the sublingual test. These tests are seldom used at the present time.

SUMMARY

Diagnostic allergy tests are usually performed in the doctor's offices. The skin is used for most of the tests, which are not at all painful. They not only assist in corroborating the diagnosis of an allergy disease, but also often confirm or determine the cause of the illness and indicate the type of treatment which should be pursued.

The most common types of skin tests performed are the scratch and intradermal. The former are most useful in infants and young children because of the ease with which they can be done. The scratch test, of which the puncture or prick test is a modification, is performed by making scratches on the skin and gently rubbing the testing substance into the scratches. The sites most frequently chosen for this form of testing are the back between the shoulder blades or the inner surface of the forearm. Intradermal, or intracutaneous, tests, so called because the testing substances are injected in solution within the layers of the skin, are considered more sensitive. The outer surfaces of the upper arms are the most frequent sites selected for these tests. All skin tests are read within fifteen minutes to half an hour and are graded according to the size of the hive and the surrounding redness (erythema) they produce.

Passive transfer employs a nonallergic subject to receive the tests. Sites on his skin are sensitized with a serum from the allergic person, and after twenty-four hours or more are tested intradermally. The tests are read and graded in a manner similar to that in which direct intradermal tests are read and graded. No transference of allergy takes place since the sites are only sensitized locally, and the sensitization is lost in a few days to a week. An advantage is that many tests can be performed at one sitting, and it has been found useful in infants and children who will not or cannot take direct skin tests. The tests are also useful for those whose skin is so highly sensitive or so changed by a skin disease that it does not lend itself to direct skin testing.

Another diagnostic test is one which employs the conjunctiva (lining of the eye). The suspected allergen in powdered or liquid form is placed in the eye and its effect noted. An unusual and exaggerated amount of redness and inflammation after the testing substance has been introduced constitutes a positive reaction. Although this test is used by some allergists, its use is limited, since only a few tests can be performed at one sitting and most people dislike the reaction which may result.

Other tests include the nasal inhalation test (sniffing the suspected substance into the nose), the instillation test (application of the suspected material in liquid form into the nose), and the bronchial inhalation test (inhalation of the testing material into the bronchial tubes). A positive test is indicated by paroxysms of sneezing, cough, or difficulty in breathing. These tests are not commonly used in the United States. They have been discontinued primarily because of the very disagreeable reactions they produce and because the simpler skin tests usually provide as much information.

The iontophoresis test and the sublingual test are other tests which are infrequently employed. In the iontophoresis test the testing solution is introduced into the skin by means of an electrical apparatus. Its effect is like that of the scratch or intradermal tests and like these tests causes no pain on introduction. The sublingual test relies upon rapid absorption of the testing substance under the tongue. Its use is limited because testing is restricted largely to foods; very few can be done at one sitting and there is no consensus of its satisfactoriness among allergists.

Diagnostic allergy tests are used in many diseases other than allergy diseases with their usefulness varying from one disease entity to another. In the field of allergy they are essential and invaluable.

Chapter Five

Pollen in Allergy

Allergy symptoms can be instigated by an allergic person's breathing in noxious substances to which he is sensitive, eating one of them, coming into contact with them, or having them injected into his body. Symptoms may also be initiated by bacteria or their products in an infectious process and by physical agents such as cold, heat, and pressure. One of the most common causes of allergy symptoms, as exemplified by the millions of hay fever sufferers throughout the world, is the inhalation of dusts originating from plants. These dusts are composed of pollen grains which, when given off in large amounts, have the appearance of dust.

BOTANICAL CONSIDERATIONS

Pollen can be identified only with the aid of a microscope. It is the male fertilizing element of the plant and can be compared with the sperm in animal life.

The *flower* of the plant is the basic structure which has been designated by nature to perform the reproductive process. The flower is a stem, generally a branch stem, bearing floral leaves which are completely different from foliage leaves. The pollen (Latin for "fine flour") is formed in the portion of the flower called the *anther,* the basic sexual organ of the male plant. The anther is located at the terminal end of a structure called the *stamen;* the female counterpart is the *pistil* which contains the ovary where the "eggs" are produced. Some flowers contain only the male elements and are designated as *staminate;* others contain only the female elements and are known as *pistillate* flowers. Flowers of only one sex are called *imperfect* while those which are bisexual are considered *perfect.*

43

Sometimes only one type of flower, either the female (pistillate) or the male (staminate), exists on one plant. Such a plant is named *dioecious;* the plant with both sexes, the hermaphrodite, is *monoecius.* Nature has determined that flowers should not fertilize themselves, although they may be capable of doing so. When they do, the result is usually an inferior fruit or a poorly flourishing plant.

POLLEN AND ALLERGY

The function of pollen is to reproduce its own type of plant, just as the function of the animal sperm is to reproduce the animal species. For this to occur the pollen must be transmitted from one plant to another. Although some plants are fertilized by artificial insemination, most are inseminated by natural means, the pollen being carried to the ova of its corresponding plant primarily by wind or by insects. The plants that are insect-pollinated are *entomophilous,* or insect-loving, while those that are wind-pollinated are *anemophilous,* or wind-loving. Since to produce symptoms of allergy in humans, the pollen grains must reach the skin, the nose, or bronchial tubes, the pollen of most concern are those which are wind-borne.

The average size of an allergenically important pollen grain is roughly 25 microns; some, however, are as small as 2.5 microns, others as large as 200. Interpreting microns in commonly used measurements, one micron is equal to 0.000039 inches. The fine dust one observes on clothes after a walk in the woods or suburbs is usually pollen. Everyone is familiar with the yellow powder, the pollen, which is left on the hand after holding a dandelion. The common dandelion produces about 245,000 pollen grains. Even this large amount is insignificant compared with the amount produced by wind-pollinated plants. For example, a single well-developed short ragweed plant, the common hay fever producer in two thirds of the United States, can generate as many as one trillion pollen grains. It has been estimated that the average city lot (one tenth of an acre) of ragweeds is capable of producing 100 ounces in a season; that is 60 pounds per acre. The actual production probably is often many times this figure. Undoubtedly, hundreds and hundreds of tons of ragweed are liberated each season in large cities such as New York, Philadelphia, and Chicago. Pollen must be differentiated from the seed of a plant. When the plant has gone to seed, the pollination is nearly always over.

Although insect-pollinated plants are not nearly as significant to allergic persons as those that are pollinated by the wind, at times they may produce severe symptoms, especially among gardeners and florists. Decorative flowers, for the most part, are insect-pollinated. Their bright color, pleasing scent, and sweet nectar attract many insects, especially bees in search of nectar. The sticky pollen of the flower adheres to their legs, wings, and body, and they can carry large amounts of pollen which often causes allergy symptoms in people who come in contact with the bees. Furthermore, their honeycombs may contain large quantities of pollen, and a sensitive person can develop symptoms merely by eating the honey. Bees usually do not carry the pollen of more than one variety of a flower at a time.

Some species of plants which grow within lakes and rivers are water-pollinated. The pollen drifts or floats in the water to reach its female counterpart, which in turn comes to the surface to meet it. Other pollen of these water plants is heavy and sinks into the female blossom for the purpose of fertilization.

Airborne pollen is exceedingly light in weight and can therefore be lifted into the air and carried long distances by the wind. Pollen has been identified hundreds of miles from its source and has been collected from airplanes as high as seventeen thousand feet above sea level. Consequently, no city is really free of pollen and no allergic city dweller is immune from respiratory allergy disease due to pollen. Nevertheless, tall buildings do tend to block the course of wind-borne pollen, whereas in the country where there are long stretches of land with no obstruction from tall buildings, pollen is distributed more freely.

Weather conditions also influence the distribution of pollen. When the air is still, pollen tends to remain where it was produced; in windy areas it is blown about actively. Rain washes pollen from the air, so most hay fever sufferers feel relieved during a rainstorm. Most plants pollinate in the early morning hours; thus allergy symptoms caused by pollen are more frequent during those hours of sleep. But if the windows of the home are kept closed at night or a filter is placed in the windows, only very small amounts of pollen enter the house. Then, only when the pollen-sensitive person leaves his home and comes in contact with the pollen-laden outside air do symptoms develop. As the day goes on and the linings of the nose or the bronchial tubes are continually bombarded with pollen, symptoms usually increase in severity. By evening these membranes may have become so irritated that almost any disturbing irritant, particulate material may affect them and cause sneezing or coughing spells.

Since pollen is sticky, it tends to collect on textiles, so in areas where clothes or bedding is hung out to air or dry, pollen may be brought into the house. Pets can collect pollen grains and carry them into the home as well.

One eminent allergist postulated these requirements for the production of significant and widespread allergy symptoms caused by pollen:

1. *The pollen must contain an excitant of hay fever.* There are numerous plants which produce profuse amounts of pollen but cause no symptoms because their pollen is nonallergenic; that is, they do not possess the exciting factor or "toxicity." Why this occurs in certain plants and not in others has not been discovered and is a continuing subject of research.

2. *The pollen must be anemophilous, or wind-borne, in its mode of pollination.* This is true except for those people engaged in gardening. In addition, decorative bouquets have been known to carry symptom-producing pollen, and can cause symptoms when kept in a closed hospital room or worn as a corsage.

3. *The pollen must be produced in sufficiently large quantities.* If a plant, no matter how allergenic, produces but a very small amount of pollen, it will not be a prime cause of inhalant allergy symptoms. A sufficient amount of pollen must reach the sensitive individual to affect him.

4. *The pollen must be sufficiently buoyant to be carried considerable distances.* This depends to a great extent upon the weight, form, and general physical character or maturity of the pollen. Presuming close and extensive contact, a person may develop allergy symptoms from the pollen, which is so heavy it does not travel far, of a plant in his backyard.

5. *The plant producing the pollen must be widely and abundantly distributed.* Certainly a plant in one's yard can cause symptoms to the person who lives there, but the pollen must be widely disseminated to produce widespread symptoms.

DISTRIBUTION OF POLLEN

Distribution of the important pollen-producing plants is a key factor in the evaluation, diagnosis, and treatment of inhalant allergy diseases. Certain plants are indigenous to given areas of the world, but with the present tendency toward suburbanization there frequently is a change in plant population from one type to another. When families move to a new location outside city limits, they often landscape the property with their favorite trees or shrubbery, use a new lawn mixture, and develop gardens with new plants. The result is a new type of vegetation with a subsequent increase in new pollen production. But plant growth is not always due to preconceived planting. Most of it, as far as the active allergy-producing plants are concerned, is accidental, the pollen being carried by the wind and taking root in a vacant lot or along a road to grow, mature, and reproduce. Some plants are native to a particular area and do not thrive elsewhere. Geographical or physical conditions such as climate, character of the soil, amount of rainfall, seasonal changes, and height above sea level are some of the determining factors.

Changes in vegetation, and therefore production of different pollen likely to produce allergy symptoms, occur continuously in every area. Years ago it was popular for hay fever sufferers to escape ragweed by vacationing in "hay fever havens," usually situated in the northern part of the country adjacent to a lake where ragweed was rare. But in due course the hotels planted grass and flowers on the grounds and many built golf courses. Inevitably ragweed sprang up. No longer were these spots the "havens" they once were.

In southern California where there are very few native trees, commercially planted walnut trees posed a problem for many years. As subdividers came and purchased the ranches of English walnut groves for future homes, they replaced the walnut trees with the faster-growing Chinese elm trees. As a result, this variety of elm is now an important cause of spring and fall hay fever in these areas. The rearrangement of the native flora which occurred in southern California is not at all uncommon in other parts of the country.

Substantial data regarding the identity and distribution of pollen-producing plants have been developed over the past fifty years. This has resulted from the collaboration of allergists and botanists of colleges, universities, and county arboretums.

A meticulous investigation begins with the identification of the plant and the determination of the pollination dates. Microscopic examination of collected pollen follows. The location and abundance of the plant must be established.

Then comes the all-important inquiry into the potential allergenicity of the plant. This step requires extracting of the principle active ingredients from the pollen, a sophisticated procedure necessitating the use of various extracting fluids. A diluted extract is then employed to perform hundreds of allergy skin tests on subjects who may or may not be allergic to the pollen. If the plant is allergenic and the extract is not merely an irritant, a small percent of the total group tested will react with the formation of a hive; these people are allergic to the plant pollen from which the extract was made. (In the event that all, or a large percentage, of the people react, the reaction is caused simply by an irritant.)

Surveys for suspected plants are repeated from time to time because of the new plants which may take root and grow. Many allergists have made it a habit to inspect the plant life as they drive through the city or country to ascertain what is pollinating at a particular time of the year. Some allergists have made it a practice to collect pollen which falls from the air onto vaseline coated slides kept on the window ledge of their offices for a twenty-four-hour period. By examining the slides under the microscope the doctors can determine which plant is pollinating at that particular time.

The pollen can also be counted to determine its concentration. A commonly used method of pollen counting is the volumetric method. Samples of air are drawn into a special device containing coated slides and the pollen is then deposited on the slides. The count, determined by a formula, is based on the number of pollen grains found in an area of one square centimeter during the twenty-four hours of exposure.

Many allergists use the informal, less accurate, though perhaps equally informative method of allowing a sheltered vaseline-coated slide to be exposed on the roof or a window ledge. Counting the number of pollen grains per predetermined unit (square millimeter) that have fallen onto the slide, the physician can compare the result to previous counts.

At one time, many large cities in the United States reported a pollen count daily during the ragweed hay fever season. It was thought that this was a valuable service to hay fever sufferers who then would have an idea of the amount of pollen concentration in the air from day to day. However, this practice, although still in existence, is now not as common as it once was, as it was learned that it actually afforded very little real information to the hay fever victim. The pollen count varies from one district to another, sometimes from one street to another, and since most of the slides are exposed high up in tall buildings, the information collected from them could be misleading. The concentration on the slides may be far less than at "nose level," which is what is important to the individual. In addition, there is usually a delay in announcing pollen counts, and the results may reflect the abundance of pollen from the previous day and not the current count. There are other factors which can lessen the value of a count, such as the technique of pollen collection and the mathematical conversion of the count, as well as the habits of the sufferer. Nevertheless, these pollen counts have helped indicate a pattern, and from their study an estimation has been made of what the pollen count might be from year to year.

Despite this, occasionally it is necessary for the physician to visit a patient's home in order to identify some unusual plants which may be surrounding it and which are of strictly local origin. Usually these plants are found to be entomophilous (insect-pollinated) and are causing trouble because the patient lives in such close proximity to them. Sometimes a patient will bring a suspicious plant to the allergist's office for identification. If the doctor does not recognize it, he can always call upon one of the national allergy societies or local botanical specialists for help.

Aside from the local alterations which have been mentioned, the basic pattern of pollen distribution throughout the United States, and indeed the entire world, has for the most part remained relatively static and has been well explored and documented. In general, the trees pollinate in the early spring, the grasses in the spring and early summer, while the weeds pollinate in the late summer and early fall. Individuals sensitive to trees, grasses, or weeds, therefore, are likely to suffer symptoms during well-delineated periods of the year. This is less clear-cut in the southern part of the United States where there is a tropical or subtropical climate. In such areas the pollinating periods of the trees, grasses, and weeds overlap, and there may be more than one distinct grass and weed season depending on the rainfall and variability of temperature. The pollinating season is thus extended, but it remains, nevertheless, somewhat predictable.

In the United States the dwarf and the giant ragweeds are the most common causes of hay fever. These weeds grow everywhere except west of the Rocky Mountains. Bermuda grass, another important hay fever producer, thrives in the southern portion of the nation. Aside from the ragweeds, the common allergy-producing weeds are pigweed, lamb's-quarters, sagebrush, and Russian thistle. The most common grasses, in addition to Bermuda grass, are June grass, rye, velvet, timothy, orchard, and redtop. The important trees are the poplar, elm, maple, oak, and walnut; there are also many others. It is common for the country to be divided into six or nine geographical areas in which the important allergenic plants are listed.

On the premise that an arbitrary line on a map is not an accurate way to demonstrate the exact distribution of pollen there is nonetheless, a chart listing the important allergenic plants in major cities of the United States and some foreign countries. The allergenicity of the plant listed under the city closest to the reader's home is graded from one plus (+) to four pluses (++++). One plus (+) indicates a plant of slight importance; two pluses (++), one of moderate importance; three pluses (+++); a plant of marked importance; and four pluses (++++), a plant of primary importance in that area.

SUMMARY

A very important cause of allergy symptoms, particularly of the seasonal variety, is the pollen of certain plants. Pollen is a microscopic dust which when inhaled by the allergic or sensitive person is likely to produce allergy symptoms. Some pollen is carried on the legs and body of insects, often those seeking nectar. Other pollen is carried by the wind from the male to the female plant. These wind-pollinated plants are the producers of abundant pollen that are the most common cause of allergy diseases.

Hay fever which occurs in most of this country during the late summer and early fall is caused by the inhalation of pollen. In the eastern part of the United States it is due to two varieties of the ragweed plant. The male ragweed plant can produce one hundred ounces of pollen in one season.

Pollen may be found miles away from its original plant source when it is borne by the wind. It has been found even thousands of feet up in the air, so one does not need to have a specific plant in the backyard to have allergy symptoms. It has been postulated that in order for the pollen of a plant to produce allergy symptoms there are certain conditions which must be met. The pollen must have a certain toxicity, an unexplained factor which distinguishes allergy-producing plants from those which are harmless. Most commonly, the pollen should be borne by the wind rather than by an insect, although insect-pollinated plants can produce symptoms when the victim comes into close contact with them. The plant should also be an abundant producer of pollen so that a sufficient amount gets into the atmosphere. For some reason a number of plants do not produce much pollen. The pollen, to be an important incitant of allergy diseases, must be light enough to be picked up by wind currents and scattered about. Finally, there should be enough growth of this plant to make it a significant factor. A plant that grows only in a small area is not an important cause of allergy disease.

Plants and their pollen, although distributed in all parts of the world, generally seem to remain in the general area where they originate. No doubt this is due to the climate of the area, its rainfall, barometric pressure, general temperature, prevailing winds, type of soil, and other factors, many of which are yet unexplained. However, there are examples of plants which have been intentionally transplanted to new locales, have taken root, and have become important causes of allergy problems in their new locale.

Many physicians interested in allergy have made surveys of plants in the vicinity of their homes and offices and have counted the pollen in the general atmosphere. The survey is often performed simply by observing which plants are growing and which are pollinating at a certain time of the year. Crude pollen counts are made by exposing a vaseline-covered glass slide outdoors for a twenty-four-hour period and microscopically identifying and counting the pollen. Although there are much more sophisticated methods of counting the pollen mathematically and quantitatively, the crude procedure, if repeated day after day, month after month, and year after year, gives adequate information regarding the type and approximate quantity of the pollen in the atmosphere.

On the basis of the more intensive botanical surveys and pollen counts performed throughout the world, tables of important pollinating plants, their seasons of pollination, and their relative significance have been established. Charts on pages 52-60 indicate the important allergy-producing plants by city and surrounding area; the information, however, is subject to change with changing botanical conditions.

52 ALL ABOUT ALLERGY

Grasses	Albuquerque, New Mexico	Atlanta, Georgia	Baltimore, Maryland	Bismarck, North Dakota	Boise, Idaho	Boston, Massachusetts	Buffalo, New York	Butte, Montana	Chicago, Illinois	Cleveland, Ohio	Dallas, Texas	Denver, Colorado	Detroit, Michigan	El Paso, Texas	Fresno, California	Kansas City, Missouri
Barnyard Grass / Echinochloa crusgalli		6-8 +	6-8 +			7-9 +	7-9 +		7-9 +	7-9 +	7-9 +	7-9 +	7-9 +	5-9 +	6-9 +	6-8 +
Beach Grass / Ammonphila																
Bermuda Grass / Cynodon dactylon	3-12 ++++	5-11 ++++	7-10 +								3-12 ++++			4-1 +++	3-10 ++++	4-11 ++
Bluegrass / Poa	5-8 +±	2-7 +	4-8 +	6-8 +	4-9 +	4-7 +	4-7 +	5-7 +	4-9 +	4-9 +	3-6 +	6-8 +	5-9 +	5-7 +	1-5 ++	4-6 +
Bromegrass, Brome / Bromus	4-6 ++		5-6 +		6-7 +		6-7 +			6-7 +	5-6 +	6-7 +	6-7 +	5-6 +	3-6 +++	
Buffalo Grass / Buchloe dactyoids	4-6 +										5-8 +			5-7 +	5-7 +	
Canary Grass / Phalaris		5-7 +	6-7 +			6-7 +	6-7 +	6-7 +	6-7 +		5-7 +	6-7 +	6-7 +		4-6 +	5-6 +
Fescue / Festuca	4-7 +	5-6 +		5-7 +		5-6 +	5-6 +		6-8 +	6-8 +	6-8 +	5-7 +	6-8 +		5-6 +	4-5 +
Grama / Bouteloua											5-7 +	6-9 +		5-9 +		
Johnson Grass / Sorghum halepense	4-9 +++	6-8 +									5-11 +++		6-9 +	4-10 +	4-9 +++	5-10 +
Kentucky Bluegrass / Poa pratensis	5-8 ++	6-8 +	5-7 +++	5-7 ++	5-8 ++	6-7 ++	6-10 ++	5-10 +++	5-8 +++	5-8 +++	3-6 ++	5-8 ++	5-8 +++	4-6 +	4-8 +	4-6 +++
Koeler's Grass / Koeleria cristata	7-9 ++			5-6 +	5-6 +		5-6 +	5-6 +	5-6 +	5-6 +	5-6 +	5-6 +	5-6 +	6-9 +		5-6 +
Maize, Indian Corn / Zoa mays	6-9 +	7-8 +	7-8 +	7-9 +					7-9 +	7-9 +	7-9 +		7-9 +		6-8 +	7-8 +
Meadow Fescue / Festuca elatior				6-7 +	6-7 +	6-8 +	6-8 +	5-6 +		5-6 +		5-7 +			5-6 +	6-7 +
Meadow Foxtail / Alopecurus pratensis	6-8 +					5-6 +										
Oats / Avena	3-6 +			6-7 +								5-6 +			3-5 ++	4-5 +
Orchard Grass / Dactylis gloerata	6-8 +	6-8 +	5-6 ++	5-7 +	6-7 ++	5-8 +	5-8 +	6-7 ++	6-9 ++	5-6 ++	5-6 +	6-8 ++	5-7 ++		4-8 +	5-6 ++
Paspulum / Paspulum	6-9 ++	6-9 +			7-9 +						4-10 +			5-7 +	5-9 +	
Redtop / Agrostis alba	5-8 +		6-7 ++	6-7 +	6-8 ++	6-8 +	6-8 +	6-7 ++	6-8 ++	6-8 ++		6-8 +	6-8 ++		6-8 +	6-8 +
Rye / Secale cereale				6-7 +							6-7 +					6-7 +
Rye Grass, Ray Grass / Lolium	3-8 ++		5-7 +			6-7 +	5-7 +		6-8 +	6-8 +	4-6 ++		6-8 +		4-6 ++++	4-6 +
Saltgrass / Distichlis	4-9 +			6-8 +							6-8 +	6-8 +		5-7 +	4-7 ++	
Sudan Grass / Sorghum vulgare	4-9 +++	6-8 +									5-11 +++		6-9 +	4-10 +	4-9 +++	5-10 +
Sweet Vernal Grass / Anthoxanthum odoratum		5-6 +	5-6 +			5-7 +	6-7 +		6-7 +	6-7 +			6-7 +			
Tall Oat Grass / Arrhenatherum elatius																6-7 +
Timothy / Phleum pratense		5-8 +	6-7 +++	5-7 +	6-8 ++	6-10 ++	6-10 ++	6-7 +	6-7 +++	5-7 +++	4-7 +	6-8 ++	6-8 +++			4-7 ++
Velvet Grass / Holcus lanatus		5-6 +	6-7 +			6-8 +	6-8 +			6 +	6-7 +					
Wheat Grass / Agropyron	6-8 +		6-7 +	6-7 +	6-9 +	6-8 +	6-8 +	6-8 +	6-8 +	6-8 +	5-7 +	5-7 +	6-8 +	5-7 +		6-7 +
Wild Rye / Elymus	5-6 +	5-6 +			6-8 +						5-6 +	6-8 +			5-7 +	

Little Rock, Arkansas	Los Angeles, California	Minneapolis, Minnesota	Nashville, Tennessee	New Orleans, Louisiana	New York, New York	Oklahoma City, Oklahoma	Omaha, Nebraska	Philadelphia, Pennsylvania	Phoenix, Arizona	Portland, Oregon	Reno, Nevada	Richmond, Virginia	Salt Lake City, Utah	San Francisco, California	Seattle, Washington	Spokane, Washington	St. Louis, Missouri	Tampa, Florida	Washington, District of Columbia
6-8 +	6-9 +	6-8 +	6-7 +	4-11 +	4-10 +	4-10 +	6-8 +	6-8 +	5-7 +	6-10 +		6-10 +		6-9 +	6-10 +	6-10 +	6-8 +		6-8 +
														6-7 +					
4-11 ++	2-11 ++++		5-11 +++	4-12 ++++		4-11 +++		5-8 +	3-12 ++++	4-9 +		3-11 +++		4-10 +++			7-9 +	3-11 +++	7-9 +
4-6 +	1-7 ++	6-7 ++	3-4 +	1 5 +	4-7 +	3 6 +	6-7 +	6-7 ++	5-8 ++	5-8 ++		3-8 +	6-7 +	1-6 ++	5-8 ++	5-8 ++	4-8 ++		4-8 +
	3-6 +++	5-7 +	5-6 ++	3-6 +	4-6 +		5 7 +	5-7 +	4-6 ++	4-7 ++	5-6 +			5-6 ++	3-6 ++++	4-7 +++	5-7 ++	5-7 +	
		6-8 +	5-7 +		4-6 +												5-7 +		
5-6 +	4-6 +		6-7 +	4-6 +	6-7 +	6-7 +	6-7 +	6-7 +		5-7 +				4-6 +	5-6 +	5-6 +	6-7 +	5-6 +	6-7 +
4-5 +	3-5 +																		
		5-7 +					6-8 +	5-7 +		6-9 +							5-7 +		
5-10 +	4-9 +		6-9 ++	4-11 ++			6-8 +	6-9 +		4-9 ++			6-8 +	5-9 +				6-9 ++	
4-6 +++	4-8 +	5-7 +++	5-7 +++	5-9 +	5-6 +++	5-7 +	5-7 ++	5-7 +++	5-8 +	5-10 +++	5-7 ++	4-8 ++	5-7 ++	4-8 +++	5-10 ++++	5-10 ++++	5-8 ++++		5-7 ++
5-6 +	4-6 +	6-7 ++	5-6 +		5-6 +	5-6 +	6-7 +	5-6 +	7-9 ++	5-6 +	5-6 +			6-7 +	5-6 +		6-7 +	6-7 +	
7-8 +		7-8 +	6-8 +	4-7 +		6-7 +	7 +		6-9 +					6-9 +		7 +	7 +		7-8 +
6-7 +	5-6 +	6-7 +		6-7 +		6-7 +	6-7 +		6-7 +	5-6 +	5-8 +	5-6 +	5-6 +	6-7 +	6-7 +	6-8 +			7-8 +
		4-5 +		5-6 +					5-6 +	6-8 +									
4-5 +	4-6 ++	6-7 +			4-6 +	6-7 +			3-6 ++	3-6 +				4-6 +++	3-6 +	6-7 +			
5-6 ++	4-9 +		6-9 +	6-9 +	6-9 +			4-9 +	4-9 +	6-7 ++		6-8 +	4-7 +	4-9 +	4-9 +				
6-7 +	6-8 +		5-9 +	4-11 +		6-8 +			6-9 ++	7-9 +	7-9 +	6-9 +	6-9 +	6-8 +	7-9 +	7-9 +	7-8 +	7-9 +	7-9 +
6-8 +	6-8 +	6-7 ++	6-7 ++		6-8 ++		6-7 ++	6-8 ++	5-8 +	6-9 +	6-9 ++	6-7 +	6-9 +	5-8 ++	5-8 +	6-9 ++	6-9 +	6-8 +	
6-7 +		5-6 +	5-6 +			6-7 +	5-6 +							6-9 +					
4-6 +	4-6 +++	5-7 +	5-6 ++	4-7 +	5-6 +	4-8 +	5-7 +	5-6 +	3-8 ++	5-8 ++++		5-7 ++	4-7 ++	5-7 ++++	5-8 ++++	5-7 +	6-7 +		5-6 +
	4-9 +	5-7 ++	5-7 ++	5-7 +	5-7 ++		5-7 ++	5-8 ++	6-8 +	5-7 +++	5-6 +	5-7 ++	5-6 +	5-8 ++	5-7 +++	5-7 ++	5-7 ++		5-6 ++
5-10 +	4-9 ++		6-9 ++	4-11 ++		6-8 +	6-9 +		4-9 ++			6-8 +	5-9 +				6-9 ++		
		5-7 ++	5-7 +	5-7 +	5-7 +		5-7 ++	5-7 ++		4-6 ++		5-7 ++		4-6 ++	4-6 ++			6-7 +	
6-7 +	6 +					6 +		6-7 +						6-7 +		6 +			
4-7 ++		6-7 +++	6-8 ++	4-6 +	4-9 ++	6-9 +	6-7 +	6-7 ++	6-7 +++	6-7 ++	6-7 +	5-8 +++	6-7 +	5-7 +	6-7 +++	6-7 +	6-7 +++	6-7 +	6-7 +++
		5-6 +					6 +		6-7 +	5-7 +			5-6 +	6-7 ++++					6-7 +
6-7 +	6-8 +			5-7 +	5-7 +	6-8 +	5-7 +	6-8 +	5-8 +	6-7 +	6-8 +	6-7 +		5-8 +	5-8 +	6-8 +			6-7 +
	4-8 ++	5-6 +		4-6 +			5-6 +		5-6 +	5-7 +	6-8 +		6-8 +	4-7 ++	5-7 +	5-7 +	5-6 +		

Each cell shows the allergy season range over the plus-sign intensity rating.

Trees	Albuquerque, New Mexico	Atlanta, Georgia	Baltimore, Maryland	Bismarck, North Dakota	Boise, Idaho	Boston, Massachusetts	Buffalo, New York	Butte, Montana	Chicago, Illinois	Cleveland, Ohio	Dallas, Texas	Denver, Colorado	Detroit, Michigan	El Paso, Texas	Fresno, California	Kansas City, Missouri
Acacia / *Acacia*															2-3 / +	
Alder / *Alnus*		1-2 / +	3-4 / +	3-4 / +	3-4 / +	3-4 / +	3-4 / +	3-4 / +	3 / +	3-4 / +	1-2 / +	4-5 / +	4-5 / +		1-3 / +	
Ash / *Fraximus*	2-5 / ++	3-5 / ++	3-4 / ++	4-5 / +	3-4 / +	5 / +	4-6 / +	4-5 / +	4-5 / +	4-5 / ++	2-5 / ++	4-1 / +	4-5 / +	2-4 / ++	3-4 / +++	4-5 / +
Basswood, Linden / *Tilia*			5-7 / +		4-5 / +	4-5 / +	4-5 / +	4-5 / +	4-5 / +	4-5 / +	4-5 / +	4-5 / +	4-5 /			4-5 / +
Beech / *Fagus*		3-4 / +	4-5 / +			4-5 / +	4-5 / +		4-5 / +	4-5 / +			4-5 / +			
Birch / *Betula*		4-6 / +	3-4 / ++	4-5 / +	4-5 / ++	4-5 / ++	4-5 / ++	4-5 / +	4-5 / +	4-5 / ++	3-4 / +	4-5 / ++	3-5 / +	3-4 / ++	3-5 / +	3-5 / +
Box-Elder / *Acer negundo*	2-3 / +	3-4 / +	3-5 / +	4-5 / +	4-5 / ++	4-5 / +	4-5 / +	4-5. / ++	4-5 / ++	4-5 / ++	3-4 / ++	4-5 / +++	4-5 / ++	3-4 / +	3-4 / +	3-4 / +
Casuarina, Beefwood / *Casuarina*															3-6 / +	
Cedar, Juniper / *Juniperus*	11-3 / ++										12-2 / +++	3-4 / +		1-3 / +		
Cottonwood, Poplar / *Populus*	1-4 / +	3-4 / +	3-5 / +	3-4 / +	4-5 / +	4-5 / +	4-5 / +	4-5 / ++	4-5 / ++	4-5 / ++	3-4 / ++	3-5 / ++	4-5 / ++	1-3 / ++	2-4 / ++	4-5 / ++
Elm / *Ulmus*	2-3 / +	2-3 / ++	3-4 / ++	4-5 / +	3-4 / +	3-4 / +	4-5 / +	3-4 / +	3-4 / ++	3-4 / ++	3-4 and 10-12 / +	3-4 / +	3-4 / ++	3-4 / +	2-3 / ++	3-4 / ++
English Walnut / *Juglans regia*															4-6 / +	
Hackberry / *Celtis*	2-4 / +	4-5 / +	4-5 / +	4-5 / +		4-5 / +	4-5 / +	3-4 / +	3-4 / +	3-4 / +		3-4 / +	3-4 / +	3-4 / +		3-4 / +
Hazelnut / *Corylus*		2-3 / +	2-3 / +			3-4 / +	3-4 / +		3-4 / +	3-4 / +	2-4 / +		2-4 / +			
Hickory / *Carrya*		3-5 / +	4-5 / ++	5-6 / +		4-5 / +	5-6 / +		5-6 / +	5-6 / +	3-5 / +		5-6 / +			4-5 / +
Hornbeam / *Carpinus*		2-4 / +	3-4 / +			2-4 / +	24 / +		3-4 / +	3-4 / +			3-4 / +			3-4 / +
Maple / *Acer*		3-4 / +	3-4 / +	4-5 / +	3-5 / +	4-5 / +	3-4 / +	4-5 / +	3-4 / +	3-4 / +	2-4 / +	4-5 / +	3-4 / +		3-5 / +	3-4 / +
Mulberry / *Morus*	3-4 / +	3-4 / +	4-5 / +	4-5 / +		4-5 / +	4-5 / +	4-5 / +	4-5 / +	4-5 / +	3-4 / +	4-5 / +	4-5 / +	3-5 / +	3-5 / +++	4-5 / +
Oak / *Quercus*	3-5 / +	3-4 / +++	3-5 / +++	4-5 / +	4-5 / +	4-5 / +++	4-5 / +++	4-5 / +	4-5 / +++	4-5 / +++	3-5 / ++	4-5 / +	4-5 / +++	3-4 / +	3-4 / ++	3-5 / ++
Olive / *Olea europaea*														4-6 / +	4-6 / ++++	
Osage-orange / *Maclura pomifera*			4-5 / +			4-5 / +	4-5 / +				3-4 / +					4-5 / +
Paper-mulberry / *Broussonetia papyrifera*			4-5 / +								3-4 / +					5-6 / +
Pecan / *Carrya illinoensis*		3-5 / +									3-5 / ++			4-6 / +		4-6 / +
Pepper Tree / *Schinus molle*															5-8 / +	
Privet / *Ligustrum*			5-6 / +												5-7 / +	
Sweetgum / *Liquidambar styraciflua*		3-4 / ++	4-5 / +			4-5 / +	4-5 / +		4-5 / +	4-5 / +	3-4 / +	4-5 / +	4-5 / +		3-5 / +	4-5 / +
Sycamore, Plane Tree / *Platanus*	3-4 / +	3-5 / +	4-5 / +	4-5 / +	4-5 / +	4-5 / +	4-5 / +	4 / +	4-5 / +	4-5 / +	3-4 /		4-5 / +		2-4 / ++	3-4 / +
Tree-of-Heaven / *Alanthus altissima*	5-6 / +	4-5 / +	5-6 / +			4-5 / +	5-6 / +	5-6 / +	5-6 / +	4-5 / +	4-5 / +	5-6 / +	4-6 / +	5-6 / +	5-6 / +	5-6 / +
Walnut / *Juglans*	3-5 / ++	4-5 / ++	4-5 / ++	5 / +	3-5 / +	4-5 / +	4-5 / ++		5-6 / +	5-6 / ++	4-5 / +	4-5 / +	5-6 / ++		4-6 / ++++	5-6 / +
Willow / *Salis*	2-4 / +	2-3 / +				4-5 / +	4-5 / +	4-5 / +	3-5 / +	3-5 / +		3-5 / +	3-5 / +	2-4 / +		3-4 / +

Little Rock, Arkansas	Los Angeles, California	Minneapolis, Minnesota	Nashville, Tennessee	New Orleans, Louisiana	New York, New York	Oklahoma City, Oklahoma	Omaha, Nebraska	Philadelphia, Pennsylvania	Phoenix, Arizona	Portland, Oregon	Reno, Nevada	Richmond, Virginia	Salt Lake City, Utah	San Francisco, California	Seattle, Washington	Spokane, Washington	St. Louis, Missouri	Tampa, Florida	Washington, District of Columbia
2-3 +														1-4 ++					
	1-3 +	3-4 +	1-2 +		3-6 +		3-4 +	3-4 +		1-4 +	2-4 +	3-5 +	4-5 +	1-4 +	1-4 +	2-4 +			3-4 +
4-5 +	4-5 +	4-5 +	3-5 ++	3-4 +	4-5 +	3-4 +	4-5 +	4-5 +	2-5 ++	3-4 +	3-4 +	4-5 +	4-5 ++	3-6 +	3-4 +	4-5 +	4-5 +	3-4 +	3-4 ++
3-4 +		4-5 +	4-5 +	4-5 +	4-5 +		4-5 +	4-5 +			4-5 +	4-5 +	4-5 +	4-6 +					4-5 +
		3-4 +		4-5 +			4-5 +				4-5 +	4-5 +					4-5 +		4-5 +
3-5 +	3-4 +	4-5 +	5 +	3-4 +	4-5 +	3-4 +	4-5 +	4-5 +		3-5 ++	3-5 +	4-5 +	4-5 ++	3-5 +	3-5 +	3-5 +	4-5 ++	4-5 +	3-4 ++
2-4 +	2-4 +	4-5 ++	3-4 ++	3-4 +	4-5 +	3-4 +	4-5 ++	4-5 +		2-5 +	3-4 +	4-5 ++	4-5 +++	3-4 ++	2-5 +	3-5 +	4-5 ++		3-5 +
	3-6 +		3-11 +											3-10 +				3-10 +	
1-3 +			1-2 +			1-2 +			11-3 +				2-3 +						
3-4 ++	2-3 ++	4-5 +	3-4 +	2-4 +	4-5 +	3-5 +	4-5 +	4-5 +	1-4 ++	2-5 ++	2-4 ++	3-5 +	2-5 ++	2-4 ++	2-5 ++	4-5 +	3-5 ++		3-5 +
3-4 ++	2-3 +	4-5 +	2-5 and 8-10 +	2-5 and 8-10 +	3-4 +	2-5 and 9-10 +	4-5 +	3-4 +	2-4 +	2-3 +	3-5 +	1-4 +	3-5 +	2-3 ++	2-3 +	3-4 +	3-4 +	2-3 +	3-4 ++
	4-6 +										3-6 +	4-5 +	4-5 +	3-6 +	3-6 +				
3-4 +		4-5 +	3-4 +	3-4 +	4-5 +	3-4 +	4-5 +	4-5 +	2-4 +		3-4 +	4-5 +	4-5 ++				4-5 +		4-5 +
		4-5 +	2-3 +		3-4 +		3-4 +		1-4 +			3-4 +		2-4 +	1-4 +	2-4 +			2-3 +
3-5 +	5-6 +	3-5 +			4-5 +	5-6 +	4-5 +					4-5 +					4-5 +	4-5 +	4-5 ++
3-4 +		3-4 +	3-4 +		2-4 +	3-4 +	2-4 +					2-4 +					3-4 +		3-4 +
2-4 +	3-4 +	4-5 +	2-4 +	2-4 +	4-5 +	3-5 +	4-5 +	4-5 +		3-5 +	3-5 +	2-4 +	3-4 +	3-4 +	3-5 +	3-5 +	3-5 +	3-4 +	3-4 +
3-4 +	3-5 +	4-5 +	4-5 +	4-5 +	4-5 +	4-5 +	4-5 +	4-5 +	3-4 +	4-5 +	4-5 +	4-5 +	4-5 ++				4-5 +	4-5 +	4-5 +
3-5 ++	3-5 ++	4-7 +++	3-5 ++	3-4 ++	4-5 +++	3-5 ++	4-5 +	4-5 +++	3-5 +	2-5 ++	3-5 +	4-5 +++	3-5 ++	3-4 ++	3-5 ++	4-5 ++	3-5 ++	1-4 ++	3-5 +++
	4-6 ++									3-5 +++				4-6 +					
4 +		4 +											4-5 +				4-5 +		4-5 +
5-6 +		4-5 +	4-5 +		4-5 +								5 +				5 +		4-5 +
3-5 +		3-5 ++	3-5 ++		3-5 ++		3-4 +				4-5 +	4-5 ++					4-5 +	2-5 +	4-5 ++
	5-9 +			5-6 +				5-7 +						6-8 +					
	5-7 +		5-6 +	5-7 +									5-7 +					5-6 +	
3-5 +	3-5 +	4-5 +	3-5 +	3-4 +	4-5 +	4-5 +	4-5 +	4-5 +		3-5 +		4-5 +		3-4 +	3-5 +		3-5 +		3-4 +
3-4 +	2-4 +	4-5 +	3-4 +	3-5 +	4-5 +	3-5 +	3-4 +	4-5 +		3-4 ++	3-4 +	4-5 ++	3-4 +	3-4 ++	3-4 ++	3-4 +	3-4 +		4-5 +
5-6 +	5-6 +	5-6 +	4-5 +	4-5 +	5-6 +	4-5 +	5-6 +	5-6 +		5-6 +	6-7 +	4-6 +	6-7 +	5-6 +	5-6 +		5-6 +		5-6 +
4-5 +	4-5 ++	4-5 +	3-5 ++	3-4 +	4-6 +	3-4 +	4-5 +	4-5 +	3-5 +	3-5 ++	3-5 +	3-5 ++	4-5 +	3-5 ++	3-5 ++	3-5 +	3-5 ++		4-5 ++
3-4 +		3-5 +	3-5 +	3-5 +	4-5 +	3-5 +	3-5 +	4-5 +	2-4 +	3-4 +	1-4 +	3-4 +	2-5 +	1-2 +	3-4 +	2-3 +	3-5 +	3-5 +	

Weeds	Albuquerque, New Mexico	Atlanta, Georgia	Baltimore, Maryland	Bismarck, North Dakota	Boise, Idaho	Boston, Massachusetts	Buffalo, New York	Butte, Montana	Chicago, Illinois	Cleveland, Ohio	Dallas, Texas	Denver, Colorado	Detroit, Michigan	El Paso, Texas	Fresno, California
Alfalfa *Medicago sativa*			5-7 +	5-7 +	5-7 +	5-7 +	5-7 +				5-7 +	5-8 +	5-8 +	5-7 +	5-9 +
Bassia *Bassia hyssopifolia*					5-7										6-8 +
Beet *Beta*					7-8 +				7-9 +						5-10 +
Burning Bush *Kochia*	6-9 +++				7-9 +				7-9 +			6-8 +	7-9 ++		
Bush Pickleweed *Allenrolfea occidentalis*	6-9 +											5-6 +	5-7 +		
Cocklebur *Xanthium*	7-10 +	6-8 +	6-8 +	7-9 +	6-8 +	8-9 +	7-9 +	7-9 +	8-9 +	8-9 +	6-8 +	6-9 +	8-9 +	6-9 +	5-10 +
Dock *Rumex*	4-8 +	4-8 +	5-7 +	5-9 +	5-9 +	5-7 +	6-8 +	5-10 +	5-8 +	5-8 +	5-7 +	6-9 +	5-8 +	4-6 +	4-6 +
False Ragweed *Franseria*	3-10 ++			8-9 ++	8-9 ++				8-9 +++			5-9 ++	8-10 ++	3 10 +	6-9 +++
Goosefoot, Lamb's-quarters *Chenopodium*	3-10 ++	6-8 ++	7-9 ++	6-9 +	6-9 +	6-9 +	6-9 +	7-9 +	7-9 ++	5-10 ++	6-9 +	7 9 +	4 8 ++	5-10 ++	5 10 ++
Greasewood *Sarcobatus vermiculatus*	5-8 +				6-8 +										
Hemp *Canabis sativa*															
Marsh Elder *Iva*	5-9 +		7-10 +	6-10 ++	5-9 ++	7-9 +			5-9 ++	7-9 +	7-9 +	7-9 ++	7-9 ++	8 9 +	7-9 +
Pickleweed *Salicornia*					6-8 +										5-8 +
Pigweed, Amaranth *Amaranthus*	3-12 +++	2-11 ++	4-8 ++	6-7 ++	7-8 ++	7-9 ++	7-9 ++	7-8 ++	7-9 ++	7-9 ++	5-11 +++	6-9 ++	7-9 ++	3-8 ++	5-9 ++
Plantain *Plantago*	4-8 +	4-8 +	4-7 ++	6-9 +	6-8 +	5-8 +	6-8 +	6-9 +	6-8 +	6-8 +	7-8 +	7-9 +	6-8 +		4-8 +
Ragweed *Ambrosia*	7-11 +	5-10 +++	8-10 +++	8-10 ++	8-9 ++	7-10 +++	8-9 ++++	8-10 +++	8-9 ++++	8-9 ++++	8-12 ++++	8-9 ++	8-9 +++	7-11 +++	8-10 ++
Russian Thistle *Salsola*	6-11 ++++			6-9 ++	5-9 +++			7-9 ++++	8-9 +		7-11 ++	5-9 +++		5-10 ++	6-9 +++
Sagebrush *Artemisia*	6-10 +++	5-6 +	7-9 +	8-9 ++	8-9 ++++	7-8 +	7-8 +	5-9 ++	8-9 +	8-9 +	7-11 ++	8-9 +++	8-9 +	4-10 ++	6-10 ++
Saltbush *Atriplex*	6-11 ++		7-8 +	6-8 +	5-9 +	5-9 +	7-8 +	5-9 ++	5-9 +		3-6 ++	6-8 +	5-9 +	5-7 ++	4-10 +++
Seablite *Suaeda*	6-8 +			7-8 +								7-9 +		5-7 +	4-9 +
Spiny Hopsage *Grayia spinosa*	4-6 +											6-9 +		4-8 +	
Western Waterhemp *Acnida tamariscina*	6-9 +								7-9 +	7-9 +	6 9 +	7-9 +	7-9 +		

Kansas City, Missouri	Little Rock, Arkansas	Los Angeles, California	Minneapolis, Minnesota	Nashville, Tennessee	New Orleans, Louisiana	New York, New York	Oklahoma City, Oklahoma	Omaha, Nebraska	Philadelphia, Pennsylvania	Phoenix, Arizona	Portland, Oregon	Reno, Nevada	Richmond, Virginia	Salt Lake City, Utah	San Francisco, California	Seattle, Washington	Spokane, Washington	St. Louis, Missouri	Tampa, Florida	Washington, District of Columbia
5-9 +	5-9 +	5-9 +	5-9 +	5-9 +			5-9 +	5-9 +			5-9 +	7-8 +		6-8 +	5-9 +	5-9 +	5-9 +	5-9 +		
		5-8 +												7-8 +	6-8 +					
		5-10 +												7-8 +						
		7-8 +					6-9 ++	7-8 +++		6-9 +++		7-8 +		7-8 +				7-8 +	7-9 ++	
									6-9 +				8-9 +	6-8 +						
8-10 +	8-10 +	5-10 ++	8-9 +	8-10 +	7-10 +	8-9 +	6-9 +	8-9 +	8-9 +	7-10 +		5-9 +	8-10 +	6-10 +	5-10 +++		6-9 +	7-9 +		8-10 +
4-10 +	4-10 +	4-6 +	5-9 +	5-8 +	3-11 +	5-8 +	4-8 +	5-9 +	5-7 +	4-8 +	4-9 +	2-5 +	4-8 +	4-8 +	4-8 +	4-9 +	4-9 +	5-8 +	4-7 +	5-7 +
		5-10 +++	8-9 +				8-9 +		8-9 +	3-10 +++		8-10 +++		8-10 +++	5-10 +			7-9 +		
5-10 ++	5-10 ++	6-10 ++	6-8 ++	6-10 ++	6-10 +	5-10 ++	6-10 ++	6-10 +	3-10 ++	5-10 ++	5-10 ++	6-10 ++	6-9 +	4-8 ++	4-9 +++	5-10 ++	5-10 ++	5-10 ++	6-9 ++	5-9 +
										6-8 +		6-10 +		7-10 +	6-10 +					
						7-9 ++												7-9 +		
8-9 +	6-11 +++	3-9 +	5-9 ++	8-10 +	8-10 ++	7-9 +	6-10 ++	5-9 ++		5-9 +		6-7 ++	7-9 +	6-10 +	6-9 +		5-9 +	8-9 +		6-9 +
		5-8 +		5-8 +							5-9 +			7-8 +	6-8 ++	5-9 +				
6-8 ++	5-8 ++	5-9 ++	6-9 ++	6-9 ++	5-11 ++	5-9 +	5-10 ++	6-9 ++	6-9 +	3-12 +++	6-10 ++	5-10 +	6-9 +	4-7 +	5-10 +++	6-10 ++	6-9 ++	7-8 +	6-8 +	7-10 +
4-10 +	4-10 +	4-8 +	5-9 +	5-8 +	3-12 +	5-8 +	4-8 +	5-9 +	5-9 +	4-8 +	5-9 +	6-7 +	4-8 +	6-7 +	4-8 +++	5-9 +++	5-9 +	5-8 +	4-8 +	5-9 ++
7-9 ++++	8-10 +++	6-9 +++	8-9 ++++	7-11 ++++	8-11 +++	8-9 ++	8-10 ++++	8-9 ++++	8-9 ++++	8-9 ++++	7-11 +	8-10 +	8-10 +	7-9 ++++	8-10 +++	6-9 +	8-10 ++	8-10 ++++	5-10 ++	8-10 +++
		6-9 +++	6-9 +++							7-10 +++	7-9 +++	6-11 +++		6-8 +++	7-9 ++++			7-9 +++	7-8 ++	
7-9 +	7-9 +	6-10 ++++	7-8 ++	8-9 ++		7-10 +	8-9 +	7-8 ++	8-9 +	6-10 ++	7-9 +	8-10 ++++			8-11 ++++	5-10 ++++		8-11 ++++	8-9 ++	8-10 +
		5-9 +++					7-9 +			7-9 +	6-11 +++			6-9 ++	6-10 ++	7-10 +++		8-10 +++		
		5-7 +	6-8 +				7-8 +							7-9 +		5-7 +		4-9 +		5-7 +
										4-6 +				1-5 +						
6-8 +	6-8 +		7-9 +	6-9 +			6-9 ++	7-9 ++	6-9 +										7-9 +	

Grass	Temperate Europe	Mediter-ranean Basin	British Columbia Alberta Saskatch-ewan	Manitoba Ontario Quebec	Central and South America
Barley *Hordeum vulgare*	6-7 +	5-7 ++			
Bent grass; Red Top *Agrostis alba*	6-8 ++	5-7 +	6-7 +	6-7 +	++
Bermuda grass *Cynodon dactylon*		8-9 +++			5-9 +++
Bristle grass *Setaria*	8-10 +	7-10 ++			++
Brome grass *Bromus*	5-7 ++	5-7 +++	6-8 ++		++
Crested Dog's Tail *Cynosurus cristatus*	6-8 ++	5-7 +			
Cultivated wheat *Triticum sativum*	6-7 ++	5-7 +	6-7 +	6-7 +	
Dallis grass *Paspalum*		8-10 ++			++
Dog's grass; Couchgrass *Agropyrum repens*	7-8 +	6-9 +	6-8 ++	6-7 +	
English Meadow grass, Annual June grass *Poa praetense*	5-6 +++	4-5 ++	6-8 +++	5-6 +++	
False Oat grass *Arrhenaterum elatius*	6-9 ++	6-9 ++	5-6 ++		
Giant Rod *Arundo donax*	8-10 +	9-10 ++			
Goat grass *Aegilops ovata*		5-6 ++			
Koeler's grass: Western June grass; Crested Hair grass *Koeleria cristata*	6-7 ++	5-6 +	6-8 ++		
Meadow fescue *Festuca*	6-7 ++	5-6 ++	5-6 +		
Millet *Panicum*		7-9 +			++
Nodding melick *Melica*	5-7 +	5-6 ++			
Oat grass *Avena*	6-8 ++	5-8 +++			
Orchard grass; Cockfoot grass *Dactylis glomerata*	5-6 +++	5-6 +++	5-7 ++	6 ++	++
Quacking grass *Briza*	6-8 ++	6-8 +			
Rye *Secale cereale*	5-6 ++				
Rye grass *Lolium*	5-8 +++	6 +++	5-7 ++		++
Sweet Vernal grass *Anthoxanthum odoratum*	4-6 +	4-6 +	4-5 +		
Timothy; Cat Tail *Phleum praetense*	6-8 +++	6-7 +	6-7 +	6-7 +++	
Tor-grass *Brachypodium*	6-8 +	6-8 ++			
Velvet grass; Yorkshire fog *Holcus lanatus*	5-6 ++	5-6 +++	5-7 ++		
Yellow grass; Golden Oat grass *Trisetum flavesens*	6-7 +++	6-7 +			

Trees	Temperate Europe	Mediterranean Basin	British Columbia Alberta Saskatchewan	Manitoba Ontario Quebec	Central and South America
Acacia *Acacia*	4-5 +	4 ++			+
Alder *Alnus*	3-4 +	3-4 +	3-4 +	3-4 +	
Ash *Fraxinus*	4-5 ++	4 +		5-6 ++	12-2 +
Basswood; Linden *Tilia*	6-7 ++	6 ++		6-7 +	
Beech *Fagus*	4-5 +			5 +	
Birch *Betula*	4-5 +	4-5 +	4-5 +	4-6 +	+
Elderberry *Sambucus*	5-6 +	5-6 +++			
Elm *Ulmus*	2-4 ++	3-4 +	4 +	4 ++	+
Hackberry *Celtis*		4 +++		5 +	+
Hazelnut *Corylus*	2-3 +	2-3 +	3-4 +	4-5 +	+
Hickory *Carya pecan*				6 +	
Hornbeam *Carpinus*		3-5 +			
Juniper; Cedar *Juniperus*				4 ++	
Maple *Acer*		2 ++	4-5 +	4-5 +	+
Mulberry *Morus*		4-5 ++		5 +	+
Oak *Quercus*	4-5 ++	4-5 +++	4 +	5-6 +	
Olive *Olea*		4-6 ++			
Paper Mulberry *Broussonettia*		4-5 +++			
Phylaria *Phyllirea*		6 ++			
Pine *Pinus*	5 ++			5-6 +	
Poplar; Cottonwood; Aspen *Populus*	2-5 +	3-4 ++	4 +	4-5 ++	
Privet *Ligustrum*		5-6 ++			
Spruce *Picea*			5-6 +	5-6 +	
Sycamore; Plane *Platanus*	4-5 ++	4-5 ++			
Tree of Heaven *Ailanthus*		5-8 +			
Walnut *Juglans*		3-4 +		5-6 +	+
Willow *Salix*	3-4 +	3-4 ++	2-4 ++	4-5 +	
Yew *Taxus*	4-5 +			4-5 +	

Weeds	Temperate Europe	Mediter-ranean Basin	British Columbia Alberta Saskatch-ewan	Manitoba Ontario Quebec	Central and South America
Allscale; Saltbush *Atriplex*	7-9 +	8-9 ++	8-9 +	7-8 +	
Bur Marigold *Bidens*	7-9 +				++
Cat Tail *Typha*	6-8 ++	6-8 +			
Cocklebur *Xanthium*	9-10 +	7-9 +			
Dandelion *Taraxacum officianale*	4-5 ++		5-9 ++		
Dock; Sheep Sorrel *Rumex*	5-8 ++	6-9 ++	8-9 +	6-8 +	
English plantain *Plantago*	5-9 +++	4-7 +	5-9 ++	5-9 ++	
False ragweed *Franseria*			7-9 +		++
Goldenrod *Solidago*	7-9 +			7-8 ++	
Lamb's quarters; Goosefoot *Chenopodium*	8-9 +	8-10 ++	7-9 +	7-8 ++	++
Nettle *Urtica*	6-8 ++	6-8 ++	7-8 ++	6-7 ++	
Pellitory *Parietaria*	6-9 +	3-10 +++			
Pigweed *Amaranthus*					
Prairie ragweed "Burweed marshelder" *Cyclachaenia*			7-8 ++		
Ragweed *Ambrosia*				8-9 ++++	++
Russian thistle *Salsola*		7-8 ++	7-9 ++	7-8 +	
Sagebrush; Mugwort *Artemisia*	7-9 +	9-10 ++	8-9 ++	7-9 ++	

Chapter Six

Inhalant Causes of Allergy
Other Than Pollen

The most prevalent and dramatic manifestation of allergy is seasonal hay fever, which results from inhalation of plant pollen. The seasonal type may last all year (perennial) in those parts of the country such as the South and certain portions of California where there is pollen in the air nearly twelve months of the year. In most cases, however, perennial hay fever (perennial allergic rhinitis) results from inhaling miscellaneous, assorted, mixed, or nonpollen dusts—a conglomeration of substances that floats about the air of the home, store, office building, or factory—in contrast to pollen, which is primarily a contaminant of the outside atmosphere. In addition to such miscellaneous allergenic inhalants, many nonspecific factors such as temperature, barometric pressure, and air pollution may perpetuate symptoms in a person whose sensitive nasal lining has been bombarded by pollen during a previous heavy pollinating season.

People spend much time in their homes. Aside from the many hours in constant contact with the cotton of mattresses, feathers, pillows, wool, blankets, upholstered furniture, and carpeting (with its underlay), they move about and come in contact with numerous other inhalant substances, the most common of which is conveniently termed house dust. In their business and social lives other contacts are made with allergy-producing substances, some obvious and others remarkably hidden from view. It is important for the allergy patient to know where all these substances may be found.

HOUSE DUST

House dust is not simple outdoor dirt, sand, or rock particles, such as may be propelled into the air by excavation or as a consequence of a sandstorm. It consists of raw cotton, bits of wool, feathers, animal hair, pesticide powder, scales of insects, mites, shreds of kapok, shreds of cellulose and other foreign material, and colonies of living molds (mildew) and bacteria. It is formed by the breaking down of practically any substance found in the home. As the bits of material become smaller they also become light enough to be suspended in the air where they tend to remain, eventually settling and forming a fine powder on the floor or any objects present.

The origin of this dust may be drapes, bedspreads, blankets, pillows, comforters, toys, pets, stored clothing, mattresses, box springs, rugs and carpets, rug pads, upholstered furniture, books, and hard shelves. Anything disintegrating, then harboring and collecting dust that eventually enters the air again, must be considered.

So it can be seen that house dust is not a single allergy-producing entity. It is possible that one patient's dust allergen may not be another's. Household dust has been extracted, refined, and fractionated but despite this reduction to the simplest possible compound it has maintained its capacity to produce allergy reactions and typical allergy symptoms.

The house-dust allergen used for treatment by the injection method for various allergies has many sources. Vacuum sweepings from a home in which pets are kept, sweepings from musty rooms, extracts prepared from the patient's own home—all have been employed. Dust allergen extracted from old mattresses and upholstery stuffing, then carefully refined, is widely used. Most allergists find that they achieve excellent results merely by using a house dust prepared from practically any source, then reinforcing it with specific substances to which the patient has shown a reaction, such as animal hair, wool, feathers, or molds.

DOG HAIR

A very difficult problem often encountered in allergy practice is excluding the cherished family pet from the house. Allergy to dog hair is to the protein material of the hair shaft, and even more, to the dandruff of the dog's skin. This dandruff consists of cast-off cells of the outer layer of the dog's skin and the oily material which is secreted by the dog's sebaceous glands. Since dogs are often allowed freedom to roam in the house, rugs, sofas, or beds collect hair and frequently become a source of allergy symptoms.

Long-haired dogs shed more hair and leave a larger amount for the allergic individual to encounter. The poodle breed has a coat which is more like that of a sheep's pelt and is somewhat thatched, therefore shedding less and leaving less hair behind. But because it may be more affectionate and spend more time in the house, the poodle is often equally responsible for allergy symptoms. There is no evidence that one breed of dogs is more allergenic than another.

There is a cross reactivity between the dog's saliva and dog hair and dander. Welts may develop on the skin of a child's arm caused by the lick of an affectionate dog whose hair produces respiratory allergy symptoms. One source of dog hair in the home often not recognized is Oriental rugs, such as Chinese and Persian rugs which are made of animal hair, including that of the dog.

CAT HAIR

Cat hair and dander are also causes of allergy. An exceedingly sensitive individual often has an allergy attack even when he enters a room in which a cat had been. The hair and dander tend to remain in the air or become attached to furniture for an indefinite period. The cat's hair is usually finer, as well as softer, than that of a dog, and it sheds more readily, resulting in greater dissemination through the house than the fur of other pets. Some breeds are more allergenic than others, primarily because they have longer hair and shed it more readily and in greater quantity, but this does not imply that a short-haired cat can be kept with impunity by an individual allergic to it.

Cat hair may be found in many manufactured articles, such as fur gloves, slippers, caps, automobile robes, and Oriental rugs. It is no longer used extensively in fur coats but still can be found in the linings of inexpensive overcoats. In purchasing manufactured products, the consumer should read the labels carefully. Under the current fur-labeling legislation, a fur coat must be classified and designated by its legitimate official name, as well as by the country of its origin. This has largely eliminated the use of brand names suggesting more expensive furs. Despite honest labeling now required by law, the purchaser can still be deluded *if he does not read and examine the label carefully.*

Allergy to the domestic cat extends to other members of the cat family. Veterinarians, zoo attendants, circus performers, and animal handlers who are allergic to cat hair are subject to occupational allergy illness. Tame ocelots as pets are becoming popular with some people and allergy to them has been reported.

HORSE HAIR

As with all animal hair, the allergy to horse hair is both to the protein material of the hair shaft and to the dander of the animal which is adherent to the hair shaft. The dander is considered by some to be the more important and many believe it is the sole cause, the hair serving only as a vehicle to carry it. Horse hair is used in many industries and is hidden in many articles, where it may be unknowingly encountered. Despite the increasing use of such synthetic materials as foam rubber, nylon, Acrylon, Dacron, and rayon in upholstered furniture, a certain amount of horse hair is still required, particularly for the arms of chairs and sofas. Ordinary men's suits have horse hair as part of the stiffening material in the shoulders. Horse hair is found in orthopedic mattresses, hairbrushes, violin bows, twine, gloves, hats, toothbrushes, overstuffed cushions in homes, buses, automobiles, and railroad cars. Other sources include rug pads, especially the waffle-type pad, sacks and bags, gloves, hairpieces, wigs, furs, inexpensive men's suits, and also toys. Synthetic fibers have replaced horse hair in some of these but not all. Pony and colt fur have been used for winter coats sometimes designated by deceptive trade names. Again, one must read the labels.

The clothing of stable workers, jockeys, mounted policemen, and horse trainers are significant sources of horse hair. Farmers who still use draft horses and others likely to come in contact with horses, are candidates for symptoms of horse-hair allergy, or they may transmit the sensitivity to others through their infested clothes. There have been reports of people so sensitive to horse hair that mere contact with horse manure used for fertilization sets off a chain of severe symptoms.

An enigma is the apparent increase of sensitivity to horse serum used in biological material, concurrent with the decreased use of the horse as an animal for general purposes. Perhaps this reflects increased diagnostic acumen in contemporary medicine. In any event, today physicians are aware of the serious and sometimes fatal consequences of horse serum preparations and withhold their use unless they are categorically required—and particularly by the "horse-hair sensitive" patients. A skin test, and a test utilizing the outer layer of the eye, administered in advance, may be helpful in anticipating difficulty, but a very severe allergy response to a biological material containing horse serum may occur despite a negative skin test. Fortunately, tetanus antitoxin made from human serum is becoming increasingly available, and it cannot produce a reaction.

RABBIT HAIR

Like other animal hair, rabbit hair produces allergy symptoms, particularly when the rabbit is alive. The cute Easter bunny, brought home as a gift to a youngster, will often be kept in the house until it grows into a heavily pelted allergenic adult. If meticulously processed to rid it of dander, it is less likely to cause trouble. Yet rabbit hair is used as an inexpensive fur, for felt hats, toy animals, robes, padding, scarves, and sweaters; it is often inadequately cleaned and therefore is likely to produce allergy symptoms. Even when thoroughly cleaned and processed, intrinsic allergy to the hair shaft may be sufficient to produce symptoms. It should be avoided by persons who are sensitive to rabbit hair.

Rabbit hair may be used in several ingenious ways which are frequently overlooked. Actors may use a rabbit's foot to apply makeup, and some people, being superstitious, may even carry a rabbit's foot to bring them good luck. Rabbit hair makes an excellent lining fur for gloves, coats, and jackets. The felt made of rabbit's hair is used not only for felt hats but also for the hammers of piano keys and for insulating material. Angora is the hair of the Angora rabbit (or Angora goat) and is used in expensive sweaters, scarves, trimming, and innumerable articles of clothing. Prior to the new labeling legislation, the misnaming of furs made of rabbit pelt was most common, probably because the ease of dyeing and processing made possible the appearance of a more luxurious product. Names which resembled expensive furs were formerly attached to garments made from rabbit hair; these included such deceptive names as Beaverette, Nutriette, Russian Leopard, French Sable, French Seal, Baltic Fox, Corey, Minkony, Electric Mole, and Sable Hair, all representing dyed and processed rabbit hair. The law allows the use of any trade name, but the true nature of the fur used and its country of origin must be clearly stated. Reliable manufacturers today purchase raw furs from breeders' associations which guarantee the quality of the fur, but the wise purchaser and especially a person sensitive to rabbit hair should still carefully scrutinize the labels.

GOAT HAIR

Goat hair is found extensively in wearing apparel. Mohair is manufactured from the hair of Angora goats and Cashmere is made from the hair of Cashmere goats, while alpaca is the hair product of a Peruvian variety of goat. Goat hair is frequently mixed with wool and under certain names is used for the manufacture of drapes, rugs, shawls, carpets, blankets, upholstered fabrics, dress goods, pillows, doll's hair, and wigs. Goat hair, as a by-product of tanning, is sometimes used in plaster, cheap blankets, kitchen mops, tropical worsted cloth, socks, and bedding. Expensive hairbrushes and paintbrushes are often made of goat hair. Vicuna is a variety of goat hair.

In common with other animal hairs, the dander or dandruff from the upper layers of the animal's skin is the most potent portion of the allergy-producing fraction. A highly processed variety of goat hair is less allergenic. Age appears to make raw goat hair more treacherous. This is true of many miscellaneous environmental substances. One of the explanations for this is that adulterants such as mold or even bacteria join with the allergen to produce increased allergenic activity. And allergy to the protein material in the processed goat-hair products may cause trouble.

WOOL

The significance of wool as an antigen may be overestimated. Sheepherders, stockyard workers, spinners in woolen mills, and others who are in intimate contact with either the raw wool on the animal or with the dust of unfinished wool in the air are candidates for wool allergy. All of us come in contact with wool in our clothing apparel, but because of the intensive processing the material is put through, it is very unlikely to be allergenic. On the other hand, wool from very fuzzy blankets and from heavy, bulk-knit sweaters will cause symptoms in sensitive individuals, since small particles of wool are easily inhaled. For that reason wool-sensitive patients are instructed to use synthetic yarn blankets or to cover their fuzzy wool blankets with a securely made cotton blanket cover. They may choose instead to use an extra sheet over the blanket as well as under it, and to fold the upper edge over.

Wool has a local irritating effect on the skin, and a sensitive skin will invariably be aggravated when in contact with it. Itching, redness, and a rash often result. This may occur in nonallergic people as well, so it cannot always be attributed to allergy. Probably it is due to the rough character of the wool yarn which is known to be harsh on a tender skin; therefore everyone should be alert to a possible reaction from wearing knit wool next to the bare skin.

Probably 50 percent of rugs and carpets in common use are made of wool, but the wool portion of carpets and rugs is not the most important allergy-producing segment. The more significant allergy aspect of carpets and rugs in general, but particularly those made of wool, is that they are great dust collectors. As such, they harbor all the elements which comprise the house-dust antigen such as animal hair, feathers, cottonseed, wool, molds, bacteria, insect emanations, and practically everything which enters the home and pollutes the air. For that reason a wool rug is not recommended for use among allergic persons. In addition, the type of padding under the rug is important. After years of usage, rug padding begins to fragment, seep through the rug, and enter the air of the room. There are four leading types of under-rug padding, known as carpet underlays in the trade. These are sponge rubber and three types of felt. There is a flat rubber type but it is not yet widely sold for home use. Another type, the sponge rubber type, is a pad with a ripple or bubble surface.

The varieties of felt are (1) the all-hair variety which is usually cattle (cow) hair; (2) the hair fiber blend, a mixture of animal hair and a fiber which is usually jute; (3) the hair fiber blend coated with rubber on both sides. The all-hair variety, although an excellent underlay, is the most allergenic, while the rubberized felt is probably the best compromise. Mold grows in both the fiber and the hair, but not in the rubber. Therefore, the sponge rubber or even the rubberized felt makes an acceptable nonallergic underlay.

CATTLE HAIR

Cattle hair, like other animal hairs, is used commercially in many hidden ways. Under-rug waffle pads contain cattle hair along with other ingredients. Oriental rugs, particularly those from China and India, contain hair from cows, as do chenille carpets and bedspreads. Hairbrushes with imported bristles, certain twine and rope, toys, felt, stuffing for furniture, artists' brushes, and coarse blankets have poorly processed cattle hair. The term "poorly processed" is used because, as in all animal hair, the more thorough the cleaning and processing the lesser the allergenic qualities.

OTHER ANIMAL HAIRS

The hide, hair, and pelt of almost every available animal are used in some way for household purposes. In rural communities hog hair may be an important cause of allergy symptoms, particularly in farmers. Hog hair is used in insulation, in mixing mortar and plaster, and in brushes; therefore those in the building and painting trades may come in contact with a considerable amount of this seemingly unimportant allergen. Before the advent of foam rubber and other materials for stuffing, hog hair was used in large quantities for stuffing furniture, mattresses, and automobile cushions. It is still found as a stuffing in antique furniture, but its use in mattresses and in automobile upholstery is now rather uncommon.

Laboratory workers who work with mice, guinea pigs, rats, monkeys and many other animals that are employed for experimentation or laboratory procedures are particularly subject to allergy symptoms if they are allergic to animal hair and dander. Allergy to human hair is uncommon but may develop in barbers and wigmakers who come in close contact with it in their work. The quip about a wife being allergic to her husband's hair or vice versa is not always a joke. It is possible, although uncommon, for a person to become allergic to another person's hair.

Workers in the fur industry have for many years been subject to what has been accepted as an occupational disease—*fur asthma*. This has always been assumed to be due to sensitivity to the actual fur which was being sheared, cut, trimmed, and made into garments, but today there is so much processing with various chemicals for dyeing and preserving the fur that the respiratory symptoms fur workers exhibit may be caused by other factors.

Imported camel hair is obtained from the Bactrian camel. It is used in the manufacture of the popular camel-hair coats and jackets as well as in fine blankets, carpets, and rugs. Expensive old shawls used to be made from camel hair and some are still used. The well-known Jager cloths are made from camel hair. The advertised so-called camel-hair brushes are sometimes made with camel hair but very often they are composed merely of squirrel or kolinsky hair. In other products supposedly composed of camel hair, wool is frequently used as an adulterant or substitute.

FEATHERS

Feathers have long been considered an important and common cause of allergy symptoms. Many physicians have had the experience of effecting a dramatic cure in a patient by merely having him eliminate his feather pillow and substitute a foam rubber or Dacron pillow, or by his covering the original pillow with a well-made rubberized pillow encasing which prevents the feather particles from passing through. Such a cover should have extra-good seams and a tight zippered opening. However, a cure does not always result, for although the sufferer's pillow has been changed, the other feather pillows in the room may not have been removed, substituted, or covered. Feathers, therefore, are still in the air. To eliminate feather contact, all pillows and upholstered furniture containing feathers must be treated in the same manner.

Poultry farmers, pet-shop employees, and veterinarians are obvious victims of allergy to feathers if they are susceptible. The feathers which produce symptoms include, in addition to those of the goose, chicken, duck, and turkey, the feathers of popular household pets, like the parakeet, the lovebird, the myna bird, and the canary.

Allergy to the feathers of only one bird species may exist, and one is not necessarily allergic to the feathers of all birds. To determine if this is the case in a certain patient, some clinical experimentation may be required. In general, it is almost axiomatic to say that the allergic individual who is sensitive to one variety of feathers should avoid all kinds of feathers as much as possible. Obviously, the amount of exposure must be considered, so people who work on poultry farms or in the vicinity of birds should be particularly wary. The feathers of a canary kept within a cage all the time, however, can hardly be compared with the feathers in a pillow on which the allergic individual sleeps eight out of twenty-four hours.

Feathers on live birds laden with dandruff and attached to the oily portion of the skin are more likely to produce allergy symptoms than the feathers of killed birds used in pillows or upholstered furniture. Feathers used in new pillows are always thoroughly cleaned and sterilized. Old feather pillows are more likely to induce symptoms than are the newly processed and cleaned ones; they may also be infested by molds and bacteria.

COTTONSEED

The culpable portion of the cotton plant is not the well-known and easily recognizable drugstore variety of absorbent cotton, nor is it the processed and polished cotton material of men's shirts and women's dresses. It is, rather, the rough, raw, grayish, dirty-looking cotton which can often be seen bulging through the seams of an old mattress. The cottonseed in the cotton produces allergy symptoms. During the process of ginning, most of the seed is removed, but some, called linters, remains attached to the short cotton fibers. Cotton linters are used in the manufacture of mattresses, cushions, pads, upholstered furniture, as batting or wadding, waterproofing material, artificial silk, drip candles, book bindings, linoleum, sleeping bags, mustard plasters, and oilcloth. Cottonseed is also ground up and used for animal feed. It is the basis for cottonseed oil used in the manufacture of oleomargerines and lard substitutes such as Crisco and Snowdrift. Wesson oil is pure cottonseed. It is unlikely that these oil products cause allergy symptoms, however, because of their high degree of refinement. Cottonseed meal is also used as a fertilizer but not as frequently as it was at one time because price prohibits this, and in addition the newer synthetic fertilizers are taking its place. Nevertheless, it is still used as feed for animals, primarily as an additive.

KAPOK

Kapok is another plant substance which in its ground-up state produces allergy from inhalation. It is composed of silky fibers which encircle the seeds of the tropical American ceiba tree. Because of its softness, silkiness, and availability, it is frequently used as a filler in pillows, especially the small variety sometimes called decorators' pillows. It is also extensively used for sleeping bags and as a stuffing for dolls and toy animals, and for life jackets. Frequently, patients who are allergic to feathers purchase kapok-filled pillows as substitutes only to find that they have just as much if not more trouble than they had with the discarded feather pillows. This, of course, may be because they are allergic to kapok as well as to feathers, but also because kapok when ground up in the stuffing of pillows provides an excellent culture material for molds and bacteria, both of which may cause allergies.

PYRETHRUM

The powdered flower of the pyrethrum plant is a very effective insecticide. Pyrethrum exterminates insect pests instantaneously. Therefore, household pesticide powders and liquids contain pyrethrum or pyrethrins, which are the oily chemical compounds derived from the plant. Usually, slower-acting insecticides are included in the same product. Insecticides containing pyrethrum are extensively used in public places such as theaters, churches, and auditoriums where there are carpeted floors and upholstered seats. Severe symptoms due to allergy can result from pyrethrum inhalation. Therefore the labels and instructions of all exterminating powders and liquids should be read carefully before using them in the house. When a commercial exterminating service is used for the home, the pest-control experts should be advised about the existence of pyrethrum allergy and they will often employ a substitute.

FLAXSEED (LINSEED)

The flaxseed extract used for allergy testing gives marked skin reactions and has been known to produce some that are very severe.

Despite its potency and ubiquitousness, its importance as a cause of allergy is questionable, except as an occupational hazard. Flaxseed or linseed is used in the manufacture of linoleum, in paints, patent-leather products, printer's ink, poultry food, varnishes, and furniture polishes. It may also be used in wave-set lotions, hair tonics, flax rugs, and insulating material. There is a question whether linseed oil, processed and extracted from the ground flaxseed, is a cause of allergy difficulty. Until there is a clear consensus, it is best for flaxseed- or linseed-sensitive individuals to avoid contact with the oil as well as the dried seed.

ORRIS ROOT

Orris root is derived from the dried root of a particular Florentine variety of the iris family. The root is fragrant, and for many years was used to supply the faint violet scent to face powders. Because of its high degree of allergenicity, cosmetic manufacturers now omit it from their products and it is seldom found in face powders today. Nevertheless, it may still be present in some perfumes and colognes of the cheaper variety. People who are allergic to orris root should suspect its presence in medicines, perfumes, sachets, colognes, shaving creams, hair lotions, tooth powders, astringent lotions, and face powders.

TOBACCO

Since tobacco smoke is intrinsically an irritant, it is difficult to separate respiratory symptoms due to sensitivity and those due to pure concentrated pollution of the immediate air which is inhaled. The validity of the allergy skin test to tobacco smoke is questionable. Nevertheless, allergic individuals are much more likely to have symptoms when in contact with tobacco smoke than are nonallergic individuals, and to develop a "tobacco cough." Nonallergic individuals are not immune to this, however.

SILK

For many years silk allergy has been considered important only for workers in the industry where silk thread is spun, processed, and manufactured. Material made of finished and polished silk is not harmful since the allergy is due to the silkworm which manufactures and stores the silk thread, leaving some of its allergenic elements adherent to it. A substance that has been indicted is the sericin glue which holds the fibers together. Processing, cleaning, and dyeing removes practically all of the allergenic material transmitted by the silkworm. Nevertheless, it is usually recommended that raw silk be avoided as wearing apparel. It is believed that individuals allergic to the silkworm may also be allergic to raw silk.

MISCELLANEOUS INHALANTS

An allergic individual is likely to react to many particles in the air; if he is not already sensitive, he invariably develops a sensitivity if exposed. The things which such a person is likely to encounter and react to are almost limitless. A few of the more common offenders are *gums and resins, soybean, glue, castor bean, flour, jute, hemp, sisal, coffee,* and *sawdust.* There are many more.

Gums and *resins* are used in hair-wave and hair-set lotions, tooth powders, toothpastes, pastes for false teeth, hand lotions, laxatives, and newsprint. They are also used as a food in the form of tragacanth, acacia, and karaya gum.

Soybean is a vegetable which, when inhaled in its whole state, is harmless. After extraction of the soybean oil, however, the residue is ground up for fertilizer and for animal feeding, and it is the ground-up soybean that is a hazard to the respiratory tract of allergic individuals. The allergenicity of soybean as a food, either as soy sauce, soybean cake, or even soy oil is controversial. It is the opinion of the majority that the soy oil because of its very refined state is not allergenic.

Glue is another substance to which allergic persons may react. Reports of glue sensitivity were described as early as 1922, but these cases were due to fish glue, not commonly used today. Nevertheless, fish glue may occasionally be encountered. It is used by some furniture manufacturers and may still be used as an adhesive in tile products.

Castor bean is a problem in allergy only when it is ground up. The castor beans themselves are very large and quite harmless, but when they are ground to be used as fertilizer after the castor oil has been extracted, the resulting finely ground powder can produce violent symptoms. Not only workers in the castor bean processing plant are subject to severe allergy symptoms, but also the inhabitants of areas in the vicinity of such plants, particularly when castor-bean dust is allowed to pollute the atmosphere. Epidemics of asthma due to castor-bean dust have been reported in neighborhoods and have ultimately been traced to castor-bean pollution of the air in the vicinity of castor-bean processing factories.

Bakers are apt to have allergy symptoms from *wheat* and *rye flour*, as are millers and others who work with very fine dust.

Jute, as well as many other fibers and materials, is found in the waffle-like padding under rugs and carpets. Some carpets utilize both jute and hemp in their backing. The bleached product soon loses its whiteness and becomes a dingy, dirty brown. Not only is this product apt to be allergenic to some people, but also, when the padding which contains jute is loosely woven, it tends to collect dust and molds in the hidden area on the underside of the rug or on the carpet floor covering. Coarse ropes and twine are made from jute.

The fiber obtained from the *hemp* plant is another product used mostly in the manufacture of twines, ropes, and cables. Hemp is also used in canvas and backing materials for carpets and is an ingredient of some newly developed plastics. Several industrial products are manufactured from hemp, notably soaps and a drying oil for plants. Farmers have found it valuable for livestock feed. It is also used as a fertilizer. A much less common use of the uncrushed hemp is as a bird feed, particularly for pigeons. Hemp, although botanically related to marihuana, *Cannabis sativa*, has no other connection. Allergy to marihuana, however, is possible and in effect is truly hemp allergy.

Sisal is a Mexican plant similar to hemp in that it is also used for making rope, sacking, twine, sailcloth, and cable insulation (because of its high tensile strength and resistance to saltwater). It is also considered an important allergen.

Coffee allergy is found among workers in coffee-roasting plants where raw green coffee is received, unpacked, roasted, and packaged. The allergy symptoms are due to inhalation of the dust of the coffee bean and must not be confused with allergy to coffee which is drunk.

Pure *sawdust* can produce respiratory symptoms in carpenters, cabinetmakers, and workers in sawmills. In most instances, this allergy appears to be specific to the type of wood used and the allergy is self-evident.

MOLDS (FUNGI)

Molds are a form of life which grow on living or decaying plant and animal material (parasite; saprophyte). These are becoming an increasingly recognizable part of the atmosphere, both in and out of the home. The mold that produces allergy symptoms does not produce disease in man as some types of parasitic growths do. The terms "fungus" and "mold" are used interchangeably, but there is a technical distinction. A fungus is a parasitic growth, while mold is the woolly material which grows on the surface. The mold, the woolly portion, breaks off to become dust, enters the air, and acts as an allergen. Allergy skin tests are performed with molds just as they are with other allergens.

Two related forms of mold, prevalent only in the grain cultivating areas of the country, are known as rusts and smuts, the latter coming from cereal grains. These are considered a disease of the plants which, although not always serious to the plant, are often the cause of allergy symptoms in people who are sensitive to them. Molds of all types are a constituent of "house dust," particularly where dampness is prevalent, such as in old homes near a body of water or irrigation ditches. They are also found mixed with pollen in the outdoor atmosphere.

The most frequently indicted molds are *aspergillus, alternaria, hormodendrum, penicillium* (*not* penicillin), *helminthosporium, fusorium, phoma, mucor,* and *claudosporium.*

INSECT INHALATION

Reactions to insect bites or stings are discussed in Chapter 10. In addition to the sting of the insect, which may be considered due to an injection of its venom, allergy symptoms can be due to inhalation of the scales, parts of the wings, and segments of the insects' bodies. These symptoms are usually much milder than those due to stings and are comparable to the symptoms produced by other inhaled allergens, such as pollen grains, dusts, and molds resulting in nasal blockage, swelling of the mucous membrane of the nose, sneezing, coughing, and wheezing.

The term "insects" is used loosely because strictly the Insecta is only one group of the larger classification of Hexapoda that is likely to cause difficulty. The best-known and perhaps the most dramatic reaction to flying insects is that caused by the *mayfly* and the *caddis fly* (sand fly). These are seen in the Great Lakes region, the Finger Lakes of New York State, along the banks of the Mississippi River, and in some of the smaller lakes in Wisconsin. They usually come in swarms, remain only a few days, and at times are so thick in the air that the atmosphere has the appearance of dense fog. This type of allergy is a local and a limited problem. The cause of this allergy is thought to be a thin membrane or sheath which the insect sheds as it flies through the air.

Aside from the mayfly and caddis fly, other flying insects have been reported to produce symptoms by inhalation in sensitive people. They have been isolated in infrequent instances. Nevertheless, they must be considered as a cause of allergy. These include the emanations from the common *housefly, bedbugs, moths, butterflies, beetles, fleas, weevils,* and *aphids.*

SUMMARY

Inhalant causes of allergy other than pollen include assorted mixed or nonpollen dusts. These include house dust, the most ubiquitous of all. House dust is formed by the breaking down of practically any substance that is in the home, including raw cotton, bits of wool, feathers, animal hairs, pesticide powder, scales of insects, shreds of kapok, shreds of cellulose and other foreign material, and colonies of living molds (mildew) and bacteria.

Animal hairs and danders (dog, cat, horse, rabbit, etc.) are frequent incitants of allergy diseases, especially of the respiratory tract. The allergy is both to the protein material of the hair shaft and to the dander of the animal which is adherent to it.

When dogs and cats are allowed freedom of the home, their hair and dander, which tend to collect in the rugs, sofas, and beds, ultimately get into the atmosphere, causing significant allergy symptoms when inhaled by one sensitive to these animals. A source of dog hair often not recognized is Oriental rugs; cat hair may be found in many manufactured articles, including fur gloves and automobile robes, as well as Oriental rugs. The cat's hair is usually finer and softer than that of a dog, and it sheds more readily, resulting in greater dissemination through the house.

Horse hair is used in many industries and hidden in many articles. Despite the increasing use of synthetic materials in upholstered furniture, a certain amount of horse hair is used, particularly in the arms of chairs and sofas. Pony and colt fur have been used for winter coats and sometimes are designated by deceptive names. One must read the labels.

Rabbit hair is fur that may be labeled by manufacturers to indicate more expensive furs. Current Federal law allows the use of any trade name, but the true nature of the fur used and its country of origin must be clearly stated. A wise purchaser of fur coats or fur-trimmed garments will scrutinize the labels.

Goat hair is found extensively in wearing apparel. A highly processed variety is less allergenic than one that is not. Age appears to make raw goat hair more treacherous, which is true of many environmental substances. Goat hair as a by-product of tanning is sometimes used in plaster, cheap blankets, kitchen mops, tropical worsted cloth, socks, and bedding. Expensive hairbrushes and paintbrushes are often made of goat hair.

Wool as an antigen may be overestimated. All of us come into contact with wool in our clothing apparel, but because of the intensive processing the material is put through, it is very unlikely to be allergenic. Even on the skin of nonallergic individuals, however, wool has an irritating effect, which may be more marked in those who are allergic and may produce a rash. Wool from the very fuzzy blankets and from heavy, bulk-knit sweaters will cause symptoms in sensitive individuals, since small particles of the wool can be easily inhaled. For that reason, wool-sensitive patients are instructed to use synthetic yarn blankets or to cover their fuzzy wool blankets with a securely made cotton blanket cover. Because wool floor coverings harbor all the elements that comprise the house-dust antigen, a wool rug may be additionally harmful to an allergy patient.

Cattle hair, like other animal hairs, is used commercially in many hidden ways. Under-rug waffle pads contain cattle hair along with other ingredients. Hairbrushes with imported bristles, certain twine and rope, felt stuffing for furniture, artists' brushes, and coarse blankets have poorly processed cattle hair which makes them more allergenic than articles made with more thoroughly cleansed and processed cattle hair.

The hairs of animals other than those already mentioned may also be a cause of allergy symptoms. Laboratory workers who work with mice, guinea pigs, rats, and monkeys may develop allergy symptoms if they are sensitive to these animals. It is even possible, though uncommon, for a person to become allergic to another person's hair. Workers in the fur industry have for many years been subject to *fur asthma,* which has been recognized as an occupational disease.

Feathers have long been considered an important factor in producing allergy symptoms. The fact that they are commonly used as a stuffing for bed pillows makes them exceedingly significant. Poultry farms, pet-shop employees, and veterinarians are obvious victims of allergy to feathers if they are susceptible. The feathers which produce symptoms include those of the goose, chicken, duck, turkey, parakeet, lovebird, myna bird, and canary.

Cottonseed is sometimes found in cotton linters and cotton that has not been highly processed. In the course of ginning, most of the seed is removed, but some may still remain attached to the remaining short fibers; this is what is termed linters. It is used in mattresses, cushions, pads, upholstered furniture, and many other household products. It is unlikely that the processed and highly polished variety of absorbent cotton found in drugstores or used in men's shirts and women's dresses is allergenic. Farmers who use cottonseed as a fertilizer or for animal feed may become allergic to it.

Kapok is another plant substance which in its ground-up state produces allergy from inhalation. Because of its softness, silkiness, and availability, kapok is frequently used as a filler for pillows; it is also used for sleeping bags, life jackets, and as a stuffing for dolls and toy animals.

The powdered flower of the pyrethrum plant is a very effective insecticide and insecticides in which this is an ingredient are often used in the home and in such public places as theaters, churches, and auditoriums.

Despite the potency of flaxseed, its importance as a cause of allergy is questionable, except as an occupational hazard. Flaxseed is used in the manufacture of linoleum, in paints, patent-leather goods, printer's ink, poultry food, varnishes, and furniture polishes. It may also be used in wave-set lotions, hair tonics, flax rugs, and insulating material.

Orris root for many years has been used to give the faint violet scent to face powders. Most manufacturers of good cosmetics have discontinued its use because of its recognized allergenicity. Yet it may still be found in cheap perfumes and highly scented colognes; in medicines, tooth powders, sachets, shaving creams, hair lotions, and astringent lotions.

Tobacco smoke is an irritant to the respiratory tract, but whether it is allergenic is open to question. The validity of the allergy skin test to tobacco smoke is still debatable.

Processing, cleaning, and dyeing removes practically all of the allergenic material transmitted by the silkworm. Nevertheless, it is recommended that raw silk be avoided as wearing apparel in those who are allergic to silk.

The miscellaneous substances which when inhaled may cause allergy in a susceptible person are almost limitless. A few of the more common are gums and resins, soybean, glue, castor bean, flour, jute, hemp, sisal, coffee and sawdust.

Molds are a form of life which grow on living or decaying plant and animal material. These are becoming an increasingly recognizable part of the atmosphere, both in and out of the home. The most common molds are aspergillus, alternaria, hormodendrum, penicillium (not penicillin), helminthosporium, fusorium, phoma, mucor, and claudosporium.

In addition to the sting of an insect, a person can be allergic to the inhalation of the scales, parts of the wings, and segments of the insect's body. The best-known and perhaps the most dramatic reaction to flying insects is that caused by the mayfly and the caddis fly (sand fly). Aside from these, other flying insects have been reported to produce symptoms in sensitive people. They have been isolated in infrequent instances and include the common housefly, bedbugs, moths, butterflies, beetles, fleas, weevils, and aphids.

Chapter Seven

The Injection Treatment
of Allergy Diseases

Doctors call the injection treatment, commonly employed in allergy diseases, *specific allergic desensitization.* The average person is apt to term it "shot treatment" or "allergy shots." None is a very good term. Desensitization means that complete neutralization of the state of sensitivity has taken place comparable to immunization against smallpox and "polio" (complete saturation of antibodies). This is accomplished in the laboratory animal by serial injections of increasing amounts of the substance which originally caused the allergy. Although the method of treatment is similar in humans and results in decreased sensitivity, it does not obliterate it entirely. A better and more scientifically correct term is *hyposensitization,* which implies that there is a reduction of sensitivity but does not imply that the neutralization is complete. Most allergists prefer to use *desensitization,* recognizing, however, that it is not precisely correct.

Among the most important considerations are the type, strength, and dosage of extract to be used in desensitization.

THEORY OF DESENSITIZATION

Allergists are not entirely sure of the exact mechanism by which successful results of desensitization are obtained. But the employment of this form of treatment for more than fifty years with repeated observations of marked relief has proved its worth to the satisfaction of all but a very few dissenters. One problem regarding the mechanism is that although complicated and exact techniques have been devised for measuring the specific type of allergic antibody (reagin) that circulates in the blood in allergy diseases, there is not yet a consensus that there is a measurable correlation between the amount that is present and the symptoms, on the one hand, and the results of treatment or the doses of antigens which may be injected, on the other. Nevertheless, several theories of desensitization have been advanced. Some are based on clinical observation and others on immunological studies.

The most widely accepted theory is the *blocking antibody* theory. It has been found that the injection of antigens, as in desensitization treatment, will produce an antibody which is detectable and is different from the usual type of skin-sensitizing antibody (reagin) that results from the ordinary or usual contact with the antigen. Although this new antibody, like the reagin, is specific for the antigen that produced it, the union of the antigen and the new antibody (blocking antibody) is harmless and does not produce allergy symptoms. This antibody competes with the skin-sensitizing antibody to unite with the antigen thus "blocking" the harmful antigen-antibody (reagin) union.

When a sensitive person receives an allergy injection, a reaction is usually produced at the site of the injection. This reaction may be so slight that it is not recognizable, or it may be severe. It has been postulated by some that when this local reaction occurs, it takes the place of a similar reaction in the shock tissue which might be produced to initiate asthma, hay fever, hives, or eczema. It has been observed that when a local reaction develops it often results in relief of symptoms at the time of the injection. Some allergists take advantage of this and deliberately give their injections intracutaneously to produce a local swelling. This theory may explain the lessening of symptoms many people experience following diagnostic intradermal allergy tests.

When, after proper sensitization, an experimental animal is given an allergy injection to produce an extremely severe reaction, there is a short period of time during which the animal is not subject to allergy reactions despite repeated injections, regardless of the size of the dose. Similarly, when a shocking dose resulting in a generalized reaction has inadvertently occurred in humans, a brief symptom-free period has subsequently been noticed. Many feel that allergy injections are miniature shocks and produce a refractory period. Others feel that there is a bombardment of the antibody-producing tissues causing lack of response, increased tolerance, and therefore fewer and less severe symptoms.

An additional theory maintains that desensitization injections foster the union of the antigen and antibody in the circulating blood rather than in the shock tissues, or given organ. Why this happens, if indeed it does, has never been adequately explained.

INDICATION FOR SPECIFIC ALLERGY DESENSITIZATION TREATMENT

Traditionally, allergy injection treatment has been employed in the treatment of allergic rhinitis, both the seasonal and the perennial forms. It is also employed in all types of allergy disease, particularly when the important causative agents are inhaled substances. Foods, although they may be a prime causative factor in an allergy disease and can be put into solutions for skin testing, do not lend themselves to injection treatment. Nevertheless, there are some physicians who attempt to desensitize against foods in this manner. One group is very enthusiastic. More than thirty years ago this method of desensitization against foods to which a person is allergic was given careful trial and consideration and generally found to be unsuccessful. It has no scientific basis and appears worthless to prominent allergists and theoretical immunologists. Desensitization to food is better performed by oral means (see Chapter 8). The substances with which desensitization is employed hypodermically are mainly the same as those that may be inhaled.

TECHNIQUE OF DESENSITIZATION

The techniques of desensitization vary in individual cases, but in general are similar. They consist of preparing an extract (tea and coffee are extracts) of the substances to which the person is sensitive as determined by his medical history and his skin tests. Treatment is begun with a very weak dilution. In order to measure the strength of an extract, chemists have utilized various standards. One is to use a given amount of the powdered material to the amount of the fluid with which the extract is to be made. For example, one part of the powdered material in 100 parts of the fluid will make a one to 100 dilution. If this is diluted ten times it would make a one to 1,000 dilution; further diluting it ten times would make a one to 10,000 dilution, and so on. This widely used method of standardization is known as the *weight by volume* method.

Another method of determining the strength of an extract is to measure the *total nitrogen* content (since nitrogen is a component of all protein) of the extract after it is prepared. A more exacting variation of this is *protein nitrogen* standardization, which is based on the concept that not all the nitrogen represents the protein portion; some may originate from other sources. There is no conclusive evidence that this is so. Perhaps in the future some other and more accurate way will be found to determine the strength of an extract.

Meanwhile, the doctor who treats a patient with an allergy disease by desensitization employs the standardization that he has found in his experience to be most satisfactory. Many doctors gauge the potency of their extracts by the manner in which their patients react to them.

There is only one reason why information regarding standardization may be important to the allergic person. When transferring from one doctor to another, one must recognize that all allergists do no use the same standardization of their extracts, but every well-trained allergist can convert from one to another in order to continue treatments without delay.

DESENSITIZING TREATMENT

Treatment always begins with a very small amount of a weak dilution. As a rule the initial dose is determined by skin tests with serial dilutions. The initial dose, customarily 1/20 or 1/10 of a cubic centimeter, is taken from the dilution just below the one that produces a positive reaction to the intradermal skin test (see Chapter 4 for a detailed description of intradermal skin testing).

As with the initial dose, the dosage schedule varies with each person's sensitivity. The ultimate object is to reach a protective dose (preferably before the pollinating season begins if pollen is being employed). This usually is a dose which will not produce any severe local reaction when the extract is injected and will not cause a general reaction. To do this, injections are given once or twice weekly. The time between injections for the most part is arbitrary and decided upon because of convenience. But experience has proved that it is wise to allow forty-eight or seventy-two hours to elapse between injections. When the proper dose is reached, it is maintained, and the intervals between injections may be lengthened. The proper dose is defined as the highest which a patient can tolerate and which relieves symptoms.

It should be emphasized that some people can tolerate a higher maximum dose than others. There are marked variations in dose tolerance from one patient to another, but this does not influence the efficacy of the protection.

REACTIONS TO TREATMENT

Two types of reactions may occur while the allergic individual is undergoing desensitization. One is the local reaction and the other is the generalized, or constitutional, reaction. The local reaction, annoying but seldom serious, takes place at the site of the injection and usually appears within minutes after the injection is given, although some local reactions are delayed and do not become manifest until several hours or even a day later. A slight local reaction consists of mild inflammation (redness) and swelling at the site of the injection. This subsides rather quickly. A more marked local reaction consists of a characteristic hive surrounded by a considerable area of inflammation. The arm may swell and be very uncomfortable. The direct application of a piece of ice is very comforting. If either type of local reaction appears after a desensitizing injection, the attending doctor should be told about it before he gives the next injection. He may wish to reduce the dose rather than increase it as he would be inclined to do when the treatment is in the increasing dose stage. Sometimes a person will have a marked local reaction, but once the dose is decreased and then slowly advanced again, no reaction will occur.

There are at least two explanations for untoward local reactions, other than an overdose. Instead of injecting the extract under the skin (hypodermically), it may have been inadvertently injected within the layers of the skin (intradermally). A second cause of large local reactions is penetration of a small blood vessel during injection. The area is likely to swell, turn black and blue, and be uncomfortable. This is traumatic, not allergic. Nevertheless, the swelling as such may also be indicative of some local reaction to the extract. Tolerance of higher doses as treatment continues indicates increased resistance.

Generalized, or constitutional, reactions do not occur as frequently as they did in the early days of desensitization therapy. Now more is known about the quality and standardization of the extracts that are being used. There is a greater respect for the potency of allergy extracts, and doses are more carefully estimated than in the past. These and many other factors have decreased the incidence of general or constitutional reactions, the causes of which are varied. Although constitutional symptoms occur much less frequently than formerly, some are unavoidable and are sometimes the result of an unsuspectedly extreme sensitivity in the patient. Fortunately today, with improved techniques, these are rare. The most common cause is an unwarranted increase in dosage caused either by failure to heed a previous local reaction (which should have been a warning) or by the lapse of too long a time between treatments. Still another cause of constitutional reactions is injection into a superficial vein in the skin. Skillful doctors are careful that this does not happen.

There are two types of constitutional reactions. One is *immediate* and the other *delayed.* The most severe reactions are the immediate ones, which often occur within a few minutes to a half hour after an injection. Because of this, many doctors request their patients to remain in their offices for half an hour after the treatment. Symptoms usually begin with a flushing of the face or itching of the palms of the hands, progressing rapidly to a generalized itching of the entire body. Giant hives and swellings may follow. The eyes may swell to the point of closing. It may become difficult to swallow because of a spasm. There may be marked sneezing, wheezing, coughing, difficulty in breathing, and sense of tightness in the chest.

A violent constitutional reaction is treated quickly and aggressively. The symptoms must be relieved immediately and additional treatment given to prevent their recurrence. Generally, the treatment is the same as that employed for any other severe allergy attack, whether it is an insect bite or a severe reaction to a drug. They are all allergy reactions with similar symptoms although different causes. The first thing the doctor usually does is to place a tourniquet on the arm where the injection was given *above* the site of the injection, between it and the heart. This is to prevent further absorption of the symptoms-producing material. Then he injects adrenalin into the site of the allergy injection producing the reaction. This shuts down the small blood vessels in the area, keeping the material localized and decreasing the rate of absorption. An additional injection of adrenalin is usually given in the other arm, to be absorbed into the body and counteract the severe symptoms. This is sufficient to control more than 90 percent of the severe constitutional reactions. As improvement takes place, the tourniquet is loosened and released. If symptoms persist, additional small doses of adrenalin may be required for their control. Rarely is more stringent treatment necessary.

To avoid recurrence some cortisone products may be injected by the doctor; antihistamines administered orally and by injection are also useful. Reactions which are delayed and may develop several or more hours after the injection are usually milder and are likely to be merely uncomfortable; these include nasal stuffiness and mildly asthmatic chest symptoms. If any swellings develop they are not of any great significance. Oral medication, such as an ephedrine tablet or an antihistamine (or both), which a doctor can order by telephone, is usually sufficient to give relief.

In some instances, reactions are more severe and require more vigorous treatment, sometimes even hospitalization. Oxygen, as well as drugs to elevate the lowered blood pressure caused by shock, may be necessary. Such reactions are exceedingly rare, and in the process of immunization, where tolerance is continuously being tested, they are virtually absent.

DESENSITIZATION TO POLLEN

Hay fever, particularly the type due to pollen, which has a sharply demarcated pollinating season, lends itself best to desensitization treatment. Treatment has been divided into *preseasonal, coseasonal,* and *perennial.* The preseasonal treatment is administered before the onset of the pollinating season of the plant or plants to which the person is allergic. Dosage, as in the injection treatment with other allergens, is always started with a very small amount of a weak dilution based upon serial skin tests. The aim of the treatment is to reach the maximum, optimum, or maintenance dose prior to the pollinating season. Treatment continued during the pollinating season is termed coseasonal. The optimum dose is continued or it may be lowered to compensate for the pollen that is circulating in the air and which the individual is absorbing through his nose.

Very often, however, a hay fever sufferer does not visit his doctor until the pollinating season has started. Coseasonal treatment may then be given in a different manner. Since there has been no build-up period, very tiny doses of a very weak dilution given at frequent intervals, perhaps daily or even several times a day, may give remarkable relief. As a rule, the injections are administered intradermally, where a local reaction may be produced. Why one receives such good results by this method of treatment is not yet thoroughly understood.

After the season is over, some physicians continue the injections through the entire year. The thought behind this is that by maintaining the effective dose, the preseasonal building-up period will be obviated. In this so-called perennial treatment, doctors lengthen the intervals between injections after the pollinating season is over to two, three, and in some cases four-week intervals. In theory this sounds like an excellent idea, and in the East and Midwest where there are many persons sensitive only to ragweed, which pollinates for about six weeks in the fall and has a clearly delineated season, it appears to work out very well. But the patient must be careful not to forget his injection date with the lapse of too long a period between the injections. If this happens, there is always danger of a constitutional reaction; or the dose must be decreased to the point of nullifying its value. Also, during the course of treatment a new extract must be substituted for the old, and these are far more potent than older extracts. One method of making the change is gradually to mix part of the new with the old. Each physician employs his own well-tried procedure.

During this process, at least weekly visits are necessary, since there is a possibility of a constitutional reaction taking place. All in all not a great deal of time is saved, and claims by some that the results are better are difficult to prove. There are many factors involved. Comparing one person's hay fever with another's and attempting to determine which form of treatment is most satisfactory is difficult, requiring a consideration of the differences in sex, age, work, play or exercise, environmental influences, emotional problems, climatic changes, and fluctuation of the amounts of circulating pollen breathed by the two people.

Perennial treatment is best used and, in fact, is necessary in locales where there are no clearly delineated plant-pollinating seasons, or where there are overlapping seasons of tree, grass, and weed pollen which may last from February to November or December—practically all year. This may be true of the Mediterranean coast, the tropics, and especially of southern California, Arizona, and southern Texas, where several of the important grasses start to pollinate in February along with the trees. Some grasses continue to pollinate into the fall weed-pollinating season and have several growths depending upon the amount of rainfall. In such instances, the allergic person must be treated at the allergist's discretion preseasonally for some pollen, coseasonally for others, and practically perennially for all.

DESENSITIZATION TO INHALANTS OTHER THAN POLLEN

People who are allergic to house dust may be desensitized by the same technique described for pollen. Usually, house-dust treatments are given all year around, although undoubtedly contact is greater during the winter months when the windows and doors are kept closed, the heat is turned on, and one spends more time indoors. Whether to include other inhalants originating in the home is a matter of the attending physician's judgment. Since house dust is assumed to be a conglomeration of all the dusts found in the home, including wool, feathers, molds, and animal hairs, it would appear that additional therapy with these inhalants should not be necessary. This is the attitude of many allergists, but others prefer to fortify their injection material with whatever other substances the person contacts in his home or work. For example, if there is a dog in the home, dog hair is added to the house dust. Since most house dusts are not usually prepared from the patient's own home, adding these materials makes the extract "tailor-made" and in many instances more effective.

WHO SHOULD GIVE THE INJECTION

Allergy injection treatments are not routine. They require altering the doses during the progress of treatment, giving the injections in a modified dose during the height of the symptoms, and being prepared to cope with any reactions that may occur, some of which may be serious. Ideally, from the therapeutic and psychological points of view, the allergist should see the patient on each visit and administer the treatments. Most do so. Personal attention is a clear necessity when treatments are initiated, when the dosage must be increased, or when a patient is very ill requiring repeated examinations and possible periodic change in medication. In the absence of these problems alternatives may be employed.

When a person lives at a great distance from the consulting allergist's offices, it is customary for the allergist to prepare the extract to be given and to instruct a local physician in its administration. Usually, a dosage schedule is forwarded with the extract together with printed instructions discussing possible reactions and how to cope with them. The patient is asked to return to the allergist when larger doses of the material become necessary or if any complications arise. In place of vials and dosage schedules some allergists prefer to furnish ampuls, each containing an individually measured dose. These ampuls are numbered in sequence. Since the entire dose is administered there is no need for measuring doses, and possible errors are avoided.

When a trained assistant or a registered nurse gives the injections, it is done under the supervision of the physician. This is a time-saving technique for both doctor and patient and is commonly employed in cases of uncomplicated hay fever or similar allergy disorders where treatments are required throughout the year and the tolerance therefore has been long established. In certain instances, particularly when a person has been taking injection treatments for a long time and is receiving a final maintenance dose, he may be taught to give his own injections. Although this is not recommended by most allergists, there are circumstances in which it may be necessary. One is when a person lives in the country where no doctor is available but treatment is required. Another is when the patient is crippled or disabled and travel is not possible. Nonetheless, this procedure involves many dangers.

Often in a company or educational setting arrangements may be made for a nurse to administer the treatments. Decisions regarding who should administer the injection and whether or not the doctor should see the patient on each visit rest with the attending physician.

TYPES OF ANTIGENS

Allergists are constantly searching for more effective material for allergy treatments. To obviate frequent injections required for effective desensitization, long-acting and slowly absorbed antigens have been studied. A substance which will enhance the activity of a medicine is called an adjuvant. Adjuvants have been used in connection with antigen extracts in several ways; some are currently under investigation and are being perfected. The addition of a highly refined mineral oil and an emulsifying agent to the antigen which is customarily made in a water medium was one of the first such mixtures investigated. The product was a so-called "water-in-oil emulsion," resembling homogenized milk in appearance. The principle behind this product was that the oil droplets would be absorbed very slowly, gradually releasing the antigen over several weeks or even months. The difficulty with this product was that nodules appeared in some individuals at the site of the injection; in others, abscesses formed. These reactions may have occurred because mineral oil is poorly absorbed and because too large a quantity of the emulsion had been injected. A fear was expressed in some scientific circles that the material might eventually produce cancer. Because of these factors and the lack of complete approval by FDA, most allergists did not adopt this form of treatment and many of those who had been using it stopped. Those who are continuing to employ the emulsion treatment are studying the results and possible side effects, keeping accurate records of each case. Another long-acting antigen that is being studied is an allergy extract mixed with Alginate (derived from seaweed). This is purely in the experimental stage.

One type of prolonged-action allergy extract which is available commercially, having been approved by the Food and Drug Administration is Allpyral. This is an extract of the allergen to which is added a chemical called pyridine. It is claimed that fewer injections are required with this type of extract and some allergists believe that this extract has great possibilities. This remains to be seen. Meanwhile, investigation is proceeding to find other products which will permit desensitization with fewer injections.

DURATION OF TREATMENT

This is a problem which must be dealt with on an individual basis. Some allergy sufferers respond to specific desensitization so well that after as little as one year's therapy they are in a remission which may last for years, or even all their lives. Others do not respond as positively; treatment must be continued indefinitely just as a diabetic needs to take insulin or some other antidiabetic agent regularly. On the average, three years is the minimum required for most patients who suffer from an inhalant allergy.

The allergy desensitization injection treatment is similar to the immunizing injections administered for polio, diphtheria, measles, smallpox, or any other well-known antiserum, with one important difference. In allergy, immunity, instead of lasting for perhaps a lifetime, wears off sometimes as quickly as one week. Nevertheless, when an injection is given week after week for many months, there appears to be a breakdown of the allergy-producing mechanism, and eventually an allergy sufferer may be relieved for weeks, months, years, and sometimes for a lifetime. This depends on the person, the type of allergy, and other factors that remain unexplainable.

The allergic person in the eastern and midwestern portion of the United States develops typical hay fever symptoms caused by ragweed from August until the frost kills the ragweed. He seldom develops immunity and may continue to require desensitization treatment season after season. Other allergy hay fever sufferers fare differently; a series of desensitizing treatments over a three-year period may result in a permanent "cure" or at least a refractory period of one to several years, until another series of treatments may be necessary. Usually, after symptoms have been absent for a year or more, treatment can be discontinued as a test. When, if ever, symptoms recur, treatment can be resumed.

SUMMARY

In addition to the use of medicines that are used for relief of symptoms, treatment of allergy diseases may be accomplished by allergy injections. The method is comparable to immunization such as that used to protect against poliomyelitis, measles, smallpox, and tetanus. It involves the "neutralization" or "saturation" of the antibody in such a fashion as to prevent its union with the antigen, which produces the symptoms of allergy diseases. Since complete protection or "neutralization" is not possible, a more scientific term would be "hyposensitization," but this is a clumsy word and "desensitization" has remained in common use.

Although this method of treatment has successfully been used since 1911, the precise manner by which symptoms are relieved is not fully understood. Several theories have been advanced, none of which is entirely satisfactory. The most acceptable theory is the blocking antibody theory.

Injection treatment is indicated in symptoms of allergy due to inhalant factors. A small group of allergists desensitizes with foods by injections.

They claim success but the overwhelming majority of experienced allergists consider it ineffective and do not use it.

Desensitization starts with the injection of a very small amount of a weak dilution of the substance to which the person is allergic. Increasingly larger doses are administered at regular intervals until the person is able to tolerate a large dose, one which prior to treatment would have reproduced his symptoms. It is thought that if the person can now tolerate this dose by injection, he can endure with impunity the amount he normally inhales. To attain this end, it is not always necessary that a very large dose be reached; often a small dose based on the patient's tolerance is equally effective.

The material used is an extract made up of the allergens to which the person has been found allergic by his medical history and skin tests. The choice of allergen and dose to begin treatment with is determined by the allergist. Allergists use several more-or-less unrelated methods of standardizing their extracts. These are weight by volume measure, and the total nitrogen and the protein nitrogen standards. If the patient knows which standardization is being used, and if he should move from one part of the country to another, he can provide his new physician with this information. Each allergist uses the standardization which suits his purpose best but he can always translate doses of one to the other.

During the course of desensitization treatment several types of adverse reactions may be experienced. One is a minor local swelling and itching at the site of the injection. Depending on the size and persistence of the reaction, the doctor will adjust his doses. The most serious reaction which can occur is what is known as the constitutional reaction. This consists of generalized symptoms which are frankly allergic, such as itching, watering of the eyes, sneezing, coughing, wheezing, and difficulty in breathing. These reactions are rare and fortunately occur within a few minutes to half an hour after the injection has been given, so that the patient is usually still in the doctor's office and can be treated promptly. Routine treatment of such reactions consists of adrenalin by hypodermic injection. Other drugs may be employed by the doctor, as necessary.

Allergy pollen injection treatment is given either before the pollinating season begins (preseasonal), during the pollinating season (coseasonal), or all year (perennial). There are definite indications for each. In certain parts of the world where plants grow and pollinate practically throughout the year, the treatment must be given perennially. In such instances, some of the injections are given preseasonally and some coseasonally as the pollinating seasons begin and end.

Injection treatment is not limited to pollen, but includes dusts and molds. Whether animal hair, tobacco smoke, wool, feathers, and other substances which may be inhaled and cause allergy symptoms should be included in an allergy treatment mixture, depends on the circumstances.

Injections are usually administered by a physician but in some instances may be given by a trained assistant or registered nurse, always on a prearranged dosage schedule. In rare cases, because of unusual conditions, self-administration is allowed.

The allergy injection material currently in popular use is a water extract of the allergen. However, studies are in progress with special vehicles which delay absorption, thereby producing a longer and better effect. Of these long-acting, slowly-absorbed extracts only one is in general use. This is an alum-precipitated pyridine extract. Others are being investigated and show promise.

The injection treatment of inhalant allergies should be continued for at least two or three years as a rule, although some people are relieved sooner. To stay well, however, the majority require treatment for many years and indeed often for the rest of their lives. No one can predict how long the treatment must last. Every person reacts differently and must be judged individually.

Chapter Eight

Food Allergy

Food allergy indicates a sensitivity to foods which may cause a number of diverse symptoms referable to many systems in the body. It is distinguished from *gastrointestinal allergy* denoting symptoms of the digestive tract which may be caused by food or other allergens. There is much disagreement among specialists about how often food allergy occurs, how important it is in the total picture of allergy disease, and how to detect it.

At one end of the spectrum are those who believe that allergy to food is extremely rampant, that it is usually overlooked by the physician, and that it may be caused by tiny amounts of food. For example, chemicals added to foods for preservation and even insecticides and fertilizers used in commercial farming operations are considered by some as important causes. At the other end of the spectrum are the physicians who feel that a hidden food allergy may cause moderate symptoms, but believe that only if the patient knowingly reacts is it important. The value and validity of various skin tests is a further subject of disagreement. Finally, one group of allergists believes that only their own test material extracted from the suspected food is strong enough to diagnose the allergy. Obviously, all of this is exceedingly confusing to the patient who may have consulted more than one specialist and received conflicting points of view.

The facts probably lie somewhere between these extremes. The greatest number of experienced physicians take the position that foods are a significant cause of allergy, but not as important a cause as inhalants. Most feel that skin tests have a definite place in the diagnostic procedure if properly performed with potent extracts and properly interpreted. But they are considered less reliable than reactions to skin tests performed for inhalants.

Understandably, allergy victims are very eager to accept a diagnosis of food allergy. Avoidance of certain foods, particularly if they are not eaten frequently, is much simpler than taking allergy injections at frequent intervals for a long time as is required in allergy due to inhalants. Yet if skin tests are positive to such foods as eggs, wheat, and milk, all of which not only are staple articles of the diet but are also found as hidden constituents of many packaged, processed, or partially cooked and canned foods, avoidance is always extremely difficult and a true allergy must be proved before prolonged avoidance is recommended. The person who develops hives, hay fever, or asthma immediately after eating lobster, for example, poses no problem. He merely avoids this food.

TYPES OF FOOD ALLERGY

Perhaps one of the reasons for the differences of opinion regarding the importance of food allergy and the value of skin tests with food extracts is that there are probably several types of food allergy, although this cannot be proved.

One well-known type is often called *permanent fixed food sensitivity.* People who have this type of food allergy constitute some 5 to 10 percent of individuals allergic to food. They do not seem to be able to build up a tolerance to the food and must avoid the food for the remainder of their lives. They develop symptoms very dramatically, often immediately after eating the food; sometimes even when eating a meal. They learn of their specific allergy early and avoid the responsible food.

In comparison to this type of violent reaction to very small amounts of food, there is a type of allergy which has been called the *cumulative* variety. Here the patient must eat comparatively large amounts of the food in order to suffer symptoms. He may also develop symptoms by eating the food every day, or several times a day for several days or a week. This type of allergy may go unnoticed for many years; or it may result in vague symptoms just short of overt allergic manifestations making the person suspect that "it is all psychosomatic." These individuals, particularly when their allergy symptoms are focused in the gastrointestinal tract, may be subjected to a great many gastrointestinal X rays and they probably are the greatest purchasers of the numerous patented antacids, laxatives, antispasmodics, and antidiarrhea medicines. This variety of food allergy is closely linked with what has been termed the *cyclic* or *dynamic* type because it varies and one can build up a tolerance for the food, then ingest it without any difficulty if not in excess.

Some allergists have reported a condition that they call *masked food allergy*. They state that just as large quantities of a certain food will incite allergy symptoms, very small quantities eaten often will result in relief of symptoms. A person allergic to wheat, for example, may have no symptoms of wheat allergy if he eats very small amounts frequently, since the symptoms will be masked by desensitization or building up of his tolerance. Avoiding or skipping the small amounts will allow the wheat allergy to reappear several days later. This is reproducible in allergies to other substances. Efforts are still being made to verify this concept.

A well-accepted observation in food allergy is that foods which cause trouble during one time of the year may be innocuous at other times. For example, a ragweed hay fever sufferer living in the East or Midwest may eat oranges, to which he may be sensitive, throughout the year without experiencing any trouble except during the ragweed pollinating season of August through October. This is explained by the thesis that when a person is allergic to many things, one allergen alone will not be adequate to produce symptoms, but if he encounters several at the same time, he will have symptoms. His immune mechanism, or his antiallergy resistance, can take care of one or even perhaps several but not a deluge of many allergies at the same time. This concept of assault on the immune mechanism occurs with other allergies. The assault need not be specific; it can also be provoked by emotional factors, intercurrent disease, barometric pressure changes, as well as other variations in weather.

As one can see from the discussion, the diagnosis of food allergy is not always easy, except perhaps for the obvious, often violent type, which the patient frequently recognizes himself. The countless intercurrent factors which can influence the symptoms of allergy, the increasing habit of eating processed and precooked foods, the difficulties in interpreting symptoms in the light of multiple exposure, and the relative unreliability of allergy skin tests, all complicate the problem.

The principal methods of investigating food allergy being currently used are (1) carefully obtained medical history from the patient, (2) allergy skin tests, (3) diet diary, (4) trial elimination diets, and (5) provocative ingestion. Additional techniques, controversial and not generally accepted, are provocative food tests by injection and under the tongue, propeptans, and the pulse-counting technique.

MEDICAL HISTORY

In food allergy an attempt is made to relate symptoms to ingestion of a particular food. A reliable history of allergy to foods must fulfill two criteria: the symptoms must be produced or aggravated by eating the food and, secondly, avoidance of this food must produce relief of symptoms. A third factor is often added; after relief is obtained, deliberate ingestion should provoke symptoms again. Meeting these criteria is often rather difficult because of the variability of the average person's diet and because of so many "hidden foods."

Some physicians submit a long list of foods and ask the patients to check off the ones which they suspect. This they call a "food idiosyncrasy list." It is not as helpful as it sounds because people rarely eat foods such as wheat, beef, white potato, or lettuce without adding something to them. Usually they are combined with other foods, sauces, and gravies to improve their taste. A hamburger may contain pork or some other beef substitute. Salads are compound foods. White bread is often fortified with vitamins, preserved with chemicals, and customarily eaten with butter or margarine, which is usually a hydrogenated vegetable oil with milk solids added. For that reason, it is not at all easy for the average person to list the foods to which he suspects he has an allergy.

The doctor is often told, "I am allergic to sweets." Probably not, because cane sugar seldom causes allergy symptoms. However, sweet jams and certain candies may cause allergy because of the fruits, nuts, or other allergenic ingredients they contain. Foods which are "bloating" or irritating to the gastrointestinal tract, and foods that cause hyperacidity or provoke symptoms of indigestion, ulcer, colitis, or gall-bladder disease, are not necessarily allergenic.

Many doctors place great emphasis on an individual's food dislikes on the theory that the aversion represents a subconscious expression of a food allergy based perhaps on an unpleasant experience in early childhood. This may be true in a certain percentage of cases; but unfortunately likes and dislikes are difficult to interpret correctly. It is not at all uncommon, for example, for a child to say, "I hate carrots." What he may mean is that he hates "mushy" *cooked* carrots. Most youngsters like raw "crunchy" carrots. Another argument against the "dislike theory" is that people avoid eating foods they dislike and therefore should have no food allergy symptoms. An exception is the person who eats foods whether he likes them or not because they are "good for him."

Despite these pitfalls, a careful history or account of a patient's eating habits to include what and when he eats is important. Sometimes this can be broken down into elementary foods he eats and can be related to the symptoms. Some people eat the same foods every day; their breakfast is practically identical, and even though their lunch and dinner may vary slightly, the basic foods they eat remain the same.

Most people, however, prefer a diversified diet and enjoy a wide variety of foods. This is particularly true of those who eat in restaurants a great deal or consume much packaged, processed, or partially precooked foods. In both instances, there are many different seasonings and other food ingredients, which in the old days the housewife rarely used.

SKIN TESTS

Virtually all allergists perform allergy skin tests with food extracts in the same manner that they perform scratch and intradermal tests to inhaled substances (see Chapter 7). Most who have had considerable experience with food skin tests agree that some positive reactions obtained cannot be verified clinically, while other negative reactions are misleading since many people have symptoms caused by a food which gives a negative test. It often depends on the food and the technique of testing.

Some allergists who feel that skin tests with food extracts are unreliable, test their patients with raw foods. Instead of preparing an extract of the foods by washing, mincing, soaking, concentrating, sterilizing, or by other processes the chemist employs to make the extract (freezing and dehydration are methods used by some) the doctor tests with a small piece of raw, unprocessed food. Usually the small of the back is used for this type of testing. The food is left there for thirty minutes. Proponents of this method claim greater accuracy and a greater parallel with clinical sensitivity. In our experience, this technique has not proved any more reliable.

One may well wonder why a reaction on the skin to a simple water extract of a raw food should reflect an allergy to a food which has probably been cooked, then acted upon by numerous complicated physiological body processes. Doctors have considered this as well and in order to duplicate a food as it finally may be absorbed from the intestinal tract, have prepared extracts with the addition of digestive juices. The objective is to obtain the allergy-producing element in a form as pure as possible and to select one of the techniques of preparing the extract which insofar as possible eliminates irritants. The results do not appear to be any different from those produced by food extracts prepared without them. What are the results? Good in many instances — worthless in others! Much depends upon the physician's interpretation of the reaction after noting the person's food preferences, habits, and suspected intolerances and untoward reactions to certain foods.

It is recognized that a positive test may indicate a past food allergy or one yet to occur rather than a present one, so it is important to keep in mind that some positive tests, regardless of how they are performed, may indict foods not currently producing allergy symptoms. There are also several incongruities in the choice of foods used for testing, which allergy sufferers recognize when they undergo an allergy survey. This is because those who do skin testing organize the procedure in a routine which will save time in setting up and recording the results. Because of this, tests are often performed with foods which are never eaten by the patient. In sum, food skin tests are of importance only if properly performed and carefully interpreted.

DIET DIARY

A simple method of tracking down food allergies is to keep a record of everything eaten during the day, with the date and time of onset of symptoms. By comparing the time of the onset of symptoms with the food consumed just previously, one can often deduce which food is the symptom instigator. If an attack of asthma occurred every Friday evening after dinner and, on examination of the food diary, it is determined that fish is eaten every Friday for dinner and every other part of the meal is variable, the correlation is evident. A more complicated case would be one in which headaches occurred at irregular intervals, perhaps once every week or two. If the diary has been rigidly maintained, it might disclose that inadvertently on each day the headache occurred, an identical food had been eaten.

This is, in fact, rarely as helpful as it appears. Unfortunately, if the patient eats in restaurants, it is difficult for him to know all the ingredients of the foods consumed, such as soup and beef stew. The best method of keeping an accurate food diary is to eat at home and restrict the diet to simple dishes without added condiments. A diet consisting of breakfast with soft-boiled eggs, toast, and coffee; a lunch of a Swiss-cheese sandwich on white bread, coffee or tea; and a dinner of beefsteak, a vegetable salad with an oil and vinegar dressing, fruit for dessert, and coffee is not difficult to follow and interpret. For gregarious people this may be difficult. It would certainly be impractical to request a hostess to give her guest the exact recipe of each dinner course. Unfortunately, while people are enthusiastic about keeping the diary for the first few days or even a week, they usually lose their interest after that.

Despite these faults, a properly kept diet diary may be an important method of discerning a food allergy which has escaped detection through the carefully secured history and routine skin tests. The diary has been found most valuable for allergy sufferers who have sporadic symptoms. When symptoms occur each day, any or all foods eaten routinely may be the cause, and the diary is worthless.

An example of a printed page of a diary is reproduced in Table I. On this chart, the person keeping the diary lists the foods he eats in the spaces at the left portion of the chart. He then indicates that he has eaten that food by making an "X" or other symbol in the column which corresponds to the day of the week. The chart is for a fourteen-day period and the blocks on the top may be dated. If the patient consumes the same foods for breakfast, lunch, and dinner each day, or for several days, he need not repeat the name of the food in the left-hand column. An "X" or other mark for that day suffices. On the bottom of the chart may be listed symptoms and the time of their occurrence, corresponding to the column indicating the time the food was eaten. Theoretically, to ascertain which food is causing trouble, all one needs to do is to read the column showing the day and time the symptoms occurred and note which foods were eaten at the corresponding time. Sometimes it is simpler for a person to keep a record of what he eats in a small notebook which fits into a pocket or purse. The foods eaten are listed after they are eaten; then any symptoms that occur are listed in the same book, preferably noted in another color. Notations can usually be made inconspicuously. The recording of complex foods should list the ingredients. Vegetable soup, for example, should list the vegetables observed. When the diet diary is completed for a week, the individual ingredients of the complex foods should be discussed in the office of the physician and instructions for the next period outlined. This technique is quite helpful.

TABLE 1

14 DAY FOOD DIARY CHART

NAME

DAYS & DATES														
FOOD ITEMS														
SYMPTOMS TIME OF DAY														
MEDICATION TIME OF DAY														

101

TRIAL DIETS

Trial diets are often called elimination diets, since they eliminate many foods from the diet of the person who is suspected of having food allergy. Though ranging from starvation to gourmet diets, most of them contain simple foods. They are based on avoidance of foods which the physician in his experience has found to be the major cause of food-allergy symptoms.

Most allergists have individual ideas of which foods are the most likely to produce symptoms. The late Dr. Robert A. Cooke, the first allergist in the United States to do skin tests, believed that the most common foods which cause allergy are egg, wheat, banana, shellfish (and fish in general), nuts, cottonseed, melon, chocolate, celery, tomato, potato (white and sweet), liver, peas, corn, oats, pork, chicken, buckwheat, and honey. Dr. Albert H. Rowe of Oakland, California, a proponent of foods as an important cause of allergy has for years been using a series of "Cereal-Free Elimination Diets." When a diet does not give the information or benefit desired, another more rigid diet is prescribed. In severe cases some allergy specialists eliminate *all* foods and place the person on a starvation diet, permitting only water or sweetened tea. In rare instances chemicals (amino acids) are prescribed to take the place of the proteins being omitted.

While all these elimination or starvation diets have merit, the person under investigation may very well be an exception to the statistical evidence. For example, assuming that Dr. Cooke's list accounts for 82 percent of the food allergies he has studied, a significant 18 percent are not encompassed. For this reason it is often preferable to utilize what might be called a *restricted* diet rather than an elimination diet. The person keeps a diary for a week or two and lists the foods which he commonly eats. If his symptoms persist, those foods on the list which he is currently eating are suspect. An entirely different diet is then substituted, consisting of foods he seldom eats and eliminating foods he habitually eats. For example, if a person eats beef every day, he should substitute lamb or pork; if he eats spinach, he should eat turnips or some other vegetable in its place.

Despite the statistics, the choice of foods is really not important, since this is a trial diet only and is restricted for a short period. To make a diet less burdensome and to accord with the hypothesis that allergies are reflected in the individual's food dislikes, it is customary, to the extent possible, to provide foods which appeal to the person's palate, which are easily obtainable and, in the case of fresh fruit and vegetables, are in season. The variety of foods is kept to a minimum. The trick is for a person with food allergy to start eating foods he seldom thinks of and making that "his" restricted diet. If food allergy is important and a sensitivity to foods is the cause of the symptoms, it can hardly be due to a food that ːne rarely eats.

The vitamins required to maintain good health must not be omitted. Calories can be supplemented by the addition of vegetable oil which contains about 250 calories per ounce. Vitamins may be added but they should not themselves be allergenic. There are nonallergenic vitamins on the market.

If all symptoms are relieved while the patient is on the trial diet, it may be assumed that food allergy caused the symptoms, but this is not absolutely conclusive. First, through deliberate production of symptoms, one must determine which of the avoided foods was the culprit. This is usually done by adding one of the patient's customary foods to the restricted diet and observing whether symptoms are provoked. Since symptoms do not always occur immediately upon eating the food, the food should be eaten daily for several days before making a judgment. After an interval of two or three days, another food may be reintroduced into the diet with similar precautions. This procedure is continued until symptoms appear after the ingestion of a food that had been avoided; this indicates unmistakable allergy. The diet is thus gradually increased until it is substantial and includes almost everything one might desire for a satisfactory diet. (This method has been termed the "escalator program" because as more and more foods are added, the individual goes up the scale to a full diet.) Usually, one or only a few foods are the cause of a food allergy. These must be avoided for the rest of one's life, if the allergy is fixed. If not, general improvement in a person's allergenic equilibrium or resistance by allergy management often improves the tolerance.

DIAGNOSTIC FOOD TRIAL (PROVOCATIVE FOOD INGESTION AND FOOD INJECTION TESTS)

The *diagnostic food ingestion test* originally proposed is rarely used at the present time. This involves visits to the doctor's office after not having eaten breakfast, then eating the suspected food and waiting for symptoms to occur, or for changes in the white blood cell count. This diagnostic food ingestion test has been largely supplanted by the *provocative food injection* tests. In this procedure a strong concentration of a suspected food is injected and the patient is observed for general symptoms such as hay fever, hives, or asthma, rather than a local reaction at the site of the injection. The proponents of this method of testing claim that if symptoms occur, the injection of a smaller dose will relieve them immediately. This method of food testing, as well as a variation in which food extracts are placed under the tongue and effects noted (sublingual test), is not accepted by the large majority of allergists.

PULSE ACCELERATION TEST

The *pulse acceleration* test is based on the theory that the heartbeat becomes more rapid when an individual eats a food to which he is allergic. The patient is taught how to count his pulse, establish and record a pattern and note any difference in rate following the ingestion of a specific food.

PROPEPTANS

Propeptans are concentrated foods treated with the hydrochloric acid and enzymes normally found in the stomach. They are dispensed in capsules. There are propeptans for each common food and the patient is instructed to take a capsule forty-five minutes before the meal corresponding to the food to be eaten. The theory is that the minute amount of predigested food will protect the person from symptoms which would ordinarily occur. Although most experience with propeptans for both the diagnosis and the treatment of food allergy has been unsatisfactory, the capsules continue to be manufactured and a few allergists still use them.

RELATIONSHIPS OF FOODS

There is always some question regarding the allergy relationship of foods. Foods that have similar names or look alike (for example, being green and leafy) may be botanically unrelated. This is only "kitchen relationship." Most physicians feel that foods which are related botanically are more apt to produce allergy than those which are not. This is not uniformly so; allergy to one and ability to eat another in the same family may coexist. In some instances food from one area of the country may produce allergy symptoms while the same food from another section of the country does not. There are, for example, some people who can eat lettuce grown in Florida without allergy symptoms, but lettuce grown outside of Florida affects them adversely. California oranges can be eaten with impunity by some who react violently to Florida oranges. Many other examples of bizarre food idiosyncrasies can be cited, but on the whole, people allergic to a particular food are allergic to the same food wherever it is grown. Foods in the same family as the one to which a person is allergic should be omitted from the diet until they have proved to be nonallergic. For this reason, it is necessary to know the families of foods. Some have strange relatives. The peanut, for example, is not a nut or a member of the nut family; it is in the pea or legume family. Almonds are closely related to prunes and peaches. Onion, garlic, and asparagus are in the lily family. Fortunately, all the cereals are not related; this allows one to be used as an allergy substitute for another. The accompanying table lists the relationships. It must be emphasized again that the rule of allergy to all members of a family is not a steadfast one, but must be investigated by diet trial.

TABLE 2

BOTANICAL RELATIONSHIPS OF EDIBLE PLANTS

FAMILY	FOODS	
Apple	Apple	Quince
	Crab apple	Pear
Beech	Chestnut	Beechnut
Birch	Filbert; hazelnut	
Buckwheat	Buckwheat	Rhubarb
Carrot (or parsley)	Carrot	Dill
	Parsnips	Fennel
	Parsley	Caraway seed
	Celery	Coriander

TABLE 2 (Continued)

BOTANICAL RELATIONSHIPS OF EDIBLE PLANTS

FAMILY	FOODS	
Cereal grains	Wheat	Rice
	Rye	Wild rice
	Barley	Corn
	Oats	
Citrus	Lemon	Citron
	Lime	Tangerine
	Grapefruit	Kumquat
	Orange	
Gooseberry	Currant	Gooseberry
Goosefoot	Spinach	Swiss chard
	Beet	
Gourd	Pumpkin	Cucumber
	Squash	Watermelon
	Cantaloupe	
Heath	Blueberry	Cranberry
Laurel	Cinnamon	Bay Leaves
	Avocado	
Legumes	Pea	Peanut
	Kidney bean	Soy bean
	Lima bean	String bean
	Lentil	
Lily	Onion	Garlic
	Leek	Shallot
	Chive	Asparagus
Mallow	Cottonseed	Gumbo *(Okra)*
Mint	Mint	Savory
	Sage	Thyme
Morning Glory	Sweet Potato	
Mulberry	Hop	Fig
Mustard	Radish	Cabbage
	Horseradish	Kale

TABLE 2 (Continued)

BOTANICAL RELATIONSHIPS OF EDIBLE PLANTS

FAMILY	FOODS	
Mustard (cont.)	Watercress Turnip Rutabaga Mustard Broccoli	Collards Brussels Sprouts Kohlrabi Cauliflower
Palm	Coconut	Date
Plum	Almond Prune Apricot Nectarine	Plum Peach Cherry
Potato	Potato Tomato Eggplant	Peppers *(red and green)*
Rose	Blackberry Raspberry	Loganberry Strawberry
Thistle	Lettuce Salsify Oyster plant Chicory	Endive Artichoke Dandelion
Walnut	Walnut Hickory	Pecan

Meat and fish do not have as distinct an allergenic relationship as do fruits and vegetables, but certain fish are related to each other as symptom producers. The most important groups are the shellfish, of which there are two varieties, the mollusks and the arthropods. The mollusks include abalone, oyster, scallop, and clam; the arthropods are crab, crayfish, lobster, and shrimp.

Eating organs or the products made from an animal is the same as eating the animal flesh itself. Beef liver, for example, is equivalent to beefsteak or roast; veal is merely immature beef. Pork allergy includes allergy to ham, bacon, lard, and many sausages. People who are allergic to egg should not eat hens; they should confine themselves to capons. Some vaccines, such as the influenza vaccine, are grown and cultured on egg media; an allergy to egg precludes their use. Many allergists believe that demonstrable allergy to feathers is tantamount to allergy to the bird that is the source of the feathers. These facts are true to a great extent in laboratory studies but usually not in clinical practice; however the hypothesis should be remembered and the food tested by trial.

Several specific food allergies should be explained. Allergy to egg is usually to the white of the egg; allergy to the yolk exists but is not as common. Milk contains several allergens. When milk is soured, it separates into two portions; the casein (or curd) portion and the whey portion, which is composed of lactalbumin and lactoglobulin. Most milk allergy subjects are allergic to the whey (the albumin and globulin segment). In that case, they may try boiled cow's milk since heat denatures the lactalbumin considerably. Other substitutes for raw cow's milk, when the person is allergic to the albumin or globulin portions, are the familiar condensed or evaporated milks. These have been subjected to prolonged heat. Simple powdered milk is less satisfactory as a substitute, as it is not exposed to heat as long as the others mentioned. Goat's milk is another substitute because there is a difference in the albumin and globulin it contains. "Milk" made from homogenized beef or lamb may be tried. If no animal milk can be tolerated, there are vegetable substitutes such as soybean, almond, and coconut milk. When a person is sensitive to the casein, or curd portion, no animal milk can be substituted because the casein segment is identical in all. The determination of which portion of milk to which a person may be sensitive is discovered by allergy skin tests. When people are allergic to beef, they may be allergic to cow's milk, as the lactoglobulin in the whey of cow's milk is related to the globulin in the serum of cattle.

An official government investigation has found that highly refined vegetable oils such as corn, sunflower seed, olive, cottonseed and safflower are not allergenic. They are thought to lose their allergenicity during the process of refinement. Although the government investigation was very thorough and expert testimony was available, some doctors continue to test their patients to these oils and instruct their patients to avoid them.

TREATMENT

A suspected food allergy must often be treated by avoiding conglomerate and convenience foods, and by not eating in restaurants where exact food contents are unknown. Careful shopping, close scrutiny of labels on cans and packages of food, and perhaps even shopping at special health-food stores or purchasing by mail order from stores which specialize in dietary problems, may be necessary. The modern housewife may have to learn to cook and bake as her grandmother did, with the use of simple recipes using fewer ingredients.

The most common foods are the most difficult to avoid since they are important ingredients of everyday cooking. These are milk, eggs, and wheat, which are also common hidden ingredients of packaged or canned foods. Pure-food laws established in most of the countries of the world require that the principal ingredients of a packaged or canned product be listed. By reading the label, the product may be found to contain "milk solids," for example. Ordinary commercial rye bread is a mixture of rye and wheat flours; this is usually printed in small type. The white of an egg is often used as a glaze in baking and is not listed.

Food technology has progressed to such a degree that unless the food labels are carefully read, the allergic person will not be aware of what the food contains. Tables 3, 4, and 5 list the more important groups of foods likely to contain the ubiquitous egg, milk, or wheat.

TABLE 3

COMMON FOODS CONTAINING EGG

TYPE	SPECIFIC FOODS
Soups	Alphabet and egg noodle soups, mock turtle soup Bouillons, broths, consommes cleared with albumen in eggs (read labels)
Meats Poultry Fish	Croquettes, loaves, patties, sausages, and meats, poultry or fish prepared with eggs
Vegetables	Any vegetable prepared with eggs
Breads	All breads, biscuits, muffins, rolls, etc. unless made at home without eggs Prepared mixes for biscuits, doughnuts, muffins, pancakes, popovers, and waffles (check labels for albumen, dried eggs, or egg powder)
Desserts	Bavarian creams, cakes, custards, doughnuts, fritters, macaroons, meringues, pies, whips,

TABLE 3 (Continued)

COMMON FOODS CONTAINING EGG

TYPE	SPECIFIC FOODS
	ice creams, sherbets unless made at home without albumen, fresh, dried, or powdered eggs
Beverages	Any beverage made from fresh eggs, dried eggs, egg powder, or egg albumen, or where eggs are used to clarify beverage (such as egg white or shell in coffee) or to produce foam (such as egg in root beer)
Miscellaneous	Candies made with eggs such as divinities; candies in which egg white is used to produce a glaze or luster (read labels on wrapped commercial candies) French toast, fritters, timbales Prepared mixes containing albumen, dried or powdered eggs (read labels) Salad dressings (read labels), egg, hollandaise, and tartar sauces

TABLE 4

COMMON FOODS CONTAINING MILK

TYPE	SPECIFIC FOODS
Soups	Any canned or dehydrated soup containing milk or milk products (read labels)
Meat Poultry Fish	All meats, poultry, or fish prepared with milk or dairy products Commercially prepared meats (read labels)
Vegetables	Any creamed or scalloped vegetable made with milk or milk products (read labels)
Breads	All breads, biscuits, muffins, rolls, etc. unless made at home without milk products Prepared mixes for biscuits, doughnuts, muffins, pancakes, popovers, and waffles (read labels)
Desserts	Bavarian creams, blanc manges, cakes, cookies, custards, ice creams and sherbets, pies, unless made at home without milk or milk products

TABLE 4 (Continued)

COMMON FOODS CONTAINING MILK

TYPE	SPECIFIC FOODS
	Prepared mixes containing milk or milk products, puddings
Beverages	Any beverage containing milk or milk products
Miscellaneous	Buttermilk, butters, cheeses, cultured milks Any salad dressing, sauce, or gravy containing milk products, butter sauces, hard sauce, cream sauce, and white sauce

Milk products include condensed, dried, and evaporated milks; casein and lactalbumin (curds and wheys), malted and powdered milks; all cheeses.

TABLE 5

COMMON FOODS CONTAINING WHEAT

TYPE	SPECIFIC FOODS
Soups	Bisque, chowder, creamed vegetable or meat soup unless prepared at home with special flour
Meat	Any meat that is breaded or stuffed
Poultry	Any poultry that is stuffed
Fish	Croquettes, loaves, and patties unless prepared at home with special flour
Vegetables	Creamed vegetable unless made at home with special flour
Breads	All breads, biscuits, muffins, rolls, etc. unless made at home with special flours Crackers, pretzels, and zwieback Prepared mixes for biscuits, doughnuts, muffins, pancakes, popovers, and waffles (check labels)
Desserts	Cakes, commercial sherbets, custards, dumplings, ice creams and ice cream cones, pastries, pies, and puddings made with wheat products Prepared mixes for any of the above (check labels)
Beverages	Ale, beer, coffee substitutes such as Postum (check labels)

TABLE 5 (Continued)

COMMON FOODS CONTAINING WHEAT

TYPE	SPECIFIC FOODS
Miscellaneous	Macaroni, noodles, ravioli, spaghetti, vermicelli Any salad dressing, sauce, or gravy unless made at home with special flour

Wheat products include bran, bread crumbs, cracker meal, farina, malt, wheat germ, and the following flours: all-purpose, bread, cake, cracked wheat, entire wheat, enriched graham, pastry, phosphated, self-rising, white and wheat.

A number of foods have deceptive names obscuring the true ingredients. There are others whose true ingredients are not disclosed. For example, frankfurters often are not made from pure beef. They frequently contain other kinds of cow meat, milk, and cereals, such as oats, cornmeal, and wheat. Table 6 lists the foods which contain "hidden" ingredients. In addition to the foods, there is a list of beverages, alcoholic and nonalcoholic, with their approximate compositions. Formulas change from time to time. When there is any doubt and the labels do not give all the information necessary, a letter to the manufacturer or distributor requesting this data will invariably be answered. Food manufacturers are always cooperative with allergic individuals.

TABLE 6

HIDDEN CONSTITUENTS OF FOOD

FOOD	HIDDEN CONSTITUENTS
Au gratin foods	Milk
Baked beans	Peas, wheat flour
Blanc mange	Egg, Irish moss, milk flavoring
Boiled salad dressing	Milk
Bologna	Beef, pork, tongue, spices
Breads (including rye, gluten,	Wheat flour, eggs, milk, and various "fillers," which might include fruit pulps, potato, nuts,

TABLE 6 (Continued)

HIDDEN CONSTITUENTS OF FOOD

FOOD	HIDDEN CONSTITUENTS
graham, wheat, whole wheat, corn, zwieback, biscuit, crackers, popovers, muffins, pumpernickel)	all cereal grains, peas, beans, lentils, peanuts, cassava roots, cooked squash, pumpkin, and sweet potato Bakers frequently glaze breads with egg white. Rye bread usually means about 25 percent rye and 75 percent wheat. Buckwheat flour is often used on the bottom of breads to keep them from burning.
Broth or consommé	Egg white (to clarify it)
Butter sauce	Wheat flour
Cakes	Wheat flour, egg, milk, nuts
Candy	Egg, milk, nuts Milk chocolate contains quantities of milk. Potato starch has been found in some chocolate creams. Egg gives luster to bonbons; it is also used for almond cakes, fondants, pastes. (Chocolate bars sometimes contain caffeine.)
Casing on meat	Egg white
Catsup	Tomato, spices, onions, sugar, vinegar
Cheeses	Practically all from cow's milk. Gorgonzola and Montasia can be made from either cow's or goat's milk; God Ost — goat's milk (gjetost), Roquefort and Romano — sheep's milk
Chicken	Wheat flour (many cooks dust chicken with flour before roasting it)
Chili con carne	Beans, wheat flour, chili peppers, spices, garlic
Cocoa or chocolate (ready to serve)	Milk
Coddled foods	Egg
Coffee	Egg white (to clarify it). See also beverage list.
Coffee substitutes	Wheat, malt, rye, rice, barley, corn, soybeans, asparagus seeds, nuts
Cookies	Wheat flour, egg, milk, nuts

TABLE 6 (Continued)

HIDDEN CONSTITUENTS OF FOOD

FOOD	HIDDEN CONSTITUENTS
Corned beef	Many spices including allspice, bay leaf, coriander, mace, nutmeg, peppers, thyme, and sage
Cracker crumbs or cracker meal	Wheat flour
Cream foods	Milk, egg, wheat flour, cornstarch
Croquettes (and all other breaded foods)	Wheat flour, egg
Custards	Egg, milk, sugar, flavoring. Boiled custards: wheat flour or cornstarch for thickening
Cream sauce	White sauce and eggs
Deviled foods	Egg
Doughnuts	Wheat flour, egg
Dumplings	Wheat flour
Escalloped dishes	Egg, milk
Fish	Wheat flour (cracker crumbs)
Frankfurters	Cow meat, beef jowls, skim milk, cereals (oats, cornmeal, wheat, etc.)
French dressing	Olive oil, vinegar, salt, pepper, spices
French toast	Egg
Fritters	Egg, wheat flour, milk
Frostings	Egg white
Gravies	Wheat flour
Griddle cakes	Wheat flour, egg, milk
Hamburgers	Wheat flour (some cooks dust the meat with flour).
Hollandaise sauce	Egg, butter, lemon juice
Ice cream	Milk, egg, flavoring. Inexpensive grades may be thickened with flour or cornstarch; some have gelatin.
Ice-cream cones	Wheat flour

TABLE 6 (Continued)

HIDDEN CONSTITUENTS OF FOOD

FOOD	HIDDEN CONSTITUENTS
Ices, sherbets	Egg white, fruit juices. The terms are often confused, although strictly speaking, ices should contain only fruit juice and water, while sherbets have egg white.
Jellies	Cornstarch
Liverwurst	Pork livers, spices
Macaroons	Egg, nuts, wheat flour
Malted drinks	Wheat and other cereal grains, egg
Malted milk	Wheat, milk
Marshmallows	Egg white
Matzoh	Wheat flour (no yeast)
Mayonnaise	Egg, olive or vegetable oil, vinegar, spices
Meat loaf	Wheat (bread crumbs or flour), egg
Meringue	Egg white, sugar
Mustard	Ground mustard, salt, vinegar
Noodles	Wheat, eggs
Oleomargarine	Milk (sometimes churned in milk)
Omelets	Milk, egg
Oat bread	Oatmeal, wheat, potato, yeast, salt
Pancakes	Wheat flour, egg, milk
Pies, pastry	Egg, flour (piecrust sometimes made with butter)
Pretzels	Wheat flour, malt, egg, onion, celery, or caraway seeds, yeast, sugar, rye
Rarebit	Milk
Roasts (beef, lamb, etc.)	Wheat flour (many cooks dust a roast with flour)
Root beer	Egg white (to make it foam), root bark, herbs, sugar, yeast
Salami	Pork, beef, garlic, spices

TABLE 6 (Continued)

HIDDEN CONSTITUENTS OF FOOD

FOOD	HIDDEN CONSTITUENTS
Sausage	Corn flour, oats, wheat cereals, potato, egg, spices, beef, pork
Sausage (pork)	Wheat flour (bread), pork, sage
Sherbet	Egg white, fruit juices
Souffle	Milk, egg, flour
Soup (including chowders, cream soups)	Wheat flour, milk
Swiss steak	Flour
Tartar sauce	Mayonnaise, capers, olives, cucumber pickles
Tortilla	Corn
Waffles	Wheat flour, egg, milk; pecans or other nuts sometimes added to the batter
Whips	Egg white or cream
White sauce	Flour, milk, butter
Wiener schnitzel	Flour, egg, cream
Yeast	Wheat
Nonalcoholic Beverages	
Cola	Caffeine, caramel, essential oils (cinnamon, coriander, lemon, nutmeg, sweet orange), glycerin, lime juice, phosphoric acid, soluble extracts of coca leaves or kola nuts, and water (carbonated)
Ginger ale	Carbonated beverage made from ginger (or ginger extract), lemon juice (or lemon oil and citric acid). Capsicum extract is frequently substituted in part for ginger
Root beer	Carbonated beverage containing caramel, sugar, and water flavored with some or all of essential oils of anise, birch, cassia, cloves, lemon, sassafras, wintergreen, coumarin, and vanilla
Sarsaparilla	Caramel, oils of anise, orange, sassafras, wintergreen, powdered pumice stone, sugar, and water

TABLE 6 (Continued)

HIDDEN CONSTITUENTS OF FOOD

FOOD	HIDDEN CONSTITUENTS
Alcoholic Beverages	
Beer (ale, stout, porter)	Fermentation of malted grain, usually barley; wheat, rye, oats, rice, and corn may be used. Hops are usually added.
Bourbon	Originally whiskey produced from corn in Bourbon County, Kentucky; also refers to a similar whiskey made from a mash or corn, sometimes with rye or malt added.
Brandy	Distilled from fermented juice of grapes. It may be made from peaches, cherries, apples, and other fruits.
Gin	Distilled from a mixture of barley, malt, rye, and corn; usually flavored with juniper berries. Following flavors may be used: angelica root, calamus, cardamom, cassia, cinnamon, coriander, fennel, licorice, and orris root.
Liqueurs	Sweet liquors made by distilling and mixing various alcohols with essential oils, flavors, and syrups.
Rum	Distilled from cane sugar products.
Vodka	A common Russian distilled alcoholic liquor made from rye, sometimes from potato, and rarely from barley. In the United States other grains are used.
Whiskey	In the United States made from rye, wheat, and corn. In Scotland and Ireland made from malted barley. Spiritus frumenti (U.S.P.) is defined as "an alcoholic liquor obtained by distillation of the mash of fermented grain (usually corn, wheat, and rye). . . ." Much liquor sold as whiskey is made by diluting strong alcohol with water and adding coloring and flavors. All grains are used.
Wines	Fermented fruit juices, usually grapes.

Desensitization to foods is impossible or unnecessary except in rare instances. When indicated, the so-called oral technique is employed. The procedure is simple. It consists of eating gradually increasing amounts of the allergenic food, beginning with a minute amount, until a normal portion is tolerated.

Although usually prescribed by the attending physician, many patients have been able to devise their own methods of oral desensitization to foods and some clinicians have made modifications of the basic principles to simplify the procedure and make it more palatable. For example, in the case of a cereal-grain sensitivity, a dry cereal may be used; one "wheaty" the first day, two the second, and so on until maximum tolerance is reached. In using cereal, care should be taken not to select one fortified with vitamins and flavored with malt.

Other methods which have been used and for the most part discarded by most clinicians specializing in this field are (a) desensitization by injection therapy, (b) desensitization by rectal instillation, (c) nonspecific shock therapy, such as the use of the patient's own blood or a mild foreign protein, (d) use of peptones, and (e) propeptans. Based on the theory that small amounts of food will mask symptoms, a group of allergists is advocating the use of food extract drops under the tongue as a "neutralizing dose." This form of treatment is not generally accepted.

The subject of food allergy is a major one and medical literature contains numerous case reports of unusual sensitivities which do not appear to follow a strict immunological pattern. Some have already been mentioned; others are even more bizarre. There is the case report of a patient who could eat raw eggs without any trouble, but could not tolerate them when in baked products such as cakes and rolls.

Such examples might encourage a defeatist attitude. This is particularly true when the inconclusiveness of skin test reactions to food antigens is considered, as well as the difficulties involved in food avoidance. Nevertheless, the results are often excellent. Good results demand a careful evaluation and a thorough understanding of the basic differences in food idiosyncrasies.

SUMMARY

Allergy to the ingestion of foods is a very important part of the total picture of allergy disease. There is a difference of opinion among allergists, however, regarding the frequency of its occurrence and the best methods of detecting its presence.

Several types of food allergies are based on the time of appearance and persistance of symptoms. These types have arbitrarily been termed the fixed food sensitivity, the cumulative variety, and the cyclic or dynamic type. A corollary to the latter is one that has been termed "masked food allergy."

The methods of investigation to determine the existence and the extent of allergy to the ingested foods are (1) carefully detailed history, (2) allergy skin tests, (3) diet diary, and (4) trial elimination diets and diagnostic deliberate trial food tests. Less-orthodox methods are the pulse-counting method, the use of provocative injection and sublingual food extracts, and ingestion of partially digested foods, marketed under the trade name of Propeptans.

The treatment of food allergy is best accomplished by avoidance. The botanical relationships of some foods may be important and the botanical relationships of fruits and vegetables must be watched. When one is allergic to one member of the family, the others should be avoided until it is proved by clinical trial which ones are safe. This is not true of biological foods such as meat, fowl, and fish, with the exception of shellfish. Shellfish are divided into two groups: the scallops, oysters, snails, and clams (the mollusk family) and the lobster, crab, and shrimp (the arthropod family). There is a marked crossed allergy within the families but not outside them. The birds and the mammals do not seem to cross-react, and the fish, other than those mentioned, are difficult to categorize.

In avoiding foods to which one is allergic, it is very difficult to determine the ingredients when the product is precooked, canned, frozen, or otherwise prepared.

Other than avoidance, the only recognized treatment of food allergy at the present time is food desensitization by oral means. This consists of eating a minute quantity of the food to which one is allergic and gradually increasing the amount daily until eventually the food can be tolerated in adequate quantities. This technique has merit and is similar to other methods of desensitization which have proved successful, but in most instances it is not necessary.

Chapter Nine

Drug Reactions

By their very nature, medicines always produce a reaction in the body. Some of these reactions are foreseeable; some are not; sometimes beneficial effects are accompanied by undesirable side effects. With the vastly increased number and types of medicines used in present-day medical science, adverse side effects have become correspondingly more frequent. The reactions may be either allergic or nonallergic. Although in many instances this differentiation may be purely academic, in others it may significantly affect the prognosis of the illness resulting from the medication and pose a problem regarding its future use.

Thus a better term for the loosely used "drug allergy" is "adverse reaction to drugs" since there are many types of unfavorable reactions or responses aside from allergy responses. The term "drug" must not be misunderstood. To the physician the word "drug" is merely a synonym for medicine. A drug is not necessarily a habituating medicine like a narcotic or barbiturate. "Drug" is defined in nontechnical dictionaries as "a substance for use in the diagnosis, cure, mitigation, treatment, or prevention of disease in man or animal." Thus aspirin is a drug; even the placebo, an inert chemical having no known physiological effect, is a drug when administered as a medicine. Oddly enough, there have been reports of adverse "drug reactions" even to a placebo, with symptoms of rapid heartbeat, headache, diarrhea, and many others, some of which can be frightening to the patient.

TYPES OF ADVERSE RESPONSES

To classify the types of adverse responses to drugs, providing some insight into the causes and mechanisms, the following terms are constantly used: *side effect, secondary effect, untoward effect, side reaction, toxic reaction, idiosyncrasy, intolerance,* and *drug allergy.* A medicine has more than one effect on the body, one of which is usually primary and is the desired one in most instances, but under certain conditions though, the secondary, the "other," or the usually undesirable effect, is exactly the one that is sought. For that reason the term "primary purpose" must not be judged by the primary purpose for which the drug was produced but rather by the usage intended for it by the doctor.

Side Effect

This is the effect of a medicine other than the one which it was specifically intended to produce. Everyone can cite examples of these. In allergy, the most prominent example is the antihistamine which, although often very effective in relieving allergy symptoms, also frequently produces drowsiness. Federal law requires that this information be printed on the package of every antihistamine sold to the customer without a doctor's prescription. Yet these very side effects are made use of in the widely advertised sleep aids, many of which are merely antihistamines. This is an excellent example of a side effect being useful. This side effect is undesirable under most circumstances (treatment of hay fever during working hours) but very desirable under others (treatment of hay fever at night). Doctors sometimes make use therapeutically of this and other "side effects," although sometimes the side effects are undesirable and must be counteracted by another medicine or otherwise dealt with.

Untoward Effect

This is a reaction which is neither expected nor usual. It is undesirable and not beneficial to the illness for which the medicine was administered.

Side Reaction

This is a less important result of a medicine or drug and may consist of several chemical reactions, which occur at the same time. Since most drugs often have more than one chemical effect on the body, when one is used to produce a certain reaction others must be expected and coped with. Not all side effects are harmful, nor are they all unfavorable (although the implication of their being undesirable is always present when the side effects are not the response sought). The difference between side effects and side reaction may be considered as one of degree only.

Toxic Reaction

This is an undesirable response to a drug that has the connotation of being "caused by a poison." Yet even toxic reactions, although frankly poisonous, can sometimes be desirable. The best example of this is the use of drugs for cancer and for leukemia. These drugs are toxic to the cancer cells, and to some extent to other cells in the body as well. It is their killing of the cancer cells that makes their use worthwhile despite their other generalized toxic effects. Fortunately, some of the newer ones are being found to be more and more toxic to cancer while less so to the normal cells.

Toxic medicines have been in use for centuries. In many instances small doses are beneficial while large ones are poisonous. The best examples of these are digitalis and curare, although there are many others. Digitalis, one of the most important medicines used for patients with heart trouble, is poisonous if given in excess.

Intolerance

Intolerance describes another type of adverse reaction to medicines. It means simply that the patient for one of many reasons cannot tolerate the medicine. Often it is merely a quantitative difference among individuals. For example, quinine in large enough doses will cause ringing in the ears in all individuals; in some, a minute amount will produce this same ringing. The latter group is considered *intolerant* to quinine.

Idiosyncrasy

This is a response to a drug which may be due to an allergy, an inborn error in the makeup of the person, his enzymes, and any other complicated chemical and physiological mechanisms involved in the complex workings of our bodies. It is an individual rather than a universal response. It may be a paradoxical response, such as wakefulness instead of sleepiness after a barbiturate, or sleepiness in place of jitteriness and wakefulness after ephedrine.

Drug Allergy

Most of these definitions overlap and some are distinguished only by degree. When the symptoms are few and merely annoying, they are considered side effects; when they are statistically rare, they are considered idiosyncrasies. Definitions are essential for an understanding of true drug allergy. Still, there are numerous adverse reactions to drugs which cannot be classified precisely even with the aid of the terminology just discussed. For example, certain medicines when taken by mouth will provoke a rash of the skin only when the skin is exposed to the rays of the sun (photosensitivity).

The types of adverse drug reactions possible are almost limitless. Some of them are difficult to classify. For example, after seventy years of use aspirin has been found to have a harmful effect on the lining of the stomach in some people and can produce internal bleeding and ulcers. Similarly, potassium tablets, specially coated so they dissolve in the small intestine rather than in the stomach, have been found to be a cause of intestinal ulcers among some people. The experience with thalidomide in Europe, where pregnant women taking the medicine gave birth to peculiarly deformed infants, is well known. Yet thalidomide is probably an excellent drug for men and for nonpregnant women.

True allergic reactions must fulfill the same criteria applied to any other allergy disease. (For an explanation of antigen-antibody reaction see Chapter 2.) Unfortunately, it is difficult or impossible to demonstrate the antibody in drug allergy, although in some instances this has been done. The usual sequence of events in an allergic reaction, beginning with sensitization by use of the drug and followed by production of antibody, with subsequent antigen-antibody reaction and ultimate release of chemicals such as histamine, is primarily assumed. The only observable fact is that the first dose usually does not produce a reaction while subsequent doses do, but even this is not uniform.

The explanation given for the inability to demonstrate the antibody in most drug reactions is that most drugs are simple chemicals and are not by themselves antigenic; thus, they are incapable of stimulating the body to produce antibodies (haptens; see Chapter 2). It has been demonstrated that the simple chemical, however, can join with a protein from the body to make an antigenic *protein-chemical complex* and that it is this complex of high molecular weight that produces the reaction. Interestingly, the part of the complex that will instigate future reactions is not the added protein but the original chemical.

DRUG REACTIONS

The most commonly observed reactions to drugs are (1) allergic or anaphylactic reactions, (2) skin reactions, (3) changes in the blood cells, (4) liver involvement, and (5) collagen diseases (described in Chapter 17). It is apparent that these reactions are not mutually exclusive. Skin eruptions, changes in the blood elements, and even liver involvement can be caused by allergy or directly by the toxic effect of the medicine. It may be extremely easy or very difficult to determine whether pure allergy is the cause of the adverse reaction to the drug. In any case, the knowledge of exact mechanisms is not always required for proper management.

Although the types of drug reactions discussed here are statistically most common, many diverse symptoms may occur. Almost any symptoms can be simulated by adverse response to any of a multitude of medicines. Many have been reported in the medical journals; most of these are probably truly allergic. Among them are shortness of breath, blue lips, increased heart rate, sleeplessness, high fever, dizziness, stomach cramps, nosebleeds, visual difficulties, and many others. Presently the adverse reactions are most commonly produced by gold salts (used for the treatment of arthritis), barbiturates (used to aid sleeping), iodides (used as expectorants in cough mixtures and in bronchial asthma), penicillin (an antibiotic), mercury drugs (used mostly in amalgum filling by dentists and on the skin as an antiseptic), quinine (used now mostly as quinidine for irregular heart action), salicylates (including aspirin, used as a pain-killer and a fever-reducing medicine), and the "sulfa" drugs (bacteria-killing agents). The most important of these today is penicillin, although antitoxins used for the prevention of tetanus and diphtheria still produce serious reactions.

Some drugs are known to be more dangerous than others. For that reason the Food and Drug Administration of the U. S. Government requires that the manufacturer list all the possible reactions, with suitable warnings on the package of all over-the-counter medicines. Sometimes the wording is more frightening to the average person than is necessary.

Samples of medicines given to patients by doctors as a trial supply also carry suitable warnings in appropriate instances. Although the government insists that any compound containing barbiturates bear the statement on the outside of the package, "Warning: may be habit forming," a doctor's prescription which may contain much more phenobarbital does not require this warning on the druggist's label. The government also insists that relevant warnings be included on all advertising copy sent to physicians by the pharmaceutical firms and in the advertisements of their product in medical journals and elsewhere.

The Allergic (Anaphylactic) Reaction

Allergy in humans is the equivalent of anaphylaxis in animals, and when severe allergic reactions occur in the human we prefer to use the term "anaphylaxis," although some use the adjective "anaphylactoid" to distinguish between the human and the animal. An allergic reaction to a drug can result in the same types of allergy symptoms that come from any other allergy contact, such as inhalants or food. These include symptoms of bronchial asthma, hay fever, hives, and eczema. The most feared type of allergic reaction is the *anaphylactoid type* or *anaphylaxis*. This reaction usually begins with itching of the body, followed by hives, asthma, running of the nose, or any other combination of allergy symptoms. A severe reaction may quickly give way to a drop in blood pressure and shock. On rare occasions this reaction results in death.

This is the same type of symptom or reaction that can occur in the very rare severe reactions to allergy skin tests and after an equally rare overdose of an allergy extract during the course of allergy desensitization. Every well-trained allergist knows exactly how to treat such a condition. Actually the treatment is simple; the most important point is that it should be performed with dispatch. This is the type of reaction a severely allergic sensitive person can suffer after being bitten by a bee or some other insect (see Chapter 10). On rare occasions it follows the use of a vaccine against lockjaw (tetanus). This severe type of reaction is known as *anaphylactic shock;* when it is less severe it is known as *angioedema* or *angioneurotic edema;* a very mild case may be called simply *hives* or *urticaria.* Lesser symptoms, such as those of hay fever and asthma, along with the others mentioned previously, occur less frequently in vaccine reactions.

Serum Sickness Type of Allergic Reaction

This is a peculiar type of allergic reaction to a medicine that occurs five to ten days (or longer) after the drug is administered. Unlike typical allergic reactions which by definition presuppose prior contact, the serum sickness type of allergic reaction may develop even when the medicine had never knowingly been used previously. There are several possible explanations. One is that prior contact may have existed but was not recognized. For example, in the case of penicillin or other antibiotic-delayed serum sickness type of allergic reactions, the reaction may occur in a person who to his knowledge has never had antibiotics. But in these days when penicillin is used for the treatment of mastitis in cows (despite laws prohibiting the sale of milk commercially for several days after the use of penicillin in the cow) there has been some evidence of human sensitization from drinking the milk. Other antibiotics are widely used in fattening fowl for the market, so that it is possible for sensitization to occur unknowingly.

Another explanation of delayed reaction following primary use of a vaccine or medicine is based on the original theory of production of allergy symptoms. Although the new antibodies are formed on exposure, prompt excretion of the antigen does not take place, and it remains in the body until an antigen-antibody union occurs five to ten days after the original exposure. Delayed excretion mimics second exposure to the antigen.

Skin Eruptions

These are given the medical term of *dermatitis medicamentosa,* inflammation of the skin due to medicines. They are the most familiar reactions to medicines but are never as serious or as severe as the allergic, or anaphylactic, reactions. Although hives are considered a skin eruption, they are usually classified under the allergic type of reaction. This classification is arbitrary since all varieties of skin eruptions can be caused by allergy. The symptoms most often observed take the form of redness of areas of the skin *(erythema),* oozing and scaling eruption *(eczema),* inflammation of the skin with peeling *(exfoliative dermatitis),* blisters *(vesiculobullous eruptions),* small hemorrhages in the skin *(purpura),* inflammation involving local gland openings *(acne),* a large miscellaneous group which are of varying shapes and forms known as *erythema multiforme,* and a type of eruption that seems to be located in the same area of the skin each time it appears (hence, called a *fixed drug reaction).* To a limited extent certain specific eruptions are characteristic of certain specific drugs.

Eczema may occur in two types of drug exposure. One is contact with the drug, in which case it is known as *eczematous contact dermatitis,* or *dermatitis venenata.* This type is exactly the same variety that occurs after contact with poison ivy, poison oak, or poison sumac or with any other contact as described in Chapter 13. A very large number of drugs can produce this type of dermatitis. Druggists not infrequently get it on their hands from penicillin powder; dentists develop rashes on their fingers from handling "caine"-type anesthetics; nurses may have rashes on their hands resulting from streptomycin; hairdressers who use chemicals may have it on their hands.

The other type of eczema seems much like eczema caused by food but the cause is drugs. In the acute and severe form there may be swelling of the area with redness and small blisters. These blisters in due course rupture and ooze a watery substance which eventually dries, forming crusts on the surface. Itching is often intense. When the reaction is not as violent, *papules* (pimples) appear, followed by some thickening of the skin with crusting. When the condition persists and becomes chronic, the entire skin becomes thick, hardened, lichenified (leathery), and often discolored. Infection of this area may occur with swelling of the adjacent glands and red streaks extending from the skin lesion to the glands ("blood poisoning"). No site on the skin is more prone than others to have these lesions. They may be present at the sites usual for classical atopic dermatitis (the folds of the elbows and knees, the neck and face), or the area involved may suggest direct contact with the antigen, as in contact dermatitis. This often poses a problem in diagnosis, but the possibility of a drug as the cause must always be considered; avoidance, with subsequent cleansing of the skin, will inevitably determine the final diagnosis. The drugs most frequently associated with eczema-type reactions are quinine products, "sulfa" drugs, penicillin, local anesthetics, and sex hormones.

Erythema, redness of the skin, is occasionally called *exanthemata* because it looks like scarlet fever eruptions. It may vary from mere redness of the skin to severe inflammation with peeling; the rash may be localized or it may be all over the body. Sometimes there are small red areas *(macules)* along with *papules* (pimples), which is called a *maculopapular* eruption. This type of drug rash can result from practically any medicine, but barbiturates and sulfonamides are most frequently incriminated by doctors.

Urticaria and *angioedema* are forms of hives ranging from those just under the skin to extreme swelling of the face, eyes, and joints, with or without fever. Itching is usually intense. Penicillin is the greatest offender.

Vesiculobullous eruptions (blisters) result mainly from the use of "sulfa" drugs. *Acneform* (acne-like) eruptions may occur after the use of iodides, ACTH (adrenal hormone), and certain medicines used to control epileptic seizures. The acne-like eruptions can progress to become *pustular* (small skin abscesses) and *granulomatous* (tumor-like but not cancerous). *Erythema nodosum* is an inflammation of the skin and the tissues underneath the skin, accompanied by the production of small, painful red masses at the sites. These sites are usually on the shins but they may be anywhere. Often there is pain in the joints and fever associated with the rash, and young adults are most affected. The lesions can occur after certain general diseases, such as rheumatic fever, streptococcal infections, cat scratch disease (a virus disease following a cat scratch or similar skin injury). But certain drugs, particularly the iodides so frequently used as cough expectorants, bromides usually prescribed for nervousness, and the "sulfa" drugs, may be precursors. Photosensitization, a tendency of the skin to become sunburned easily, may follow the use of "sulfa" drugs, certain antibiotics, quinidine, or the thiazides used for high blood pressure and to accelerate elimination of excess fluids from the body.

Abnormalities of the Blood

Purpura is the medical term for small hemorrhages under the skin. They occur for no ascertainable reason, or they may be the first sign of a serious systemic disease. It is also not an uncommon type of reaction to drugs. When there is no decrease of platelets or thrombocytes (certain elements of the blood necessary for clotting) it is often called *nonthrombocytopenic* purpura. The drugs most commonly found to be the underlying cause of this type of drug reaction are the barbiturates, quinine and its derivatives, phenacetin (often used in headache remedies), gold salts (used for rheumatoid arthritis), and certain drugs used in the treatment of epilepsy. In some instances, drugs can also produce the *thrombocytopenic* purpura in which there is a decrease in the platelets or thrombocytes necessary for the blood clotting. Whether either or both of these purpuras is a true allergy phenomenon is still in question.

The drugs most frequently associated with thrombocytopenic purpura are arsenic (less commonly used today than in the past), aminopyrine (formerly a very popular headache remedy), thouricils (used in hyperactive thyroid condition), iodides, gold salts, and mercury (formerly commonly encountered in skin antiseptics).

Aplastic anemia is a severe disease resulting from depression of the red cell manufacturing capacity of the bone marrow. This may occur dramatically after the use of certain drugs. It has been reported after the use of gold salts, arsenic, some antibiotics (notably chloramphenical), sulfonamides, sources of radiant energy such as X rays, atomic explosions, and medicines employed for the control of epilepsy. Granulocytopenia, a marked reduction in certain white blood cells normally found in the bloodstream, may also result from many of these, as well as several other drugs. Many of the drug reactions overlap and have a more pronounced effect than others. The U. S. Food and Drug Administration consistently warns physicians by issuing bulletins and requiring pharmaceutical manufacturers to disseminate the information to the medical profession.

Liver Disease

The liver is occasionally involved as part of an adverse reaction to the ingestion or injection of drugs. There are at least two types of response. In one there is a toxic reaction with damage to the cells of the liver; in the other there is a swelling of the small ducts through which bile flows; this swelling is more commonly an allergic reaction. In either case, the primary sign is jaundice. Over the years serious disease and even death from liver involvement have been reported following the use of such drugs as arsenic, the "sulfa" drugs, penicillin, quinine derivatives, and some medicines used for epilepsy. Fortunately these are not common and every physician is well aware of the possibilities. One tranquilizer which is also effective for nausea and vomiting (Chlorpromazine) has been implicated in producing the allergic type of swelling of the bile ducts. This reaction has put the average doctor on his guard and made him more careful in using medicines of the chemically related phenothiazine group, but since they are all excellent therapeutic agents they are usually prescribed when they are indicated and necessary. Any reaction is easily recognized and reversible; some in the group are safer than others.

Penicillin Reaction

Penicillin is undoubtedly the most common cause of adverse drug reactions. Allergic reactions to penicillin occur in 5 to 10 percent of the patients to whom it is administered and constitute about 10 percent of the reported adverse drug reactions in the United States. It is the most common cause of anaphylactic shock. It is estimated that in the United States between one hundred and two hundred people die yearly from anaphylactic shock brought on by penicillin. One of the reasons for this is the large amount of the drug that is used. In 1943, 29 *pounds* of penicillin were produced; in 1959 this had increased to 790 *tons*. Since then, there have been numerous new penicillin compounds and derivatives manufactured which have a much increased and broader range of usage and effectiveness. The newer penicillins are also likely to produce allergic reactions.

How do penicillin allergic reactions occur in some people who have never to their knowledge taken or been given the drug? One way in which it may have been taken into the body is by foods (such as cow's milk, previously described) and viral vaccines. Polio vaccines and others have penicillin added to them to prevent the growth of bacteria, and a person can inadvertently become sensitized from their use. Another method is that described under Serum Sickness Type of Allergic Reaction where the antigen remains in the body days or even weeks after the introduction of the penicillin. The penicillin antibody initially produced can later unite with the leftover antigen.

Allergy to penicillin can manifest itself in numerous ways, ranging from a mild itchy rash to severe anaphylactic shock. The rash may be hives, in a spectrum of severity from superficial wheals on the skin to swelling of the face, arms, eyes, and even the joints (angioedema; angioneurotic edema) to blisters, black hairy tongue, and peeling of the skin with inflammation. Any symptom characteristic of any other allergy disease can occur. Manifestations such as noted for other drugs can also result. These include hemorrhages into the skin, anemia of the blood destruction variety, increase of eosinophiles in the blood, and decrease in other types of circulating white blood cells. Collagen diseases may result from penicillin reactions; these include *systemic lupus erythematosus, periarteritis nodosa,* and other types of inflammation of the blood vessels with destruction of the walls *(necrotizing angiitis).* These are identical with those discussed in Chapter 18. Other reactions that have been seen resulting from the use of penicillin are drug fever, liver disease, jaundice, and kidney disease. Reaction to penicillin has sometimes been called the "Great Imitator," since it can mimic almost any disease.

A special type of reaction to penicillin is the "id" reaction (described fully in Chapter 13). Penicillin can produce typical "id" reaction lesions which may appear as red blisters on the hands and feet and in the groin.

This type of dermatologic involvement often persists for a long time, even after penicillin has been discontinued.

Unfortunately it is not always possible to predict whether or not a person is going to have a penicillin reaction; skin tests used to predict penicillin reactions are not conclusive. The skin test performed carefully with penicillin, much as one performs a skin test with pollen or dusts, will be positive if the person is very allergic to it and indicates that there is a greater probability of a severe reaction if a regular dose is employed. However, a negative skin test does not guarantee that a severe reaction will not occur. Some doctors routinely do a scratch test with soluble penicillin using a solution of 20,000 units in each cubic centimeter; others perform an intradermal test with weaker dilutions. Others place a drop in the eyes and watch for redness, swelling, and itching.

Recently, a more promising test which seems to involve less chance of error has been suggested. A breakdown product of penicillin called PPL (penicilloyl-polylysine) is used as the antigen in the skin testing procedure. However, this material is not easily obtained and in addition does not guarantee absence of a severe reaction. The exact mechanism of penicillin hypersensitivity continues to be explored; eventually more precise tests will be devised.

The general rule observed by doctors is that if a penicillin reaction had occurred on previous occasions, sensitivity is assumed to exist and the drug must not be used, or used only when it is indispensable, and then it must be administered with great caution. Penicillin given by mouth is less likely to produce a reaction than that given by injection. When given by injection, prolonged action type (procaine penicillin) is much more likely to cause a reaction than the aqueous solution which must be injected every four to six hours. Reactions also are much more likely to occur when the penicillin is given infrequently, rather than at regular intervals. For example, the person with rheumatic heart disease who must take penicillin as a preventive measure month after month and year after year is less likely to have a reaction than the person who receives but one or several injections a year.

Other Antibiotics

Sulfa drugs can also produce reactions. The newer "sulfas" are not as dangerous as the earlier ones, and the combination of three sulfa drugs has proved to produce still less reaction. Some of the reactions involve the kidneys by causing obstruction of their small tubes (tubules). Water must be taken plentifully and often. Although reactions may include nausea and vomiting, hives, all types of rashes, fever, blood in the urine, and decrease in white blood cells, most of these are uncommon and do not occur until the patient has been taking the drug for a long period. The long-acting sulfas have been implicated in many cases.

The *tetracyclines* are the most commonly prescribed antibiotics, as they have a "broad spectrum" of activity and destroy a greater variety of bacteria than many of the other antibiotics. At times a culture is made of the secretions resulting from an infection, and a "sensitivity test" is done to indicate which antibiotic the principal organisms will respond to. Any of the several tetracyclines dispensed by prescription can be recognized by the suffix "mycin" as the last part of the trade name (such as Achromycin, Terramycin, Aureomycin). When reactions do occur, they are often secondary effects such as diarrhea and itching of the rectum due to overgrowth of yeast and nonpathogenic organisms (organisms which do not produce disease). Skin rashes, as well as inflammation of the tongue, may occur, but true allergic reactions characterized by hives or shock are rare.

Erythromycin has a surprisingly low incidence of reaction, although compounds may cause liver involvement in rare instances. As with any drug, rashes and minor allergy may occur in sensitive persons. *Lincomycin* has the tendency to produce diarrhea in some people. It can safely be given even to a penicillin-sensitive person. *Chloramphenical* (chloromycetin) is an unusually excellent antibiotic, but like all drugs it must be used cautiously, as it may cause severe, serious, and even fatal blood abnormalities.

Miscellaneous Drugs

It is not feasible to list all the reactions. Aspirin is interesting because it is so commonly used. A peculiar type of asthma occurs in some people who take aspirin who also have small tumors in their noses (polyps). It is claimed that this is not a true allergy to aspirin but has a mechanism different from typical bronchial asthma from other causes. Still, it may be a specific type of drug reaction.

In rare instances aspirin sensitivity can be connected with sensitivity to certain trees and foods as well as drugs, flavorings, and suntan lotions. The chemical term for aspirin is acetyl salicylic acid. In effect, allergy to aspirin is a reaction to the salicylic portion of the compound, the salicylate. Although some doctors deny this and produce evidence to support their view, the evidence that the salicylate is at fault seems more cogent.

Antitoxins are considered drugs. When made of horse serum they may be severely allergenic to some people. In addition, vaccines used for the prevention of influenza and poliomyelitis can cause adverse reactions; for example, if cultured on egg media, people sensitive to egg (perhaps to chicken feathers, as well) will have an allergic reaction. Other vaccines contain penicillin to kill certain organisms while still others employ a mercury compound for the same purpose. People allergic to either eggs, chicken feathers, penicillin, or mercury can have a reaction to the vaccine of corresponding or related content. Oddly enough, even antihistamines, which are used to treat allergic reactions, can in rare instances produce untoward symptoms, in addition to drowsiness. After long usage some may have an effect on the white blood cells in the body. Rashes due to antihistamines have been reported.

Insulin has been known to produce allergic reactions. Since it is usually derived from beef or pork, the allergy is usually specific to the animal source rather than to the hormone itself. Often a change from one source of insulin to another is effective in preventing the reaction. Reactions can be local, a fairly common phenomenon, or general. The general reaction may be evidenced simply by the insulin's failure to accomplish its purpose of lowering the sugar content in the bloodstream, or in other cases by typical itching, rashes, hives, runny nose, and asthma.

Certain enzymes are frequently used for therapeutic purposes. Two often prescribed are reputed to relieve swelling and other effects of an injury, such as a swollen black and blue eye following a blow. The proteolytic enzymes used for this purpose are *trypsin* and *chemotrypsin,* both of which are potent sensitizing agents and can produce severe allergic reactions. Other enzymes used for this and similar purposes are less sensitizing.

Local anesthetics, contrary to general belief, do not often produce severe drug reactions. They are rarely the cause of allergy to the patient. However, the well-known Novocain (procaine) and other "caines" or injectables can produce a shocklike state and a drop in blood pressure, a feeling of faintness, and dizziness. This is believed to be due to a reaction on the blood vessels of the body. Slow injection and avoidance of penetration of the anesthetic into the blood vessels may well prevent this. Some feel that the delayed and prolonged pain in the mouth and gums that occasionally follows local anesthetic use in the dentist's office is due to a delayed reaction to the anesthetic. It is true that this occurs more often with some anesthetics than with others, but the allergic nature has not been substantiated.

Mercury has often been mentioned as a cause of drug reactions. Mercury, once commonly employed in medicine is still used in some diuretics (medicines to increase urine output). It is also used by dentists as an amalgam filling and is a constituent of many antiseptics that have replaced the old-fashioned tincture of iodine.

Although *arsenic* is rarely used now, contact with it can occur by the inhalation of insecticide and with the use of *Fowler's solution,* an old medicine still used by some doctors in the treatment of anemia. *Iodides,* which in some people produce acne-like pimples, often pustular, are used primarily as an expectorant. They will also cause swollen glands and runny nose as well as decrease in thyroid secretion in some people.

The *excipients* are supposedly inert material added to tablets or capsules containing only a small amount of medicine to make them bulky enough to see, count, and swallow. Pills also usually contain a dye to make them distinctive. The dye and the excipients are considered harmless substances, nonallergic and nontoxic to the majority of people. Milk sugar is an example of a "harmless" excipient, but to the person with milk allergy, it is far from harmless. Other fillers used are gum arabic, syrup, lanolin, and starch, all of which can in rare instances be the cause of an adverse reaction, difficult to diagnose.

Dyes used in drugs are usually those which have been examined and approved by the Food and Drug Administration. Reactions to these dyes are rare, but they do occur. There is a case reported of a severe reaction to a green-colored cortisone derivative tablet, but not to the same drug in a tablet colored yellow. Any drug or chemical compound ingested or injected is capable of producing a reaction in some individuals.

DIAGNOSIS

The diagnosis of an adverse reaction to medicines is made primarily by analyzing the sequence of events preceding the onset of the symptoms with an understanding of the possible reactions one may expect. The appearance of the rash, the symptoms displayed, and knowledge of the drug used are important clues. The patient may be able to contribute useful clues to the physician, particularly in the case of an allergic reaction with characteristic hives or swelling. The even more common practice of wearing identification bracelets or necklaces, or carrying identification cards stating allergy or idiosyncrasy to penicillin or other drugs, has been helpful in emergencies. This removes a hazard to a large number of individuals.

TREATMENT

The best treatment is avoidance of the suspected or incriminated drug. This is known as *prophylactic* or preventive treatment. Once a reaction has occurred, the obvious treatment is to discontinue the medication. With most skin rashes or temporary damage to internal organs this is all that is necessary. When itching, hives, or pain in the joints is caused by drugs, it is treated as it would be if the cause were any other allergen. Jaundice caused by drug ingestion is managed much as any nonsurgical type of jaundice.

The most adverse reaction that needs vigorous treatment is the severe allergic reaction with or without shock. The treatment of this is the same as that for any other allergic reaction and is discussed in the appropriate sections of Chapter 4 (Diagnostic Allergy Tests), Chapter 7 (The Injection Treatment of Allergic Diseases), and Chapter 10 (Reactions to Biting and Stinging Insects).

The medicines used for allergic reactions are epinephrine (Adrenalin) for immediate relief of severe symptoms and antihistamines for relief of itching and swelling and reduction of allergic inflammation. If these are not adequate, the cortisone products are used and the amount given, whether by injection or by mouth or by both, depends on the severity of the reaction. Asthma occurring as a symptom of an allergic reaction to a medicine is treated in the same way as asthma caused by any other allergen. This includes the use of aminophylline intravenously and by rectum. When blood pressure drops to a dangerously low level and the patient is in shock, medicine to elevate the blood pressure (Aramine, Levophed) must be used. In many instances a person notices a rash on the skin or an itching of the body and suspects a reaction to a medicine that he has been taking. In such a case, particularly if the reaction is not a severe one, it is safe to take an antihistamine, even one with a "nasal decongestant," to stop the itching. But if the symptoms persist, a doctor must be consulted. Even though there may be no immediate danger, there is a possibility of the symptoms' persisting for a very long time.

When a penicillin reaction occurs and persists, it is evident that some molecules of penicillin are still present in the body. In this event, *penicillinase*, an enzyme which destroys penicillin, may be beneficial. Some of the newer penicillin compounds are known to be "penicillinase resistant," but it has been found that sufficiently large doses of pencillinase enzyme will also destroy these. Although penicillinase does not necessarily relieve the severe allergy symptoms for which antihistamines, epinephrine, and cortisone are used, it reduces the severity of the symptoms and often the duration of the reaction.

As is true of all drugs, even those used for the treatment of drug reactions, there have been several reported cases of allergic reactions to penicillinase. Most of the reactions have been of a minor nature, such as fever, chills, hives, and pain at the site of injection of the drug. Anaphylactic shock has been reported, but only rarely, after using penicillinase. This enzyme, although theoretically an excellent adjunct to the treatment of penicillin reactions, has been found wanting by many specialists, perhaps because the patient is seen too late by his physician and treatment is delayed.

SUMMARY

"Drug allergy" is a term that is loosely used to describe all types of adverse drug reactions. Since allergy, as we have formally defined it, does not cause all these reactions, a better term might be "drug reactions". These adverse reactions are produced inadvertently when a drug is given for some different effect.

A distinction can be made among adverse reactions known as side effects, secondary effects, untoward reactions, side reactions, idiosyncrasies, intolerances, and true drug allergy. Many of these terms overlap. Several types of reactions to drugs cannot be classified under any of these categories.

A true allergic reaction must be produced by an antigen-antibody union. Unfortunately, in drug reactions it is usually difficult, even impossible, to demonstrate the presence of an antibody. The allergy skin test is not as effective in the demonstration of drug allergy as it is in other allergy diseases.

The most commonly observed untoward responses to drugs are the true allergic or anaphylactic (anaphylactoid) reactions, skin eruptions, changes in the blood cells, liver involvement, and collagen diseases. Virtually any physical symptoms can be duplicated by the results of adverse response to drugs.

The most frequently encountered symptoms of the allergic type are hives or angioedema, as described in other chapters of this book, accompanied by swollen joints and high fever. Asthma, running of the nose, and eczema may also occur. The most dangerous reaction is shock accompanying these symptoms, followed by a drop in blood pressure and unconsciousness. This is treated with epinephrine (Adrenalin), anti-histamines, and blood pressure elevating drugs.

Delayed serum sickness type of reaction occurs five to ten or more days after the use of the drug. The symptoms are usually hives with swellings. Severe shock rarely occurs, but there may be persistence of symptoms. Skin eruptions following the use of drugs include hives, erythema (redness of the skin), exfoliative dermatitis (inflammation of the skin with peeling), vesiculobullous eruptions (blisters), purpura (small hemorrhages in the skin), acne, and recurrences of the rash at the identical site (fixed drug eruption), as well as erythema multiforme (a nondescript red irregular area of many configurations). Contact dermatitis or dermatitis venenata may follow contact with a drug and is similar to the rash one sees after exposure to poison oak, poison ivy, and poison sumac.

Use of drugs can produce certain abnormalities of the blood. Purpura may be of two types. One is associated with a decrease of certain elements in the blood necessary for coagulation (platelets); in the other there is no decrease in these elements. Severe anemias may also occur. Liver involvement with jaundice as the main symptom may result from an adverse drug reaction. Periarteritis nodosa is a comparatively rare collagen disease affecting the tissues between the cells in many organs of the body; it may be produced by certain drugs.

The most common cause of allergic drug reactions is penicillin. Although a person must have previous contact with an allergen (in this case the drug), reactions to penicillin have been reported without any known prior contact. This is explainable by any one of several theories. Reactions to penicillin are usually of the hive and angioedema type, but severe shock and even death may occur. Several tests have been devised to determine whether one is likely to have a severe reaction or not.

Unfortunately, a negative reaction to these tests does not preclude the possibility of a reaction. A history of previous adverse reaction to penicillin is usually an indication for either avoidance or extreme caution in the use of penicillin.

Other antibiotics are less likely to produce allergic reactions. They do, however, produce secondary effects as well as side effects. "Sulfa" drugs may involve the kidneys, but most doctors are aware of this danger and advise the patient about prevention. On rare occasions the "sulfa" can also produce a decrease in the blood cell elements, nausea, hives, rashes, and fever. Allergic reactions to the "mycin" drugs are infrequent. One type of adverse reaction that may occur with tetracyclines and other antibiotics is the secondary effect of diarrhea and itching of the rectum.

Aspirin (acetyl salicylic acid) sensitivity is common. It can readily cause irritation of the lining of the stomach with bleeding and ulcers. As a true allergen it can cause hives, asthma, and any other known allergy manifestations. Aspirin allergy is considered by most to be due to the salicylate radical of the compound. There may be a concommitant allergy to natural plants that contains this radical.

Allergy can occur to insulin, antitoxins, vaccines, and virtually every other medicine. Allergy to local anesthetics, except as in contact dermatitis, is rare. The type of "drug" that is often overlooked as a cause of an adverse reaction is the "filler" (excipient) used to make a tablet or capsule large enough to swallow. This may contain milk sugar among other materials. Another factor is the dye often used.

The U.S. Food and Drug Administration has strict labeling laws requiring specification on the label of the main adverse reactions that may be produced by medicines sold without a prescription. In the case of prescription drugs the physician and the pharmacist are similarly informed.

The best treatment of drug reactions is avoidance of the suspected medicine; in most cases after discontinuation the symptoms disappear. Antihistamines may be safely taken by mouth in suspected reactions, and soothing lotions and creams applied to the skin. Severe and violent reactions must be vigorously treated by a doctor in the same manner that other severe allergic reactions are managed.

Chapter Ten

Reactions to Biting and Stinging Insects

All persons are affected to some degree by bites from such insects as mosquitoes, fleas, and bees. In the normal individual the reaction is primarily that of a mild prickling sensation, localized swelling, and varying degrees of inflammation. Some people, however, feel the effect of an insect bite much more intensely than others. They are allergic to insects and, in addition to the pain, localized swelling, and inflammation, which usually are intensified, they may develop a mild constitutional reaction consisting of flushing and swelling of the face and neck, fits of sneezing and watering of the eyes (hay fever), a cough, and difficulty in breathing (asthma). Generalized hives and swelling of the entire body may occur. If the reaction is not halted, signs of "anaphylactic shock" may appear. This consists of a marked drop in blood pressure, a weak, almost unobtainable pulse, abdominal pain, nausea, vomiting, and at time involuntary evacuation of the bladder and bowels. The lips, fingernails, and skin may become bluish (cyanotic). Loss of consciousness and even death may ensue unless treatment is promptly given. The symptoms will be recognized as identical to other allergy symptoms and indicate the presence of specific allergic antibodies (reagins).

Those in the animal kingdom of the class *Insecta* that are most likely to cause these serious reactions are in the order of Hymenoptera. These comprise wasps, yellow jackets, hornets, bees, and ants. Second is the order Diptera, consisting of mosquitoes, house flies, gnats, deer and horse flies, and stable and black flies. Fleas belong to the order Siphonaptera, and although they are seldom known to produce a violent reaction, they are nevertheless a considerable nuisance. The same is true of the order Hemiptera, which includes bedbugs, box elder bugs, and kissing bugs. The latter are becoming better known as a cause of allergic reactions in certain areas of the country. Sucking lice, spiders, scorpions,

139

mites, ticks, cockroaches, and unidentified insects are responsible for only a relatively small number of severe reactions.

CAUSES OF REACTION

Reactions are caused by sensitivity or allergy to the body protein of the insect. This was originally proved by experiments with mosquitoes. When given allergy skin tests, patients allergic to mosquito bites gave as marked positive reactions to the venomless male mosquito as they did to comparable extracts of the venom-equipped female mosquito. But only the female mosquito can bite. This, as stated, really doesn't constitute proof incriminating the body protein. It merely excludes the venom as the sole cause while leaving an open X factor as part of the cause. What was thus proved true about sensitivity to the insect's body protein of the mosquito has also been proved true for the wasp, bee, yellow jacket, and hornet. There have been many studies to determine why some persons are more susceptible to insect bites than others. Although body odors, perspiration, and even carbon dioxide tension have been incriminated, the fact remains that severe reactions are due solely to an allergic reaction.

INCIDENCE

Recently, an attempt has been made by the Insect Allergy Committee of the American Academy of Allergy to compile a registry of persons allergic to insect bites or stings. In about three years, 2,606 persons registered; of these, 114 reported unusual reactions to more than one type of insect. The types of response varied from localized swellings to generalized reactions involving the entire body. Six hundred and thirty of the general reactions were life-threatening with 392 of these patients experiencing unconsciousness, severe difficulty in breathing, swelling in the throat, or, in effect, anaphylactic shock for which prompt measures had to be instituted to prevent death. In many instances the reactions were delayed an hour or more. In some individuals the reaction was merely an annoying local swelling with some pain at the site, but others had pain in several joints, abdominal cramps, and diarrhea with accompanying fever. About one-third of all people who react in this violent manner to stinging insect bites reported they had experienced some unrelated type of allergic disturbance, such as hay fever, eczema, or asthma, earlier in life. Occasionally, a severe reaction to a stinging insect causing rapid death may be confused with a heart attack, when for example a man collapses on the golf course and it is not known that he was stung. Men are more frequently affected than women since they live a more outdoor life. Similarly, the incidence of insect bites is higher in younger people. Most severe insect bite reactions reported in medical journals occur in individuals under thirty years of age. This is a reflection of exposure, not a lower incidence of immunity.

THE COMMON INSECTS

Wasps have a square head shield. Their great jaws (mandibles) are short and toothed at the tips. At rest, the wings fold longitudinally against the egg-shaped body. Yellow jackets are marked with black and yellow stripes and are quite easily recognized. Their abdomens are like those of the hornets, broad and robust. They build large nests which shelter a great many individuals. Bees' tongues can sip nectar from flowers. Their heads and thoraxes are covered with fine feathery hair, and their hind legs or feet are spread out.

There are some fifteen hundred varieties of bees, ranging from the intelligent honeybees to the parasitic bees of virtually no intelligence. The worker, the honeybee, sinks its barbed stinger into the skin of a victim so that it cannot be withdrawn. As the bee attempts to escape, the tug disembowels the bee. The stinger with the bowel, muscles, and venom sac attached are left behind and the bee dies.

The order Diptera, although the largest group of insects that bite and cause reactions, seldom produce generalized reactions, and the most annoyance is caused by the itching that they produce at the site of the bite. Sometimes, however, horseflies and deerflies as well as stable flies do cause considerable local pain. Black flies, frequently called buffalo gnats, may initiate several large and painful swellings on the face, where they are likely to bite. These flies are quite common in the northern portion of the United States and in southern Canada. Insect repellents, easily obtained at any pharmacy or supermarket, can be used on the body and are very effective in keeping these insects away.

The fleas are Siphonaptera and there are many species. These vigorous wingless insects have bodies covered by a strong armor of fine scaly plates, and mouth-parts which are designed for sucking. These parasites of man and domestic animals flourish wherever they are not disturbed—on rugs, mats, or in the straw or litter on which infested cats and dogs have slept. The flea most annoying to human beings is the *Pulex irritans*, which infests dogs, cats, and other mammals. The best protection against fleas is having rugs swept vigorously and cleaned and aired from time to time. Mattresses, pillows, or blankets on which a pet sleeps should also be cleaned and aired. Dogs can be medicinally bathed to eliminate fleas with one of the many excellent preparations on the market. Cats, on the other hand, are harder to bathe and it is more difficult to rid them of these pests.

A problem in the West is the kissing bug, also known as the assassin bug, *Triatoma protracta*. They have been reported in Mariposa County, California, where the Bureau of Vector Control of the California State Health Department listed at least 110 persons who in the past few years had one or more allergic reactions to the bite of this bug. They have been found in Texas, Arizona, and New Mexico, as well. Allergic reactions are quite severe in susceptible individuals, and the bite is painful. One South American variety is the carrier of Chagas' disease, characterized by fever, swollen glands, and swelling of the face. The North American kissing bug has not produced this or any infectious disease in humans, but the result of its bite is itching at the site, followed by itching and hives over the entire body. Loss of consciousness accompanied by nausea and vomiting occurs in some instances; in others, there may be swelling of the eyes as well as the tongue and throat, causing difficulty in swallowing, speaking, and breathing.

Biting insects of the Heleidae family are variously known as punkies and sand flies. They flourish primarily in the South, but are found elsewhere as well. Small and difficult to see ("no see-ums"), these pesty insects are annoying to bathers and hikers, but seldom cause more than a prickly sensation when they bite.

Most people fear being stung by a dragonfly, mosquito hawk, or devil's darning needle. Their names, to be sure, are terrifying but they hardly ever cause any trouble. None of these insects sting and the possibility of a collision with a person is unlikely, since they are swift, agile, and precise in their flight.

Usually, when a person has experienced a serious reaction, subsequent stings produce reactions of even greater intensity. Fortunately, this is not always true and there are some individuals who report diminished reactions over the years. It is by being stung repeatedly that professional beekeepers often build up a natural resistance to the beesting. Since it is impossible to predict precisely the type and severity of symptoms that may develop, persons who know they react to stinging insects should use every effort to avoid them. If the location of the nest is known, it should be eradicated.

ERADICATION

The eradication of the nests and living quarters usually requires skill, specialized knowledge, and experience. The sensitive individual who attempts to destroy them amateurishly may be letting himself in for more trouble that he anticipates.

Wasps build their open-comb nests in all sorts of out-of-the-way, hidden, protected areas—under eaves of houses, porches, carports, barns, behind shutters, and in shrubs. The trained exterminator destroys these nests by knocking them down with a long wooden pole such as a broom handle, by hosing them, or by scraping or slipping them into a container which is quickly covered with a tight lid. For three consecutive days thereafter he jet-sprays the area with a powerful insecticide, usually in the form of a gas.

Whereas wasps most often build their homes off the ground, yellow jackets build theirs in the ground or behind rocks. They leave small holes through which they emerge during the daylight hours and return at dusk. Since they are seldom in their lairs during the day, eradication of their nests must be performed at night. The usual method is to mark the outlet during the day with a thin stick and at night pour gasoline or kerosene freely down the hole. It need not be lighted. Lye can be used the same way. This process is repeated for two consecutive nights, which is usually sufficient to kill them. People who have a lawn and prefer to water at night should be unusually careful not to point the stream of water from the hose at the entrance to the yellow jackets' nests. This agitates them, and they may come out in large numbers, unmercifully stinging the intruder.

The nests of hornets are situated in hives, usually in shrubs or high up in the branches of a tree. The hives are gray, pyriform or football-shaped, and are easily recognizable. A flaming torch is usually used to destroy them, although an experienced and professional pest remover may clip the branch with the hive on it and quickly thrust it into a container, then close it. If the hives cannot be reached with a flame and clipping is not feasible, it may be necessary to spray that portion of the tree where the hive is located with poison gas.

The methods applicable to hornets' nests may also succeed in removing honeybees while they are swarming about or nesting in a hollow. County agents, in counties where there is such an official, have been noted for their willingness to assist in eradicating pests of all kinds. Despite nest eradication, wasps, yellow jackets, hornets, and bees are likely to seek out the same place later to build another home. We are told by patients who have had such an experience that products used to spray furniture to keep dogs off are very effective in keeping these insects from returning. This may be worth trying.

PREVENTION MEASURES

One reason that stinging insects are so prevalent around camps where there is out-of-door cooking is their attraction to food. The following precautions should be taken when food is served outside. First, it should be kept tightly covered until it is served. Second, immediately after use—even during the meal—utensils should be rinsed, washed, and put away. Garbage cans should be kept tightly covered, and an insecticide should be liberally sprayed around the entire garbage area. Patios should be sprayed freely with an insecticide during the day as well as at night when they are lighted. With the advent of electric tools such as power lawn mowers and hedge clippers, the possibility of accidentally breaking into the nest of stinging insects has increased. When this happens the insects are startled, and frequently attack.

Not only food but odors attract insects. They like perfumes, and, in fact, prefer some to others. Scented hair tonics and hair sprays, suntan lotions, face and body powders and creams lure them. Some bees are attracted by colors and are drawn to clothing of gaily colored, dark, and coarse material. They are more indifferent to white clothing with a hard finish. Bees are most likely to sting on bright warm days, particularly if they are bothered while collecting nectar. They also become agitated and aggressive if a heavy rain has washed away the nectar from the flowers, and they may resort to stinging people.

If a man sensitive to stinging insects is in an area where bees are likely to be prevalent, he should keep his body well covered by wearing a long-sleeved shirt and long trousers. Women should also keep their arms and legs well protected. Children should not be allowed to go barefoot while walking on country roads, in grassy areas, not even on a sandy beach. Above all, one should keep his eyes open for the nests of insects. A good rule for insect-sensitive individuals to follow is to look before touching. Children, especially, should be cautioned not to kick objects carelessly while walking on country roads. They just might kick a rock which conceals a nest of yellow jackets and set them free in a fury.

PROPHYLACTIC (PREVENTIVE) TREATMENT

The results of desensitization have proved very beneficial, and anyone who has suffered a severe reaction from the bite of a stinging insect should, if possible, avail himself of this form of treatment. Since there is some cross-antigenicity among the wasp, hornet, yellow jacket, and bee, it is customary to use a mixture of the allergy extract prepared from the bodies of all four in desensitization. There are, however, some allergists who prefer to treat only with an extract of the insect which stung the patient. But because most people are rarely able to recognize the insect which stung them, this is seldom practical.

Individuals sensitive to stinging insect bites must first have a skin test performed to determine the desirable and safe starting dose of the insect extract (technically referred to as the antigen). Serial dilutions are used in the tests and only a minimal amount is placed within the layers of the skin (an intradermal test). Treatment is begun with a very small amount of the dilution which fails to give a reaction. Sometimes the dilutions must be as high as one part in 100,000,000. Hypodermic injections of this antigen are given in slowly increased amounts and strengths until the individual notices a hive or area of redness (local reaction) persisting at the site of the injection.

Doctors differ as to whether the treatments should be continued weekly, every two weeks, every three weeks, or monthly. Much depends on the patient's susceptibility and whether or not he frequents places inhabited by stinging insects. Although there is no perfect guideline for terminating treatment, most physicians believe that after three years the individual may be sufficiently immunized to withstand any future sting, but he cannot be certain. However, persons who have nearly died as a result of a sting understandably may prefer to remain on treatment indefinitely.

EMERGENCY SELF-TREATMENT

Some doctors make up an emergency kit for their patients sensitive to stinging insects; others suggest that they procure such a kit from a pharmaceutical concern. There are several kits on the market.* Although they vary somewhat in composition, they are similar. In general, they contain two hypodermic syringes with needles attached. These have been sterilized and the needles protected from contamination by a plastic cover. One syringe is filled with Adrenalin (a trade name for epinephrine hydrochloride), in the proper strength and quantity for hypodermic injection. The other syringe is filled with an injectable antihistamine also in proper strength and quantity for treatment. Upon being stung, the individual is advised to immediately cleanse the outer surface of the upper arm with an alcohol sterile pad, which is supplied with the kit, and have someone inject the contents of the syringe containing the Adrenalin into the area, rubbing it vigorously to facilitate absorption. If the person who has been bitten has no companion to give the injection, he must administer it himself. In that case, it may be easier to use the thigh as the site for the injection. Adrenalin, the same drug that doctors use for emergency treatment of this sort, acts rapidly.

The contents of the second syringe containing an antihistamine should be administered immediately after the Adrenalin. Antihistamines relieve

---

*Emergency kits for treatment of insect bites may be procured on a doctor's prescription from the following laboratories: Center Laboratories, Inc., Channel Drive, Port Chester, N.Y. 11050; Hollister-Stier Laboratories, 2030 Wilshire Blvd., Los Angeles, Calif. 90057; Purex Laboratories, Inc., 346 Broadway, Staten Island, N.Y. 10310. There are probably others.

itching and help prevent anaphylactic shock. As soon as the injections
have been given, the area of the sting should be carefully examined. If
the stinger is still present, the honeybee can be assumed to be the culprit
since that is the only stinging insect that leaves its stinger behind. This
should be very meticulously removed with a tweezer, sharp knife blade,
or fingernail, using a scraping action. Care must be taken to avoid
squeezing venom from the sac into the wound as might occur by pinching
the stinger between the thumb and forefinger.

A tourniquet is usually included in the emergency kit. This should be
placed on the leg or arm, between the site of the bite and the heart to stop
the flow of blood through the artery and prevent absorption of the insect
material. It must be applied tightly. However, it should never be left on
too long and should be loosened every three to five minutes. As soon as
the symptoms disappear, the tourniquet should be removed. Ice packs
and cold towels, if they are available, may be placed on the sting. This
helps to slow the rate of absorption and reduce the discomfort and
swelling.

Some emergency kits contain a tablet to be placed under the tongue,
instead of the hypodermic injection of Adrenalin. This is for those who
are squeamish about having someone give them a hypodermic injection
or taking it oneself. The drug commonly used (isoproterenol) is
unquestionably easier to administer than Adrenalin, but the speed of its
action and its efficacy are not nearly so great. Adrenalin may also be
introduced into the system by way of a spray or nebulizer. This, like
Adrenalin injected hypodermically, serves to open the bronchial tubes. It
can be purchased without a prescription in any drugstore. In some kits,
other tablets to be taken by mouth are included (antihistamine,
ephedrine, and cortisone derivative tablets), but their action is much
slower and less predictable than medication administered directly by a
hypodermic injection or even absorbed under the tongue. If the reaction
has not subsided within ten minutes, a second injection of Adrenalin is
advisable, and during this period every effort should be made to locate
the nearest physician or hospital facility.

SUMMARY

Reactions to insects can be serious and even fatal. The most common
insects responsible for grave reactions are the stinging insects, specific-

ally the wasps, yellow jackets, hornets, and bees. In general, bites of mosquitoes, stable flies, fleas, ants, bedbugs, and other similar ubiquitous insects are merely a source of irritation and annoyance. The itching and local swellings caused by these insects are easily relieved by soothing lotions, creams, and ointments, or the application of cold packs.

The cause of the reaction is allergy to the body protein of the insect and not to the venom. The symptoms of insect allergy vary from a simple itching rash with moderate or severe localized swelling to hives over the entire body, watering of the eyes, running or congestion of the nose, cough, and difficulty in breathing. In extreme cases there is actual shock with loss of consciousness.

Avoiding or eradication of the insects is in effect the best "treatment" of the allergy. If that is not possible, emergency therapy is used immediately after one is bitten. A special emergency kit providing medication that anyone can administer should be carried by every person who has ever experienced a severe allergic reaction to the bite of an insect. For prophylaxis, the sensitive individual can be desensitized by injections of an extract prepared from the body of the insect, or group of insects, to which he is allergic. This, fortunately, is very effective preventive therapy; it must be performed by a physician who is experienced in the technique .

Chapter Eleven

Hay Fever — Seasonal and Perennial

TERMINOLOGY

The disease was originally called hay fever in England because it was most prevalent during the haying season and produced "fever" (then understood in the sense of malaise, not elevated temperature). We now know that hay is not a causative factor. The correct scientific nomenclature is *allergic rhinitis.* "Allergic" refers to the underlying cause of the illness, and "rhinitis," derived from the Greek, means inflammation of the lining of the nose. Then "allergic rhinitis" means swelling of the lining of the nose caused by sensitivity to some substance.

Allergic rhinitis can actually be divided into two types: *seasonal,* which appears only during certain seasons of the year, and *perennial,* which lasts throughout the year. Most people still prefer to call the seasonal type "hay fever"; in this discussion, hay fever, seasonal hay fever, and seasonal allergic rhinitis will be used interchangeably. In like manner, perennial hay fever and perennial allergic rhinitis will be considered synonymous, and will be used when discussing the type that lasts throughout the year. This is in conformity with the most widespread usage.

Allergic rhinitis has also been called allergic coryza, rose fever, pollinosis and vasomotor rhinitis. Both seasonal and perennial allergic rhinitis display similar symptoms and the treatment is much alike.

GENERAL DISCUSSION

Of all diseases of allergy, allergic rhinitis is by far the most common, the seasonal variety (hay fever) producing the most violent symptoms. Although not serious in the sense of shortening the life of the sufferer, it nonetheless contributes to many unhappy hours and days in the life of the afflicted person. It is a major illness responsible for millions of

149

workdays lost in industry, and many hours of inefficiency in the performance of skilled jobs. In addition, there is an increased awareness that more serious illness, such as bronchial asthma, also caused by allergy, may follow if the condition is left untreated.

Hay fever, like all violent types of allergy diseases, is less common in the aged than in the young. Scientists have attempted to explain why this is so and have presented several possibilities. Some think it is caused by changes in circulation such as a decreased blood supply that takes place in a person's tissue structures incident to the aging process. It is also thought that in youth there are more opportunities for intimate exposure to allergenic substances, particularly pollen. Whatever the explanation, seasonal allergic rhinitis occurs most frequently between the ages of twenty and thirty.

It is generally assumed that the seasonal variety is caused by inhalation of pollen, while the perennial type is due to inhalation of household dusts, such as house dust, feathers, wool, animal hairs, and cotton (see Chapter 6). Of course in southern areas like subtropical regions of the United States (for example, Florida, Arizona, and southern California) the plants pollinate throughout the entire year. This can obviously produce symptoms all year, but the resulting disease can be called seasonal, since there are different plants pollinating during various overlapping seasons.

SYMPTOMS

The symptoms of a violent attack of hay fever, such as might occur in an area where the seasons do not overlap (as in the ragweed areas of the Midwest and East) are generally known and readily observed. Usually itchy, red, watering eyes, attacks of incessant sneezing, an itching, clogged, or runny nose predominate. In addition, many persons complain of itching of the roof of the mouth and of the ear canals. In advanced cases, the bronchial tubes are affected, producing symptoms of asthma, such as heaviness of the chest, difficulty in breathing, wheezing, and annoying cough. The repeated paroxysmal fits of sneezing, during which the sufferer sneezes explosively, are commonly the most obvious symptom, an attempt on the part of the body to expel the watery mucus which has accumulated in the nose. This is true also of the cough which develops in some persons with hay fever; it is an attempt of the body to rid itself of the mucus which has collected in the bronchial tubes. Often the sneezing attacks are precipitated by a change of temperature or the inhaling of smoke, dust, or other irritants. Even bright sunshine has been known to provoke an attack of sneezing, but inhalation of pollen to which the person is sensitive is the primary cause. Although blowing the nose succeeds in clearing the head temporarily, the nasal passages do not remain free of secretion for very long. For that reason hay fever sufferers, despite their constant sneezing, find it increasingly difficult to breathe through their noses.

In describing his attacks of hay fever, Henry Ward Beecher wrote: "Your handkerchief suddenly becomes the most important object in life. The slightest draught or wind sets you to sneezing. If the door is open, you sneeze. If a panel of glass is gone, you sneeze. If a little dust rises from the carpet, or the odor of flowers is wafted to you, or the smell of smoke, you incontinently sneeze. It is a riot of sneezes. First, a single one like a leader in a flock of sheep chasing over, in twos, in fives, in bunches of twenty." To one who is afflicted with hay fever, Mark Twain's lines on seasickness may be very appropriate: "First, you feel a little sick, then you feel very sick. Then you don't care if you live or die. Then you just wish you would die."

The common complaint, in addition to the usual fits of sneezing, is clogging, stuffiness, or congestion of the nose, which prevents free breathing. This sense of obstruction may alternate with episodes of seemingly incessant flow of thin watery secretion. Constantly wiping and rubbing it because the tip itches so intensely produces the red, swollen nose, so embarrassing to the hay fever sufferer. Often before the nasal symptoms begin, the eyes are affected. They itch and water, burn and smart, and become red and swollen. After the sneezing begins, other annoying symptoms may develop. Of these, itching of the roof the mouth and the ear canals are the most common. Frequently there is a swelling of the nasal membrane and accumulation of mucus; this blocks the openings of the sinuses into the nose, and sinus headaches develop. Because of this accumulation of mucus in the nose and the swelling of the lining of the nose, most hay fever victims breathe through their mouths. This eventually irritates the back of the mouth, the throat, and the upper windpipe, adding to the discomfort. Later on, as the hay fever season progresses, the bronchial tubes themselves may become affected by pollen coming in direct contact with them; a cough with wheezing, accompanied by difficulty in breathing, develops.

The symptoms include fatigue and often depression. Patients have difficulty in carrying on their daily duties; children find it hard to concentrate and their schoolwork suffers accordingly. Sometimes exhaustion is mistaken for a separate illness. In perennial allergic rhinitis, the symptoms differ only in degree. Much, of course, depends on the area where the individual lives and the concentration of allergen he encounters.

ETIOLOGY (CAUSE)

Pollen

The cause of hay fever (seasonal allergic rhinitis) is primarily pollen sensitivity, not just to one plant, as a rule, but to several, perhaps as many as five, ten, or more. Pollen (see Chapter 5) is the main fertilizing element of the flower. When these grains come into contact with the cells of the lining of the nose, they act as antigens, joining with their appropriate antibodies to form antigen-antibody union and release certain chemicals, such as histamine, among many others. (See Chapter 2.) The chemicals released produce swelling and excess mucus secretion in the nose, and have a similar effect on the bronchial tubes, accompanied by spasms of the bronchi. Contact with the membrane of the eyeballs and eyelids produces characteristic eye symptoms. Since plant pollen is in the air only while the plant pollinates, the symptoms of hay fever due to pollen fade away and disappear when the pollinating season is over. In some parts of the country the pollinating season of allergy-producing plants is brief and sharply delineated; in others, the season is prolonged. In most areas there are at least three separate pollinating seasons, one for trees, one for grasses, and another for weeds. The table at the end of Chapter 5 outlines the most important allergy-producing plants in and around the large cities of the United States and some foreign countries, together with the usual dates of pollination and their relative degrees of importance.

Because of the ease with which the pollen can be brought into direct contact with the lining of the nose, the wind-pollinated (anemophilous) plants are the principal agents causing hay fever. Hay fever from insect-pollinated (entomophilous) plants usually develops only when these plants are kept in a hospital room or bedroom, or maintained as a floral decoration in an enclosed room where pollen may drift into the atmosphere. Gardeners, florists, and nurserymen may be particularly exposed to direct contact with insect-pollinated plants.

During the period of pollination, wind-pollinated plant pollen is found as far as four hundred miles from its source and as high as seventeen hundred feet above sea level. This is because it is very light in weight and is produced in abundance. Since the time of pollination of trees, grasses, and weeds can be determined by consulting a chart such as the table in Chapter 5, it is often possible for the doctor or hay fever victim to determine which plant is causing the symptoms. Special factors influencing the onset of symptoms are fully described in Chapter 5.

The general rule that allergy symptoms which occur all year around are probably caused by materials within the house is a valid one. But in areas where plants pollinate throughout the year, symptoms may be due either to pollen or to household dusts, or both. Other factors, such as an overheated home in the winter months with decreased ventilation, more dust from the furnace and excessive drying of the nose, may be contributory.

Food allergy may also be involved in producing or aggravating allergic rhinitis. Some allergists feel that food allergy is the single cause in most cases, but inhalant allergies appear to be much more significant, with food allergy perhaps contributing to aggravation of the symptoms. Molds (mildew) can cause hay fever both seasonally and all year around. Nearly everything in the air has been implicated, including butterfly wing scales, sand flies, and even the common housefly. Some cases have been ascribed to human hair and human dander. It frequently takes perseverence and ingenuity to identify the responsible agent or agents, particularly in the perennial type of allergic rhinitis.

SKIN TESTS

In order to ascertain more exactly which pollen or other inhalants are responsible, allergy skin tests are performed. There are several ways of performing these tests; none are painful and they are fully discussed in the chapter entitled Allergy Skin Tests (Chapter 4).

Molds '

In certain parts of the country and of the world fungus or mold spores (mildew) pollute the atmosphere and can produce attacks of hay fever indistinguishable from those due to plant pollen or other dusts. As in seasonal allergic rhinitis, symptoms vary in accordance with the quantity of fungus spores the person encounters and their concentration in the atmosphere. Allergy to molds is seasonal when the molds are only in the outdoor atmosphere and may be perennial when the mildew infests a household article such as a pillow or the heating system of an old, damp house. (For a further discussion of molds, see Chapter 6).

Non-Specific Causes

There are other agents which, although not a direct cause of hay fever, may influence the attacks. Change in weather is one of these. Some people find that their hay fever is worse on damp, cold, foggy days; others describe an aggravation of their symptoms on warm or hot, dry, sunny days. More symptomatology on hot, windy days can readily be explained—a larger quantity of pollen may be in the air and blown about by the wind. It is more difficult to hypothesize why symptoms are worse during the cold, damp days; allergic nasal mucous membrane may be affected, swell, become boggy and less able to resist airborne pollen. Some hay fever patients may be affected on entering an air-conditioned room, or by the draft of an electric fan. They may have similar difficulty in the winter months when entering a warm, steam-heated building after being outside in the cold. Again, an explanation is difficult; the most probable is that temperature changes affect the small blood vessels in the nasal mucous membrane. The term "vasomotor," meaning control of blood vessels, is applicable; some physicians, particularly nose and throat specialists, use the term *vasomotor rhinitis* to designate symptoms unexplained by allergy, or even instead of the term "allergic rhinitis".

Miscellaneous Inhalants

Since house dust is an irritant, in addition to being a true allergen, most hay fever patients are made worse if they come in contact with large amounts of house dust. This also applies to strong scents and odors, powders and detergents, and animal hairs. There are even some people who find that certain foods which they can eat with impunity at any other time of the year will cause an aggravation of their hay fever symptoms when these foods are eaten during the hay fever season. The explanation for this is that these people have a mild food sensitivity which by itself is negligible, but when added to pollen sensitivity, increases the hay fever symptoms by a cumulative action.

DIAGNOSIS

The diagnosis of hay fever is not difficult to make. It is based mainly upon a history of the characteristic symptoms which appear at the onset of a pollinating season and disappear when the season is over. Examination of the nose reveals a gray, boggy, swollen membrane with a large amount of watery secretion. High up in the nostril there may be translucent, shiny, glistening tumors called polyps. Occasionally the common cold is confused with hay fever, but the successive stages of a cold—the mild sore throat at the start, an aching sensation, a slight rise in body temperature, and fits of sneezing, followed in a day or two by nasal blockage and thick secretion which soon begins to crust—serve to differentiate it. In a cold, the lining of the nose has a beefy red appearance in contrast to the grayish color of the allergic membrane. In the perennial type of hay fever the appearance of the lining of the nose is also pale but it is not always swollen.

In order to differentiate the diagnosis of allergy from infection, a nasal smear is sometimes obtained. Some of the secretion is carefully swabbed from the nose, placed on a glass slide, and specially stained. The specimen may also be obtained by blowing the mucus from the nose directly into a piece of cellophane. The number of blood cells in the secretion is counted. A high percentage of eosinophile cells indicates that the condition is probably due to an allergy. If cells such as the *polymorphonucuear neutrophile* are in the majority, it suggests that the condition is more likely due to an infection since in infections these cells predominate. These findings are not foolproof, for seldom does allergic rhinitis exist over a period of time without a superimposed infection of some degree.

Physicians oriented to analytical psychology have reported that people with emotional difficulties may develop fits of sneezing which may be confused with hay fever. According to these doctors sensations such as fear, apprehension, grief, or anguish , which do not involve conflict, may also alter the membrane lining of the nose so that it resembles the changes seen in hay fever. Other emotions, such as those reflecting resentment, animosity, anger, vexation, and humility, which are the result of conflict, can give rise to nasal blockage and swollen membranes like those observed in hay fever. The rationale for this theory is that the emotions act upon certain nerves; the emotions involving conflict act upon one type while the emotions not caused by conflict act upon another. Some people certainly suffer from transient sneezing or nasal congestion when they are emotionally upset. But the *en masse* sneezing of millions that begins in the East during August when ragweed pollinates is a different matter.

TREATMENT (THERAPY)

Avoidance

The ideal treatment of hay fever would be to avoid or eliminate pollen. Efforts have been made in some communities to eradicate ragweed, the main cause of hay fever in a large part of the United States. The attempts not only were very costly but never proved effective. Clearing an area one season did not prevent a new growth the next. Furthermore, since airborne pollen can travel many miles from its source, little protection was afforded the hay fever sufferer by merely clearing the nearby lots.

Filters

While total removal of the patient from pollen to which he is sensitive is impractical, filtering the air has been suggested and is in use in many homes. The purpose is to filter the air which comes in from the outside, and to filter the air already in the home. For outside air, keeping the windows closed is a simple technique of preventing entrance of pollen, another is to use a screening, matting, or filtering air conditioner. To filter the air already in the home, an electronic air filter is most desirable. This can be portable and obtained in a size suitable for the size of the room, or installed in the return vent of the recirculating portion of the air conditioner or furnace.

Air filters, of course, are of value only when the person is in the room or rooms which are being filtered by them. All too often the claims made by some of the manufacturers of these devices are not substantiated in practice. Some machines lack an effective filter, and the fans with which they are provided do not propel enough air to be of any value. No filter, regardless of how efficiently it operates, can remove all pollen or dusts from a room since no room is ever perfectly sealed; airborne pollen can always find its way in. But when the amount of allergen is reduced in a room, it will benefit the hay fever sufferer to some degree. The bedroom, in which most consecutive hours are spent, should be selected as the site for the single filter.

There are two main types of filters used: (1) the impingement type, and (2) the electrostatic precipitating type. A third type, an absorbing filter utilizing activated charcoal capable of removing vapors of molecular weight greater than nitrogen and oxygen, filters cigarette smoke, smog, and odors but is of no practical value in hay fever. When combined with the electronic type, it may impede the air flow.

The impingement type is a mechanical trap to catch pollen or dust particles. A simple fine-wire window screen designed to keep out flies is actually a crude filter of this type. Since for the control of allergy symptoms exceedingly small pollen or dust particles must be trapped, the best filters are those with the most delicate mesh. Those in common use are: (1) glass wool impingement filters with varying efficiencies based on the size of the filters used, (2) five-ply "air mat" filters, and (3) glass rug filters. These vary in efficiency from 60 to 95 percent in filtering pollen from the air, provided there is adequate force to propel the air through the small openings in the fine screens. A filter whose intake rate is fifty cubic feet of air per minute in a room of average size such as 12 x 14 x 18 is considered effective. The window air-conditioning unit is an excellent filtering device since it traps up to 75 percent of the important allergenic pollen. Of all the impingement filters mentioned, the glass wool impingement filter is the least effective.

The two-stage electrostatic precipitator is an excellent filter, probably the best of all. It operates on the principle of attracting ionized particles by means of oppositely charged collections of wires or plates. Air enters the filter and is ionized by an electrostatic field; it then passes on to another electrostatic field where the ionized particles in the air are attracted to the oppositely charged wires or plates, which act as collectors. Theoretically, the air passing out of this electronic filter is free of particles. Its efficiency depends on an adequate flow rate, which determines the velocity of the air propelled through the unit. Several technical engineering and electrical principles are important in the manufacture of this type of filter; namely, the size and length of the wires or plates, and the spacing between the plates. The United States National Bureau of Standards has set up standards of efficiency as well as methods of testing electronic filters. These have been adopted by air-processing engineers.

If the forced-air furnace that is generally employed in the home is equipped with an impingement filter and kept clean, it governs the room temperature and keeps the pollen count low. During the summer, the heat may be turned off but the fan can be turned on. If there is adequate recirculation, it will also minimize dust. This depends on what percentage of the air entering the furnace comes from out-of-doors and what percent is recirculated. The popular window refrigerated air conditioner is equipped with an impingement filter. If the room is properly cleaned and all windows and doors are kept closed, as much as 75 percent of allergy-producing pollen which would enter the room is eliminated. It should be realized, however, that the 25 percent of pollen not eliminated will collect in the room and in a short time may become a large accumulation. For this reason, the electronic filter which picks up particulate matter in the room, filters it, and then recirculates the air is a very fine adjunct to the ordinary air conditioner and has the added advantage of filtering household dust.

Another excellent system of air conditioning and cleaning the air is one which combines refrigeration and heating with a two-stage electrostatic filter. This must recirculate a sufficient percentage of the air in order to eliminate house dusts. Addition of a gas-absorbing medium is still another improvement. However, depending upon the size of such a filter, the cost might well be prohibitive for the average private home. An electronic air cleaner can be installed in a forced-air heating system without much added cost. In summer, as with impingement filters, the fan alone can be used. If there is adequate recirculation, it will also reduce dusts. A minor adjustment may be necessary for some furnaces.

Filters which can be worn in the nose and filter out pollen have been tried but have never gained acceptance primarily because those that cover the nose give one a grotesque appearance. The smaller ones devised to fit inside the nose have been uncomfortable and inefficient. Neither completely filters out the pollen.

Of course with all filtering devices, pollen, dust, and other allergens which are implanted in rugs or which have settled on furniture and drapes cannot be filtered until they are dislodged and become airborne. Even with an air filter, frequent and thorough cleaning of a home is still required.

Some advertised filters produce ozone by passing electrical discharges or ultraviolet light rays across the flowing air. The ozone odor makes many people think these filters are effective. Ozone may be useful in industry as a bactericide or a water disinfectant, but it is toxic to man in the range of bacterial concentrations, and when it "deodorizes" it does so mainly by producing a temporary paralysis of the smelling (olfactory) apparatus. It does not remove pollen, mildew, or dust to any measurable degree.

There also are some advertised filter devices which produce negative ions. It is asserted that negative ions are beneficial in relieving hay fever symptoms even though no pollen is removed from the air. These claims have never been substantiated.

DESENSITIZATION

Desensitization (hyposensitization) is the specific treatment for hay fever and is mainly prophylactic. It is employed primarily to prevent the onset of symptoms rather than to treat them after they develop. Occasionally, however, it is used successfully to ameliorate symptoms after the pollinating season has begun. (See Chapter 7 for a full discussion of this method of treatment.)

Symptomatic Treatment

Relief can also be obtained by using medicines. This is *symptomatic* treatment. Until the advent of the antihistaminic drugs, little could be done to relieve the symptoms of hay fever quickly other than use of nose drops or advising the sufferer to take a vacation in a place free of pollinating plants. Nose drops and sprays commonly employed in the past continue to be used but in a very limited fashion.

Nose Drops and Sprays

The drugs used in nose drops or sprays give some comfort but the relief is limited and brief; even more severe congestion soon returns. The drugs contained in hay fever nose drops or sprays are for the most part local vasoconstrictors. Many are advertised and on the market. Most can be secured at drugstores without a doctor's prescription. The hay fever sufferer also soon finds out to his dismay that he is addicted to the nose drops or spray and must carry the medication around with him constantly for repeated use. The action of the vasomotor drugs in the common hay fever nose drops and sprays is first to constrict the tissue lining of the nose to allow more breathing space. After a little while, often only a few hours, a secondary effect takes place. The lining of the nose begins to swell and the breathing area becomes just as narrow or narrower than before the nasal medication was applied. This is the "rebound phenomenon." When this happens, the victim reaches for the drops or spray to use again. A vicious cycle is set up which is hard to break. The dependency on nose drops or sprays in hay fever has been likened to true drug addiction in that the person using the drops or sprays cannot do without them. Actually, symptoms comparable to the withdrawal symptoms of the narcotic addict have been observed in some people trying to discontinue use of the local nasal vasoconstricting agents.

In addition to nose drops and sprays, nasal inhalors have been placed on the market. These contain medication similar to that of the drops. The ease of administration recommends them; also they can be carried about easily in a pocket or purse. However, the effect of the volatile vasoconstrictor is just as brief as the one in liquid form in nose drops or sprays and there is also the same tendency to use them too often.

Many of the nose drops and sprays have had added to their original formula antibiotic drugs, and the user often is likely to believe that these have special merit. This is not the case since hay fever is caused by an inhalant sensitivity or inhaled allergy and not a bacterial infection. If hay fever should be complicated by infection, antibiotics, if indicated, would be prescribed for use by mouth or injection. Some people, especially those who are allergic, can develop a sensitivity to an antibiotic even in a nasal preparation. In any event antibiotics should only be taken under a doctor's supervision. Other ingredients that may be found in nose drops and sprays are added primarily to lessen their irritation and make them more acceptable. Except in special cases most doctors have stopped prescribing any medication to be applied directly to the nasal membrane.

Antihistamines

The *antihistamines*, as their name implies, are directed at neutralizing the histamine which is released in the nose. Inhalation of the substance to which the person is allergic initiates an antigen-antibody union, in turn releasing histamine. This is described fully in Chapter 2. Antihistaminic drugs are exceedingly effective in some people and ineffective in others. Also, some persons can tolerate a large dose of this type of medication with no side effects, while only a small dose will cause drowsiness, dizziness, dryness of the mouth, and other bizarre disturbances in others. Much also depends upon which antihistaminic drug is prescribed. The chemical structures of some are identical or slightly altered, but others have an entirely different chemical structure and this, to some extent, determines the side reactions noted in some individuals.

In popular radio, TV, and newspaper advertisements, little mention is ever made of drowsiness, the main side effect of most antihistaminic preparations. But careful scrutiny of the label will disclose a warning about this and it should be always kept in mind, especially when taking an antihistamine during the day. Automobile accidents have been reported as caused by the driver having taken an antihistaminic pill and falling asleep at the wheel. Children taking antihistamines often complain of sleepiness and interference with their concentration at school. Other reactions have been reported, including nervousness, irritability, wakefulness, nausea, fatigue, headache, vomiting, blurring of the eyes, and palpitation of the heart.

Antihistamines, when tolerated, relieve the nasal congestion in most people and have some effect on the sneezing paroxysms. Their most constant pharmocologic action is to dry up the secretions in the nose. When some secretion persists in the nose, the sneezing bouts are seldom relieved since sneezing is nature's way of getting rid of the excess mucus. At the present time many of the antihistaminic drugs may be purchased without a prescription. The syllable "hist" is commonly used within the trade name. The general rule of the Federal Government is that the average antihistamine may be sold without a doctor's prescription if it is not more than one-half the physician's usually recommended dose and if the product is properly labeled.

In the following table, some of the commonly prescribed antihistamines are listed with their generic (official chemical) name. The list indicates the different brand names for identical antihistamines as well as compounds containing them. Many of the compounds are "cold remedies"; some are prescribed to relieve or prevent seasickness and still others have been used as "sleep aids." Law provides that all medication sold over the counter in a drugstore must list the contents therein. By consulting the following table and reading the contents printed on the outside of the package, a purchaser will be able to discover if he is buying one antihistamine identical to another sold under a different trade name. He will also be in a position to know whether a new doctor's prescription is for an antihistamine he may have had prescribed for him under another name. Antihistamines most commonly sold without a doctor's prescription in the United States are marked with an asterisk.

In addition to the antihistaminic tablets or capsules that may be prescribed to be taken every few hours, there are a number of so-called prolonged-action preparations. These are very popular, for surely it is

TABLE OF ORAL ANTIHISTAMINES FREQUENTLY PRESCRIBED*

GENERIC (official chemical) NAME	BRAND NAME AND MANUFACTURER OF ANTIHISTAMINE	BRAND NAME AND MANUFACTURER OF MIXTURE WHICH CONTAINS THE ANTIHISTAMINE
GROUP I. In this group drowsiness is marked.		
1. Diphenhydramine	Benadryl *(Parke-Davis)*	Ambenyl *(Parke-Davis)* Benadryl with ephedrine *(Parke-Davis)* Benylin *(Parke-Davis)* Hydryllin *(Searle)*
2. Doxylamine	Decapryn *(Merrell)*	
3. Bromodiphenhydramine	Ambodryl *(Parke-Davis)*	Ambenyl *(Parke-Davis)*
4. Carbinoxamine	Clistin *(McNeil)*	
5. Dexcarbinoxamine	Twiston *(McNeil)*	
6. Phenyltoloxamine	Bristamine *(Bristol)*	Algic *(Spencer)* Anfac *(Pharmafac)* Contramal CP *(Phys. Prod.)* Ephoxamine *(Spencer)* Naldecon *(Bristol)* Sinutab *(Warner-Chilcott)* Toldex *(Pitman-Moore)* Tristacomp *(Phys. Prod.)*
GROUP II. These are mildly sedative.		
1. Tripelennamine	Pyribenzamine *(Ciba)*	Dibistine *(Ciba)* Multihist *(Dorsey)* Plimasin *(Ciba)* Pyribenzamine with ephedrine *(Ciba)*
2. Clemizole	Alecur *(Roerig)*	
3. Thenylpyramine	Histadyl *(Lilly)* Thenylene *(Abbott)*	Corenil *(McNeil)* Co-Pyronil *(Lilly)* Histaclopane *(Lilly)* Histadyl and ASA Comp. *(Lilly)* Histadyl with ephedrine *(Lilly)* Hista-Vadrine *(First Texas)* Isoclor *(Arnar-Stone)* Neo-Rhiban *(Kendall)* Pentryl *(Chilcott)*

GENERIC (official chemical) NAME	BRAND NAME AND MANUFACTURER OF ANTIHISTAMINE	BRAND NAME AND MANUFACTURER OF MIXTURE WHICH CONTAINS THE ANTIHISTAMINE
		Palohist *(Palmedico)*
		Propahist *(Blue Line)*
		Semikon *(Messengill)*
		Thenylene APC *(Abbott)*
4. Pyrilamine	Neo-Antergan *(Merck Sharp & Dohme)*	Citra Compounds *(Boyle)*
		Contramal CP *(Phys. Prod.)*
		Duadacine *(Lloyd Bros.)*
		Histalet *(Scott-Lee)*
		Multihist *(Dorsey)*
		Nalertan *(Neisler)*
		Napril *(Marion)*
		Neocafotan *(Premo)*
		Palohist *(Palmedico)*
		P.P.A. *(Dorsey)*
		Propahist *(Blue Line)*
		Pyma *(Testagar)*
		Pymadex *(Testagar)*
		Restamine *(Strasenburgh)*
		Rynalert *(Neisler)*
		Rynatan *(Neisler)*
		Super Rhi-Lief *(Walker Corp. & Co.)*
		Triaminic *(Dorsey)*
		Tristacomp *(Phys. Prod.)*
		U.R.I. *(Sig: Inc.)*
		Ursinus *(Dorsey)*
5. Thenyldiamine	Thenfadil *(Winthrop)*	Neo-synephrine Comp. *(Winthrop)*
6. Antazoline	Antistine *(Ciba)*	Dibistine *(Ciba)*
7. Thonzylamine	Neohetramine *(Warner-Chilcott)*	

GROUP III. These may cause nervous stimulation.

1. Pheniramine	Trimeton *(Schering)*	Pyma *(Testagar)*
		Pymadex *(Testagar)*
		Triaminic *(Dorsey)*
2. Chlorpheniramine	Chlor-Trimeton *(Schering)* Histadur *(Wynn)* Teldrin *(Smith Kline & French)*	Algic *(Spencer)* Aristomin *(Lederle)* Contramal *(Phys. Prod.)* Coricidin *(Schering)* Coricidin-D *(Schering)*

GENERIC (official chemical) NAME	BRAND NAME AND MANUFACTURER OF ANTIHISTAMINE	BRAND NAME AND MANUFACTURER OF MIXTURE WHICH CONTAINS THE ANTIHISTAMINE
Chlorpheniramine (cont.)	Histaspan *(U.S. Vitamin)*	Cortiforte *(Schering)*
		Coryban-D *(Roerig)*
		Covanamine *(Van Pelt & Brown)*
		Demazine *(Schering)*
		Duadacin *(Lloyds Bros.)*
		Histadur *(Wynn)*
		Histalet *(Scott-Lee)*
		Hista-Vadrin *(First Texas)*
		Metreton *(Schering)*
		Naldecon *(Bristol)*
		Nalertan *(Neisler)*
		Napril *(Marion)*
		Nolamine *(Carnrick)*
		Novahistine *(Pitman-Moore)*
		Ornade *(Smith Kline & French)*
		Palohist *(Palmedico)*
		Phenate *(Mallard)*
		Prednaman *(Dome)*
		Propoahist *(Blue Line)*
		Pyma *(Testagar)*
		Pymadex *(Testagar)*
		Pyrroxate *(Upjohn)*
		Rynalert *(Neisler)*
		Rynatan *(Neisler)*
		Super Rhi-Lief *(Walker Corp. & Co.)*
		Tirstacomp *(Phys. Prod.)*
3. Dexchlorpheniramine	Polaramine *(Schering)*	Guaiamine *(Sutliff & Co.)*
4. Tripolidine	Actidil *(Burroughs Wellcome & Co.)*	Actifed *(Burroughs Wellcome & Co.)*
5. Pyrrobutamine	Pyronil *(Lilly)*	Co-Pyronil *(Lilly)*
6. Brompheniramine	Dimetane *(Robins)*	Dimetapp *(Robins)*
7. Dexbrompheniramine	Disomer *(White)*	Disophrol *(White)*

GROUP IV. These are related to the tranquilizers.

1. Promethazine	Phenergan *(Wyeth)*	
2. Isothipendyl	Theruhistin *(Ayerst)*	Kryl *(Ayerst)*
3. Methdilazine	Tacaryl *(Mead Johnson)*	

GENERIC (official chemical) NAME	BRAND NAME AND MANUFACTURER OF ANTIHISTAMINE	BRAND NAME AND MANUFACTURER OF MIXTURE WHICH CONTAINS THE ANTIHISTAMINE
GROUP V. Many of these are seasickness medicines.		
1. Chlorcyclizine	Di-Paraline *(Abbott)*	Emprazil *(Burroughs Wellcome & Co.)*
	Perazil *(Burroughs Wellcome & Co.)*	Fedrazil *(Burroughs Wellcome & Co.)*
		Histalet *(Scott-Lee)*
2. Meclizine	Bonadoxine *(Roerig)* Bonine *(Pfizer)*	
3. Phenindamine	Thephorin *(Roche)*	Nolamine *(Carnrick)* Thephorin AC *(Roche)*
4. Buclizine	Bucladin *(Stuart)*	
5. Dyphenylpyraline	Diafen *(Riker)* End Allergy *(Amfre-Grant)* Hispril *(Smith Kline & French)*	
6. Dimethindene	Forhistal *(Ciba)*	

*(Adapted from Harris, M.C., and Shure, N., *Sensitivity Chest Diseases*, F. A. Davis Company, Philadelphia, 1964.)

far more comfortable to take medication only once every eight or twelve hours instead of every three or four. They are widely sold as "over-the-counter" medicines in drugstores and are prescribed by most physicians. However, there are disadvantages that must be considered along with the obvious advantages. Certainly, when one has trouble during the night a long-lasting medicine is helpful since awakening to take another dose is an unwelcome interruption of sleep. During the day, however, it is not difficult to take additional doses; short-acting ones that wear off quickly may be all that are necessary because the symptoms may not persist. Further, the effect is not always exactly predictable. In some people they last for eight hours, in others for twelve, and in others for four or even less A few years ago, forty-five thousand tablets of a prescription drug that was said to release its ingredients over a twelve-hour period were seized by the Food and Drug Administration after it was determined that the ingredients were released in only two hours. It is always wise to observe your reactions to these "long-acting," "sustained release," and "timed release" medicines before using them regularly.

For many people who suffer from hay fever, the eye symptoms are as severe or worse than the nasal symptoms. Although antihistaminic drugs may give some relief of the nasal symptoms, they seldom do much to relieve the itching and tearing of the eyes, or injected blood vessels of the conjunctiva. For the relief of these symptoms, local medication is often necessary; eyedrops are usually prescribed. Most of them contain a vasoconstrictor drug that will shrink the blood vessels of the surface of the eyeball. Occasionally, a special ophthalmic cream or ointment is prescribed for this purpose. None of these should be used without supervision of a doctor for they may be harmful, particularly if an eye disease already exists. Some tend to raise ocular pressure or tension. This is particularly true of hydrocortisone and other cortisone derivatives.

Steroids (Cortisone)

Corticotropine and corticosteroids are an extremely important class of drugs used for nearly all allergic diseases. They are used sparingly and only when all other measures fail absolutely to give much needed relief. They have many different side effects, some of which can be serious. The most used corticosteroids at the present time are prednisone, prednisolone, dexamethasone, betamethasone, triamcinolone, methyl and fluprednisolone and paramethasone. They are marketed under various trade names but none should be taken without a physician's order or supervision. A more detailed discussion of the corticosteroids is presented in the chapter on bronchial asthma, a condition in which they are much more frequently prescribed than in hay fever.

Miscellaneous Treatment

All told the outlook has become much brighter for the hay fever patient in recent years, and the measure of relief that can be obtained with current methods is very great.

A group of *miscellaneous measures* has been suggested, particularly for the treatment of perennial allergic rhinitis. Among these is the use of a bacterial vaccine. This is claimed to be of value for the perennial type in which the boggy nasal membrane has persisted for a long time, permitting bacterial infection to take place. Most allergists who employ this form of treatment use a vaccine that is already prepared and which contains the organisms commonly found in chronic infections of the nose, sinuses, or respiratory tract. Some allergists prefer an autogenous vaccine, one that is specially made up for the person being treated and contains only the organisms recovered and cultured from the area of infection. Bacterial desensitization is performed in much the same manner as that described previously in desensitization with pollens and household dusts. There is some disagreement among physicians whether large or small doses of the vaccine provide better relief of symptoms or, indeed, whether bacterial vaccine therapy is of any value at all, but each doctor uses the type of treatment and the dosage which in his experience has proved effective.

Cauterization of the nasal lining by carbolic acid or actual electric cautery has had some degree of popularity, more in the perennial type of hay fever than the seasonal. It is still used by some nose and throat specialists but not often by allergists. The burning of the nasal membrane provides but temporary relief and cannot be repeated frequently. Injection of cortisone derivatives directly into the nose is at times effective.

A special diet is useful only in the presence of a food allergy which has been proved to be a cause of, or to aggravate, the allergic rhinitis. Irritating, although nonallergenic substances should be avoided by the allergy sufferer. These include dusts of all kinds, strong odors and scents, tobacco and other types of smoke, and strong household cleaning chemicals.

SINUSITIS

Although nasal sinusitis and nasal polyps are the most common complications of both seasonal and perennial allergic rhinitis, they are more common in the perennial form. The frontal sinuses are paired cavities located in the forehead skull bone just above the eyes. They are connected to the nose by a mucous membrane which is a continuation of the nasal cavities. They also drain into the nose through these openings (ostia) which, when they are closed by secretions, cause the frontal sinuses to become swollen. This produces a headache just above the eyes, and if infection occurs, may cause chills, elevation of temperature, and a general feeling of discomfort and mental sluggishness. Discharge from the nose may be increased and thicker than usual, as well as discolored. The discharge is greater when the head is held upright and usually is more abundant in the morning than in the afternoon.

Vasoconstricting nose drops or sprays help shrink the tissues and allow more adequate drainage of the sinuses but the hazards and disadvantages of this form of treatment have already been stressed. The inhalation of steam often relieves the symptoms of frontal sinusitis. One of the oldest remedies is steam from compound tincture of benzoin, one teaspoonful to a pint of boiling water. The steam is inhaled by placing the face directly over the escaping vapor. Usually a towel is placed around the head and the vessel to prevent any leakage of the steam. But if any relief is obtained it is probably due to the moist heat rather than to the benzoin.

The application of heat or heat rays from an ordinary heat lamp (which is nothing more than an electric bulb and reflector) gives great comfort and helps allay pain. Excess use may cause a burn.

When pain in the face and the head is unusually severe, analgesics such as aspirin and codeine may be prescribed by the physician after he has made certain that there is no history of a sensitivity to the drug being prescribed. Very often an attempt is made to isolate the organisms responsible for the infection and to use an effective and suitable antibiotic. Antibiotics are only valuable when infection is present. In many cases of frontal sinusitis accompanying or complicating allergic rhinitis no infection is present, and since it is purely an allergic sinusitis, antibiotics should not be employed.

Nose and throat specialists often use negative pressure in frontal sinusitis to cleanse the nose of secretions and to promote drainage from the sinuses. After suction, the lining of the nose may be treated with an oily spray which leaves a protective layer to give a sense of coolness and clearness in breathing. This is pleasant but nothing more. In severe cases of infective frontal sinusitis, surgery for the drainage of pus is indicated but it is never resorted to in purely allergic disease where there is no evidence of infection.

The maxillary sinuses may also be involved in allergic rhinitis (particularly in the perennial type). They are located in the cheekbones on either side of the nose. In contrast to frontal sinusitis, usually just one side becomes infected. The discharge, which is profuse and increases when the head is held in the dependent position—either hang head over side of bed or bend it far backwards while sitting, is more abundant in the afternoon than in the morning. The pain of maxillary sinusitis is usually like neuralgia but at times may be sharp and referred to the frontal area above the corresponding eyebrow. Treatment is similar to that of frontal sinusitis: promotion of drainage, application of heat, and the use of antibiotics if infection is present. Sometimes it becomes necessary to wash out the maxillary sinuses. This is not a complicated procedure but is best done by a nose and throat specialist. Draining them through the normal opening (ostia) is uncomplicated; however, puncturing the sinuses through the maxillary bone is much more painful. In rare instances more radical surgical measures may be required.

The ethmoid sinuses on either side of the upper part of the nose behind and between the eye sockets, may also be involved as a result of pansinusitis, in which all the sinuses are infected. Fortunately, proper antibiotic therapy and adequate drainage of the more accessible sinuses usually make it unnecessary to treat these inaccessible sinuses. Use of bacterial vaccines made from organisms recovered from washing the frontal and maxillary sinuses has been advocated by some. If surgery is performed, the bacterial growth found on the mucous membranes may be used in vaccine preparation. Vaccine treatment is of uncertain value.

POLYPS

Polyps are present in nearly every case of severe allergic rhinitis. They are somewhat more common in the perennial than the seasonal type. Polyps develop when the secretion under the tissues lining the nose is increased and succeeds in loosening and stretching the lining to such an extent that it separates from the bony structure of the nose, producing a thin-walled pouch, which hangs down and protrudes into the nasal cavity, obstructing passage of air through the nose. They are classified as tumors, but are not serious and never malignant. Typically they are moist, smooth, glistening, and pearly gray in appearance. They seldom appear singly, tending to form in clusters high in the nose and in the sinuses, where they cannot be seen. When desensitization treatment is successful in relieving allergic rhinitis, polyps often shrink and disappear. When polyps persist as a major obstacle to breathing through the nose their surgical removal must be considered. The operation is not difficult and may be an office procedure, but if desensitization treatment is unsuccessful, polyps are likely to recur, requiring repeated operations.

As the polyps are being removed during surgery, more and more polyps which had been held back may fall into view and must be removed. For this reason, many surgeons prefer to perform the operation in a hospital. Polyps may be considered the often irreversible end result of allergic rhinitis. The preventive treatment for their recurrence is vigorous allergy management.

SECRETORY OTITIS

Several complications of allergic rhinitis are particularly important in children. The eustachian tube connecting the back portion of the nose with the inside of the ear just behind the eardrum equalizes pressure between the nose and ear. Especially in children, swelling at the opening of the tube or the accumulation of mucus which closes it will produce increased pressure and can cause fluid to collect behind the eardrum. The moist, boggy lining of the nose caused by allergic rhinitis in children and adults is an excellent breeding spot for bacteria to settle and grow so that it is not unusual for repeated infections, not only of the nose and sinuses but also of the middle ear, to occur. The combination of infection and fluid behind the eardrum may lead to hearing difficulty. Frequently the drum must be lanced and a plastic tube inserted to let the fluid escape.

Another complication of allergic rhinitis is asthma accompanied by infectious bronchitis. This may be a flare-up of allergic asthma or merely asthma due to infection.

SUMMARY

Allergic rhinitis is inflammation of the lining of the nose due to allergy. Most allergists use the term hay faver (scientifically, a misnomer) for the seasonal variety of allergic rhinitis which occurs only during those times of the year when pollen is in the air. Perennial allergic rhinitis lasts throughout the year.

The symptoms of allergic rhinitis are watering and itching of the eyes, paroxysmal attacks of sneezing, itching of the nose, and in some cases itching of the roof of the mouth and ear canals. The symptoms of both the seasonal and perennial types are more or less the same except in degree. There is likely to be less violent sneezing, eye symptomatology and itching in the perennial type but more nasal stuffiness and dryness.

The cause of both types of allergic rhinitis is primarily allergy to some inhaled substance or substances. Sometimes foods may be important. The seasonal variety is due to pollens which pervade the atmosphere at the time of pollination. Perennial allergic rhinitis is more likely to be caused by allergy to household dusts or fungus spores inhaled through the year. In a cold climate, symptoms may be worse in the winter with its principally indoor environment than in the summer.

If the sufferer lives in a southern region, in the United States or elsewhere, he may encounter pollen all year around and his perennial allergy may be due entirely to pollen. Many people who are allergic to both pollens and house dusts have some symptoms continually, no matter where they live.

In order to determine the exact cause of the illness as well as to confirm the diagnosis of allergy and treat the illness specifically, allergy skin tests are frequently performed. These are painless and principally of two types, the scratch test and the intradermal.

Treatment of allergic rhinitis consists first of preventing the attacks from occurring and second, prescribing of medication to relieve the symptoms. The first form of treatment is specific; the latter, symptomatic. Specific treatment involves eradication or avoidance of the agents responsible for the attacks, or desensitization. Since most persons with allergic rhinitis are allergic to pollen or other substances which cannot be completely eradicated or avoided, desensitization usually becomes necessary. This consists of a series of hypodermic injections of the responsible troublemakers (allergens).

Avoidance of the allergenic agents can also be accomplished by filtering the air which enters the home or place of business, a procedure which is helpful in cases of seasonal allergic rhinitis. Electronic cleaning of the atmosphere within the home or business is an aid to those who have perennial allergic rhinitis and are allergic to household dusts. There are several air-cleaning machines available, both portable and fixed, the most efficient of which are those connected with refrigerated central air-conditioning units or furnaces.

Medicines which are used for the relief of symptoms of allergic rhinitis are primarily nose drops and sprays, antihistaminic drugs, and nasal decongestants prescribed by a doctor. In extreme cases, the cortisone products and derivatives, a potent gland extract, may be required. All medication should be taken only under the strict control of a physician. Nevertheless, many efficient antihistamine preparations and nasal decongestants can be purchased in drugstores without a prescription. Some of them correspond to those prescribed by doctors but the "over-the-counter" dose is about half of that prescribed by the physician.

The complications of hay fever or allergic rhinitis are for the most part sinusitis, ear infections with subsequent hearing loss, and polyps. Children with a nasal allergy are likely to become mouth breathers, and orthodontists believe that mouth breathing contributes to irregular formation of the teeth. The danger of infection is greater in children and adults with allergic rhinitis because the boggy moist lining of the nose provides an ideal medium for the growth of bacteria.

Chapter Twelve

Bronchial Asthma

DEFINITION

Webster's definition of *asthma* is quite acceptable: "Labored breathing, either continued or paroxysmal, accompanied by wheezing, a sense of constriction, and often attacks of coughing or gasping, caused by conditions which interfere with the normal inflow and outflow of air in the lungs (as swelling of the mucous membrane of the bronchi or constriction of the bronchial walls with resultant narrowing of the lumen)." In the definition of *bronchial asthma,* the dictionary attempts to distinguish between asthma as a symptom and bronchial asthma as a disease state by defining bronchial asthma as "asthma resulting from spasmodic contraction of bronchial muscles, with constriction of the lumen of the bronchi and accumulation of mucus in the respiratory passages, due to psychosomatic, allergy, or other causes."

A more precise and meaningful definition of bronchial asthma is really impossible to set forth since it would have to include or expand the cause, mechanism, symptoms, and the ultimate result of the disease. The cause varies in every case; in the opinion of most physicians and certainly all allergists, bronchial asthma is caused primarily by allergy. Other factors such as infections and emotional problems, merely aggravate, precipitate, or prolong the condition.

The term *extrinsic* refers to those causes of bronchial asthma which originate outside the body. Pollen that is inhaled, foods that are ingested, and medicines injected into the body are extrinsic examples of allergens that may cause bronchial asthma. The term *intrinsic* suggests that there are processes within the body, such as infections that may cause the cough and difficulty in breathing. A disturbed emotional state may likewise produce such symptoms, but as our knowledge of the disease grows the intrinsic factors are gradually becoming less significant. Most physicians today regard asthmatic symptoms produced by intrinsic causes as not true bronchial asthma; that is, the symptoms are not dependent upon an allergic (antigen-antibody) reaction.

173

THE BREATHING APPARATUS (ANATOMY OF THE LUNGS AND MECHANISM OF BREATHING)

In man, the lungs are the principal organs involved in breathing. In the lungs oxygen is taken from the inspired air, absorbed by the blood, and delivered to the body tissues. In the tissues a chemical process takes place whereby the carbon is oxidized to form carbon dioxide which is then transported back to the lungs where it is eliminated in the expired air.

Air enters the respiratory system through the nose where it is warmed. It is passed down into the lungs through a series of tubes connecting the nose and mouth with the bronchial tract. The bronchial tract, or bronchial tree, as it is often called because it has the physical resemblance to a tree turned upside down, begins as one large tube about six inches long in the center of the chest. This is the *trachea*. Lower down, the trachea divides into two main *bronchi,* one going to each lung. The bronchi immediately divide into smaller bronchi which ramify into millions of microscopic *bronchioles*. Each bronchiole ends in a small balloon-like air sac. It is the mass of these millions of small air sacs (cells) that constitutes the lung tissue. These air sacs are medically termed *alveoli (alveolus* in the singular). The alveoli are enmeshed in a tightly packed maze of small blood vessels. They completely cover the small bronchial tubes which connect them to fill the entire chest cavity.

The mechanics of air entering and leaving the lungs can be said to resemble that of a sponge, which also is a mass of closely compressed small air cells or empty holes. When the sponge is squeezed it expels water; when the pressure is released and the sponge expands, it sucks water in. Similarly, the mass of air cells or alveoli of the lungs expels carbon dioxide gas when it is squeezed and soaks up oxygen-rich air when the pressure is released. The squeezing and relaxing actions are performed by the muscles and the ribs of the chest wall and in particular by the diaphragm, which is a large dome-shaped muscle separating the abdominal cavity from the chest cavity. When the chest expands, the diaphragm descends, and air enters the mass of bronchial tubes, eventually finding its way to the individual air sacs that make up the lungs. When the chest wall contracts, the diaphragm rises and air is expelled. This is like the action of old-fashioned leather bellows: when the handles are pushed together the bellows contract and air is expelled; when the handles are opened, air rushes in.

The exchange of gases takes place through the extremely thin-walled blood vessels which surround the similarly thin-walled alveoli. Subtle mechanisms govern the rate of breathing necessary to bring sufficient oxygen into the bloodstream.

The bronchial tract, from trachea to bronchioles, is lined with a very smooth mucous membrane, similar to that of the nose and mouth. This mucous membrane contains glands which secrete *mucus,* a soft gelatinous-like material which, as a lubricant, aids the passage of air through the tubes. The bronchi themselves have muscular walls which contract. They are also rich in elastic tissue which allows for their recoil during respiration.

MECHANICS OF ASTHMA

The mechanics of asthma involve constriction of the muscles in the walls of the bronchi with increased production and accumulation of mucus. To this may be added a drying-up of the mucus which further interferes with breathing. There may also be swelling of the lining of the bronchial tubes (edema of the membrane), which acts as an additional barrier to the free flow of air. Contraction of the walls of the bronchial tubes can be compared to squeezing a soft rubber hose through which water is flowing. Just as this would interfere with the stream of water, so does contraction of the muscles of the bronchial tubes impede the flow of air. The large bronchial tubes are generally not involved in the symptomatology of asthma, but rather the small ones deep in the lung tissues and close to the bronchioles leading into the air sacs. In these areas, the muscles are wound around the tubes like a rubber band so any slight pressure or interference with normal action can produce spasms.

Some mucus is necessary to permit the air to pass through the tubes with a minimum of friction. It acts like a lubricating oil but like oil, if it is in excess or too thick, it hinders rather than helps. The excessive mucus produced in bronchial asthma tends to dry up, harden, and ultimately become a thick, viscid, sticky material which further impedes the flow of air.

There are additional changes in the lungs, particularly in the small bronchial tubes, which can be seen only by cutting small slivers of the organ and examining the tissue under the microscope. These include thickening of one of the layers of the bronchial wall and the presence of eosinophiles, a type of white blood cell. One striking finding that is not seen very often, because people do not usually die during a severe attack of uncomplicated bronchial asthma, is extreme ballooning of the lungs, known as hyperinflation. In this condition, all the small alveoli are filled with air and stretched to their capacity because the obstruction prevents normal emptying. This obstruction is caused by constriction of the cordlike muscles which wind around the terminal bronchioles just prior to the point where they empty into the air sacs. Hyperinflation occurs frequently among people who have had bronchial asthma for a long time; with the relief of bronchial asthma in which there are no complications, hyperinflation is relieved and the air sacs return to normal.

CAUSE OF BRONCHIAL ASTHMA (ETIOLOGY)

Bronchial asthma is a disease resulting from bronchial spasm, swelling of the lining of the bronchial tubes, excess production of mucus by the bronchial glands, and thickening or hardening of this mucus, all due to allergy. Emotional problems and nonspecific infections may produce similar changes in the bronchial tree and asthmatic symptoms. The distinction must be made between asthma as a symptom and bronchial asthma as a disease.

As an example, an individual with severe bronchitis (inflamed and infected bronchial membrane) or an infant with bronchiolitis (inflammation of the terminal ends of the bronchi) caused by infection, may cough and even wheeze as a result of swelling of the lining of the bronchial tract and of increased mucus in the hollow portion of the tube. Such a patient may have asthmatic symptoms but may not necessarily have bronchial asthma.

On the other hand, people with psychological problems and with bronchial infections can also have bronchial asthma; one does not preclude the other. If one has bronchial asthma any additional interference with the patency of the bronchial tubes will produce an asthmatic attack.

Allergy to anything, including a medicine, can produce true bronchial asthma. It is felt that aspirin can cause asthma, without true allergy, under certain circumstances.

SYMPTOMS

The symptoms of bronchial asthma may be minor, perhaps taking the form of a mild heaviness in the chest and the feeling that all one need do is to clear one's throat or cough to secure relief. However, they may be as severe as an incessant, unproductive cough with struggling for breath and cyanosis (blue coloration of the lips and face). On the whole, the primary symptoms in either mild or severe cases are difficulty in breathing (dyspnea), accompanied by wheezing.

Difficulty in breathing caused by asthma generally involves breathing out rather than breathing in. This is true largely because during the normal process of expiration (which should be effortless) there is a constriction and shortening of the bronchioles caused by muscular contraction and the pressure of the lungs. When a person has asthma and these mechanisms are exaggerated, expiration or exhalation is unusually difficult. Yet severely ill patients may have both inspiratory and expiratory wheezing due to contraction in both cycles. Limited wheezing localized to one section of the lungs, detectable on examination and sometimes recognized by the patient, is most commonly due to causes of local obstruction other than true bronchial asthma. In true bronchial asthma there is diffuse wheezing because of the widespread constriction of the bronchial tubes. But even here, there may be an accumulation of more mucus in one segment of the chest than in another. When this happens the wheezing may be limited to one area despite the fact that diffuse bronchial changes are present. In such instances, a sharp cough will often dislodge the small plug of mucus and stop the wheeze.

Bronchial asthma may be constant or periodic. When it is constant, there is persistent wheezing, often with accompanying attacks of mild coughing which become worse on exertion. For the chronic sufferer, constant wheezing may become a way of life; he becomes adjusted to it and may not even notice it. There is a large degree of variability in people's reactions to shortness of breath and wheezing, just as there is to pain. Some are exceedingly unhappy and uncomfortable with what might be considered mild wheezing; others may be perfectly at ease with a marked degree of respiratory difficulty and wheezing. Some chronic asthmatics, particularly those whose lungs retain a great deal of air, have a large lung capacity and learn to expel air very slowly. There are actors and lawyers with severe chronic bronchial asthma who have acquired this knack and are able to speak at length without taking frequent breaths.

More often, bronchial asthma occurs episodically with periods of complete freedom from attacks (remissions). During the interval of freedom from attacks, a physical examination will seldom disclose any sign of the disease. Even measurement of lung function by machines devised for that purpose will often not indicate any breathing impairment. This indicates that bronchial asthma is a reversible disease; that is, unless permanent changes have taken place in the lungs and in the bronchial tract (changes which usually occur over many years and are frequently due to additional factors, such as repeated infection) bronchial asthma can be treated successfully.

The severity of the disease is often described in terms of its response to medication. The mild case will be improved by medicines taken by mouth or by inhalation. Many of these are available at drugstores without a doctor's prescription. When such simple medication relieves the attack (which may not occur again for some time) the condition is considered "mild" even though this so-called mild asthma may consist of a violent attack with severe breathlessness. How can a violent asthmatic attack be considered a mild case of bronchial asthma? An example is a person who develops a severe bronchial allergy attack on coming in contact with a cat. He is relieved of his attack by swallowing a pill and may never have another one unless he encounters another cat.

In considering the natural history of the disease, this person's bronchial asthma is, indeed, mild in comparison to one who is allergic to something which he cannot readily avoid, and who requires constant medication, while having only incomplete relief between attacks. Such persistent and repeated attacks occur when one is allergic to something ubiquitous like house dust, or to perennially present pollen.

Several terms applied to bronchial asthma have ominous connotations. One of these is *status asthmaticus;* another is *intractable asthma.* They really are the same, except perhaps in degree. Status asthmaticus refers to a constant state of persistent bronchial asthma, while intractable asthma refers to asthmatic attacks which are resistant to treatment. Both indicate unresponsiveness to treatment.

Very often these terms are used too loosely. Status asthmaticus, particularly, should be reserved for severe bronchial asthma in which the decrease in oxygen reaching the bloodstream results in gas volume changes in the blood and in the body tissues. In such severe cases, where there is increased acidity of the body, there may be an increase in the number of red cells in the bloodstream. A decrease of oxygen supply to the tissues of the body may develop, and if this condition persists for a long time, not only alteration in the acid-base balance but also heart failure may result. Because of newer medicines and methods of treatment, this extreme state is seldom reached.

Asthmatic attacks seem to occur most commonly at night or in the early morning hours. In allergy this may be due to changes in the barometric pressure or room temperature, which affects the sensitive lining of the bronchial tract. Posture may be a factor, since there is a decrease in lung volume resulting from additional blood accumulated by the lung in the recumbent position. Another possibility is low natural hormone (cortisone) production of the adrenal glands late at night and in the early morning hours. During an attack the person usually feels better sitting up in bed or on the edge of the bed.

The cough is dry and usually unproductive; when there is expectoration the sputum is thick and gelatinous, some looking like small pearls or thick barley. When sputum is coughed up, the attack is frequently relieved. When pain in the chest occurs it is most often a muscle pain due to the strain of coughing. Some asthmatics will have no symptoms unless they exert themselves. This may indicate that the disease process is limited, or it may also mean that in exercise the requirement for air is increased and the bronchial tubes are not capable of transporting it. The wheezing indicates that more air is inhaled than can be coped with. But once an attack — no matter how severe — is over and the patient gets some rest, he usually returns to relative normalcy with very little fatigue or debility.

COMPLICATIONS

The complication which most people fear most is *emphysema*. In the common, uncomplicated attack of asthma, hyperinflation of the lungs, or ballooning of the air space, is reversible. In emphysema the walls of the air sacs (alveoli) lose their elasticity, can no longer recoil, and resume their normal position. In addition, the walls of the air sacs are torn, and several individual sacs become one large "room," or sac, with poor walls. The air is then trapped in the alveoli and the lungs remain inflated permanently. Consequently, a complete exchange of air during each breathing cycle does not take place, and during each expiration a certain amount of stagnant air is left behind.

Some doctors believe that uncomplicated bronchial asthma does not lead to emphysema; they insist that infection must be present to destroy the sac walls and ruin their elasticity. The most prevalent view is that emphysema occurs more often with chronic bronchitis than it does with bronchial asthma and that only when bronchial asthma and chronic bronchitis coexist does emphysema develop. Most allergists conclude, however, that asthma, even without infection, can produce emphysema, although when it does, structural changes may take a long time to occur. In addition, they have found that even severe, infrequent asthmatic attacks are less likely to produce emphysema than mild attacks which are chronic. In an attack the lungs have ample time to revert to their normal state; thus, the small air sacs maintain their elasticity. But in chronic asthmatic attacks, even though mild, the air sacs remain constantly inflated and lose their elasticity. Infection often occurs with asthma, contributing to the production of emphysema.

The symptoms of emphysema are often difficult to differentiate from those of bronchial asthma. Difficulty in breathing may be the main symptom, and the individual may be conscious only of gradually increasing shortness of breath, persistent cough, wheezing, and decreased ability to exercise without panting, all of which may occur in bronchial asthma without emphysema. Certain tests performed by the patient, such as blowing in and out of a specially constructed instrument (pulmonary function test) aids in the diagnosis long before the X ray shows the characteristic picture of increased air in the lungs and widening of the spaces between the ribs. Although a person with emphysema may have an enormous amount of air capacity in his lungs, he cannot move it in and out efficiently. This efficiency can be measured by pulmonary function machines (respirometer). Many extreme changes are mirrored in the acidity of the blood and the quantity of the oxygen and carbon dioxide volume in the arterial blood.

Other, and fortunately uncommon, complications of bronchial asthma include collapse of the lungs, fractured ribs, and rupture of air cells from overdistention with consequent escape of air into the tissues of the chest wall (interstitial emphysema), any of which may follow a severe coughing spell. Long-standing bronchial asthma like other chronic respiratory diseases may produce a strain on the heart. It may be that an element of infectious bronchitis must be superimposed to produce this complication. Deaths resulting from cardiac complications of bronchial asthma are very rare.

Of interest is the effect of pregnancy on bronchial asthma. Usually a pregnant woman is free of her asthma symptoms; yet some are worse. In many instances a woman will be well during one pregnancy and sick during another. The adrenal gland hormones are thought to be responsible for this change. Some women have intensified asthmatic attacks during their menstrual period, again indicating a hormonal effect. Asthma may be worse during menopause. Exercise aggravates asthma, particularly when the threshold of the symptoms is low. These phenomena are not really "complications."

TREATMENT

During an asthmatic attack immediate treatment is essential in order to relieve the attack so that the person struggling for breath will breathe normally again. Institution of a regimen to prevent further attacks is equally important. Treatment designed to give immediate relief is *symptomatic;* treatment to prevent subsequent attacks is *prophylactic.*

SPECIFIC (PROPHYLACTIC) TREATMENT

Specific treatment in bronchial asthma may be directed at avoiding or destroying when possible the substances to which the person has been found to be allergic. One method of avoidance of airborne asthma-producers is by the use of air filters in the home or occupational setting. (These are discussed in detail in Chapter 11.) But it is practically impossible to avoid primary sensitization since we live in a world surrounded by so many substances that are likely to make us allergic. Inherited susceptibility compounds the problem. Nevertheless, avoidance is attempted to some extent in the case of infants who are likely to develop an allergy. The infant child of allergic parents, during the first year of his life, is kept away from materials such as wool, and foods such as eggs, which are considered highly allergenic. He is given new foods gradually and in small amounts, rather than a full diet within a few months. The theory is that a child will build up his own immune protective mechanism if not overwhelmed by a large amount of allergenic substances at one time.

If sensitization has taken place and the individual is already allergic,

avoidance is practiced to as great an extent as possible. The impractica-
bility of weed and grass eradication is discussed in Chapter 11.
Avoidance of dust, wool, feathers, animal hair, kapok, insect ex-
terminators, and other inhalants and contactants as well as any
implicated foods that may cause bronchial asthma should be practiced.
When inhalant substances to which an allergy is apparent cannot be
avoided, the treatment is desensitization. This is fully discussed in
Chapter 7.

Usually after three years of treatment, the asthmatic — if he is allergic
to inhalant allergens and has undergone desensitization — will be free of
symptoms and treatment may be discontinued. Of these, perhaps 80
percent do not have recurrence of symptoms. Perhaps another 10 percent
will return in a few years with recurrence of symptoms and will require
additional treatment for several months as "booster shots." There is
probably a remaining 10 percent who do not seem to be able to maintain
their immunity and need injections for many years or for the rest of their
lives.

SYMPTOMATIC TREATMENT

Treatment of symptoms is directed against the pathological effects that
occur in the bronchial tract as a result of the chemicals that are liberated
during the allergic reaction. Histamine is the principal chemical which is
liberated during the allergic reaction and one would expect antihistamines to be exceedingly useful for the control of an attack of asthma.
Unfortunately, this is not true and antihistamines are not only useless in
the average case but may in fact be harmful. They have a drying action,
and harden even further the mucus which is already becoming thick and
obstructive to air flow. Attempts have been made with questionable
results to neutralize some of the other chemicals which are liberated
during the allergic reaction causing bronchial asthma. The most
successful treatment of the acute attack is the use of medicaments which
will stop the spasm of the bronchial muscles, reduce the swelling of the
lining of the tubes, and thin the mucus. There are several medicines that
effectively accomplish this.

Epinephrine, better known under its trade name of Adrenalin, is
given by hypodermic injection and produces rapid relaxation of spastic
muscles of the bronchial tubes. The amount to be injected varies with the
person who is ill and with the severity of the attack. The only side effects
are pounding of the heart, rapid pulse rate, and a feeling of jitteriness,
which usually wear off in about fifteen or twenty minutes.

Since the therapeutic action of epinephrine is likely to last only an hour or two, there have been attempts to prepare the same material in a prolonged-action vehicle. The most popular has been epinephrine in oil. Because of the heavy oil vehicle, this preparation must be given deep within the muscle. The only other successful product that has survived is a commercial suspension known as Susphrine, which can be administered hypodermically and usually relieves an asthmatic seizure for eight to twelve hours.

Epinephrine is also employed as a spray which is inhaled so that the drug can be absorbed by the linings of the bronchial tubes, under which there are many blood vessels. This is very effective and widely used. To reach the terminal bronchioles, medicament particles must be exceedingly small, having a diameter of three to ten microns (.000039 of an inch). Nebulizers used as spray vials have been devised to produce particles of this small size. Plastic models now available are unbreakable and can be carried in a pocket or purse with ease; they also produce a measured dose of the medicine. Because of the rapid relief afforded by nebulization, the sprays have become very popular, but too frequent use may cause addiction. With the asthmatic this is more of a dependency than a true addiction, so that he fears to leave home without the comforting presence of the nebulizer in pocket or handbag. Nebulizers should be used only under a doctor's supervision.

There is also a gas-propelled nebulizer which has become inordinately popular because of its small size and portability. This new spray device, unlike the bulky, conspicuous type, can be held in the hand and the medicine sprayed into the lungs almost without notice. The principle of the device is the same as that of paint-spray and insect-spray cans; it utilizes gas under pressure. Its simplicity has encouraged too-frequent use, and the gas in the sealed container often irritates the throat and bronchial tubes. Though they are effective, their use should be limited.

Isoproterenol: This is a variation of the chemical complex of epinephrine, or Adrenalin, and has a similar and an even better effect. Technically, it is the isopropyl form of norepinephrine. Unlike epinephrine, which is only effective by inhalation or injection, isoproterenol may be taken in a liquid medicine to be swallowed; it can be held under the tongue until it is absorbed; or it can be inhaled, in either liquid or powdered form. Consequently, it is marketed by many firms under different trade names, among which are Isuprel, Norisodrine, Medihaler-Iso, Aerolone, Brondilate, Isufranol, and Nephenalin.

Although epinephrine can usually be purchased without a doctor's prescription, isoproterenol requires one, so people with bronchial asthma often use nebulizers containing epinephrine or one of the epinephrine compounds. Among the most popular are Medihaler-Epi, Vaponephrin, Asthmanefrin, Breatheasy, Selrodo, Primatine, and Episcorb.

Ephedrine: This medicine has an effect similar to epinephrine, reducing the swelling of the lining of the bronchial tubes and relaxing the spasms of the bronchial muscles. Since it can be taken orally, mixed with other medicines, in capsules, tablets, and in liquid, it is the most common medicine used for the relief of asthma. Ephedrine is a component of practically every asthma pill, tablet, or medicine on the market. Like Adrenalin, it too has the side effects of jitteriness and pounding of the heart. They are not as severe as with epinephrine but to prevent them the drug is usually compounded with a sedative.

Theophylline: The most widely used compound of theophylline is *aminophylline.* It is effective intravenously (injected into the bloodstream), by mouth, rectally in a retention enema or rectal suppository, injected intramuscularly (deep into the muscle), and even when inhaled. It is used for the most part by rectal instillation, orally, and by intravenous injection.

The effective action of theophylline depends on the concentration maintained in the bloodstream. A large dose must be taken orally to achieve this effect, but theophylline has an irritating effect on the lining of the stomach and many people cannot tolerate therapeutically effective doses. To counteract this adverse effect an attempt has been made to combine the drug with antacids and to change its chemical configuration. This has been partly successful in such products as Choledyl, Brondecon, Cardalin, and Aminodrox. Theophylline dissolved in a weak solution of alcohol has been found successful in some cases. Such products as Quibron, Theokin Elixir, Lixaminal, and Elixophyllin are popular liquid preparations of theophylline.

Theophyllines should be given under a doctor's supervision and effective doses usually cannot be purchased without a prescription. For home use when the oral medication is not effective, the rectal form may be employed and is usually very effective. It can be secured as a rectal suppository with or without a sedative included, or in a disposable small rectal enema-like container filled with the rapidly absorbed theophylline solution. For those who have severe bronchial asthma it is often wise to have several of the rectal suppositories on hand for emergency.

Mucus thinners: These help thin the excess mucus in the bronchial tubes and make it easier to expectorate. For this reason they are sometimes called *expectorants*. Asthmatics are encouraged to drink as much water and other fluid as they can. They should consume a minimum of seven to ten glasses of water daily. Most anti-asthmatic medications are diuretic, so that fluids not only serve to thin out the mucus but also prevent dehydration. At least 75 percent of asthmatics who must be hospitalized are dehydrated and require fluids intravenously. Dehydration can be avoided by drinking as much water as possible. A rule of thumb is to drink a glass during each waking hour.

Steam inhalation, a simple home remedy, is an excellent procedure. It directly softens the dried mucus and moistens the lining of the bronchial tubes. An elaborate apparatus is not necessary; a teakettle on an electric hot plate placed beside the bed is often adequate. However, automatic electric steamers are safer, more convenient, and designed to provide twelve hours of steam without refilling the canister with water. Of the several medicines used to help thin or liquefy bronchial mucus, the best and most generally employed is iodide of potassium. This can be taken in the form of drops dissolved in water or fruit juice, as tablets, or mixed with medicines. Mild complications, such as skin rash and swelling of the glands of the neck, occasionally occur but are not serious. When these are encountered the medicine should be stopped. A rare complication is enlargement and diminished activity of the thyroid gland. While these complications must be considered they should not be a contraindication to trial use of this important medicine. There are several more palatable types of iodide, one of which is Organidine. For children a syrup is available (syrup of hydriodic acid).

Another widely used expectorant is glyceryl guiacolate. Although it is not a very good substitute for the iodide, it is helpful and is frequently prescribed when iodide cannot be taken. A very popular cough medicine which can be purchased without a doctor's prescription is Robitussin. This is merely glyceryl guiacolate and is often recommended as a tonic-like medicine to help keep the bronchial secretions thin. Many asthma compounds contain this medicine.

Anti-Asthma Mixtures: These are usually capsules, tablets, or liquids, most containing medicines that have been described, with some minor variations. In Table 7 are listed those most frequently prescribed. Their similarity is apparent. The common formula is ephedrine, a theophylline salt, and a sedative, usually a barbiturate, in varying doses. In some products theophylline is omitted since it may be irritating to the stomach. Some have potassium iodide; others have vitamin C.

TABLE 7 COMMON ANTI-ASTHMATIC COMPOUNDS
OF A SIMILAR COMPOSITION

Anti-asthmatic compounds as a class contain the three following ingredients: ephedrine (acts like adrenalin but can be taken orally), theophylline (usually in the form of aminophylline), a barbiturate (to counteract the side effects of the ephedrine), isoproterenol (acts like ephedrine). All are effective. The exceptions and modifications are indicated. These medicines usually require a doctor's prescription.

TRADE NAME	MANUFACTURER	ADDITIONAL MEDICATION OR MODIFICATION
Aladrine	Table Rock or Merit	No theophylline
Amesec	Lilly	
Amodrine	Searle	
Brondilate	Walker	Isoproterenol; no theophylline
Bronkotab	Breon	Thenyldiamine (antihistamine) Glyceryl guiacolate (expectorant)
Dainite	Irwin Neissler	With or without potassium iodide (expectorant)
Deltasmyl	Roussel	Prednisone (cortisone)
Ephedrine with Amytal	Lilly	No theophylline
Ephedrine with Nembutal	Abbot	No theophylline
Ephedrine with Seconal	Lilly	No theophylline
Ephoxamine	Spencer	A tranquilizer instead of a barbiturate
Franol	Winthrop	
Hyadrine	Searle	No barbiturate
Isufranol	Winthrop	Isoproterenol in outer layer of tablet (for rapid absorption under tongue)
Luasmin	Brewer	
Marax	Roerig	A tranquilizer instead of a barbiturate
Mudrane	Poythress	Potassium iodide (expectorant)
Nephenalin	Leeming	Isoproterenol in outer layer of tablet (for rapid absorption under tongue)
Phyllophed	Rexall	
Quadrinal	Knoll	With or without glyceryl guiacolate (expectorant)
Tedral	Warner	Potassium iodide (expectorant)
Thephesin	Wilcox	Chlorpheniramine (antihistamine) Glyceryl guaiacolate (expectorant)
Verequad	Knoll	Glyceryl guaiacolate (expectorant)

Most of these compounds are obtainable by prescription only. Federal laws prohibit the sale of compounds over the counter which contain more than one-eighth grain of barbiturate. Many states, California and Pennsylvania among them, prohibit the sale of any medicine containing any phenobarbital without a doctor's prescription. That makes practically all products in Table 7 unobtainable over the counter. Some compounds are sold only on prescription in some states but may be purchased over the counter in others.

Since bronchial asthma is a very common disease, there are a large number of anti-asthmatic compounds which are advertised and promoted directly to the public. Table 8 describes some of those that are best known. Although most of them contain the usual ephedrine-theophylline-barbiturate mixture, some include older medicines which are no longer in common use. For example, glycyrrhiza is now a seldom used expectorant. Sodium bromide is a mild tranquilizer, or sedative, not nearly as powerful or effective as those we have today. Formulas are changed from time to time, and the terms "new" or "improved" are added.

TABLE 8 POPULAR ANTI-ASTHMATIC NON-PRESCRIPTION REMEDIES

Many of the advertised anti-asthmatic remedies that can be purchased without a doctor's prescription are identical with those that are prescribed by doctors. Some are old remedies and although they may be considered obsolete, they still enjoy a certain amount of popularity. In several states, any mixture that contains phenobarbital cannot be sold without a doctor's order. Rapidly changing rules of the U.S. Food and Drug Administration also have an effect on available medicines. Undoubtedly, there are many more anti-asthmatic non-prescription remedies than are listed below. This table contains only those that are taken by mouth or used as sprays and powders for inhalation.

TRADE NAME	MANUFACTURER	INGREDIENTS
A.E.P. Tablets	Stayner Corp.	Aminophylline Ephedrine Phenobarbital
Aerometer Asthma Spray	Rexall Drug Co.	Epinephrine
Allergyn	Alva Laboratories	Ephedrine Acetanilid Methapyrilene Ascorbic acid Hespiridin Niacinamide Iron Calcium lactate Vitamins A, D, and entire complex from liver and yeast concentrate

TRADE NAME	MANUFACTURER	INGREDIENTS
Amatin Tablets	Coastal Pharmaceutical Co.	Ephedrine Pentobarbital Phenobarbital Theophylline
Ascatco Liquid	Ascatco Laboratory	Stramonium Chlorobutanol Alcohol
Anthaphylline Capsules	Medico-Chemical Corp. of America	Aminophylline Anthallan
Asthmador	R. Schiffman Co.	Belladonna Stramonium
Asthmanefrin	Thayer Laboratories	Epinephrine
Asthmarel	The Falkenhainer Co.	Ammoniated glycyrrhiza Potassium iodide Caffeine
Azma-Tabs	Bryant Pharmaceutical Corp.	Ephedrine Phenobarbital Theophylline
Brater's Powder	John K. Brater Div. Cooper & Cooper	Lobelia Potassium nitrate Stramonium
Breatheasy	Breatheasy Co.	Epinephrine
Breatheasy Tabs	Breatheasy Co.	Ephedrine Methapyrilene Theophylline
Bronitin (improved)	Whitehall Laboratory	Ephedrine Methapyrilene Theophylline Glyceryl guiacolate
Bronitin Mist	Whitehall Laboratory	Epinephrine
Bronkaid	Drew Pharmacal Co.	Ephedrine Theophylline Thenyldiamine Glyceryl guiacolate
Consolidated Midland Corp. Asthmatic Relief (mild)	Consolidated Midland Corp.	Ephedrine Phenobarbital Theophylline

TRADE NAME	MANUFACTURER	INGREDIENTS
Consin Capsules Consin	Wisconsin Pharmaceutical Co.	Ephedrine Chloropheniramine Phenobarbital Theophylline
Dr. Guild's Green Mountain Asthmatic Compound	J. H. Guild Co.	Belladonna Potassium nitrate Stramonium
Dr. Whetzel's Liquid Prescription	Myers Laboratories	Potassium iodide Salicylic acid Cardamom compound Gentian compound
Dr. Whetzel's Powder	Myers Laboratories	Lobelia herb Stramonium leaves
Episcorb Inhalant	Pallab Pharmaceuticals	Ascorbic acid Epinephrine
Eptine	Nemow Co. Div. Commerce Drug Co.	Ephedrine Phenobarbital Theophylline
Feiler	S-K Research Laboratories	Ammoniated glycrrhizin Caffeine Potassium iodide
Haysma Capsules	Haysma Co.	Aspirin Acentanilid Caffeine Ephedrine
Himrod's Powder	Himrod Manufacturing Co.	Anise Oil Cedar oil Potassium nitrate Stramonium
Kellog's Relief	Myers Laboratories	Lobelia Potassium nitrate Sassafras Stramonium Sugar
Kingco	King Chemical Products Co.	Epinephrine
Leavens	Leavens Products Co.	Alcohol Belladonna Potassium iodide Sarsaparilla Sodium bromide Syrup

TRADE NAME	MANUFACTURER	INGREDIENTS
Lergenex Capsules	Marion Pharmacal Laboratories	Aminophylline Ephedrine Phenacetin Potassium chloride Stramonium
Magair Tablets	Cosylor, Inc.	Ascorbic acid Calcium Methapyrilene Potassium iodide Theophylline
Medihaler-Epi	Riker Laboratories	Epinephrine
Meditabs	Medicone Co.	Atropine Ephedrine Phenobarbital Theophylline
Mendaco	The Knox Co.	Aminophylline Potassium iodide Pyrilamine
Nephron Inhalant	Nephron Co.	Epinephrine
Parasma	Charles Raymond & Co.	Aminophylline Ephedrine Sodium bromide
Phas-Ted	Superior Pharmacal Co.	Ephedrine Phenobarbital Theophylline
Powers Relief	E. C. Powers Co.	Mullein leaves Stramonium
Primatene (new)	Whitehall Laboratories	Ephedrine Methapyryline Theophylline
Primatene Mist	Whitehall Laboratories	Epinephrine
Ralex	Partola Products Co.	Alcohol Belladonna Aromatic Spirit of Ammonia Potassium iodide Cinchona Comp.
Selrodo	Stansbury Chemical Co.	Epinephrine
Templeton's Rax-mah Greys	Templetons, Inc.	Aspirin Caffeine Euphorbia pilulifera

TRADE NAME	MANUFACTURER	INGREDIENTS
T. E. P.	Towne, Paulsen & Co.	Theophylline Ephedrine Phenobarbital
Thalfed	The S. E. Massengill Co.	Ephedrine Phenobarbital Theophylline
Thenotal Tablets	Veltex Co.	Ephedrine Phenobarbital Theophylline
Theodrine	Success Chemical Co.	Ephedrine Phenobarbital Theophylline
Theofedrine	Physicians Drug & Supply Co.	Atropine Ephedrine Phenobarbital Theophylline
Theofel	Physicians' Drug & Supply Co.	Ephedrine Phenobarbital Theophylline
Vapo Mist Inhalant	S. K. Rinard Laboratories	Epinephrine
Vaponephrin	Vaponefrin Co. Division of U.S. Vitamin Corp.	Epinephrine

MISCELLANEOUS MEDICINES

Asthma powders and asthma cigarettes consist of old-fashioned remedies, namely, stramonium leaves or potassium nitrate. When the powder or cigarette is burned and the fumes inhaled, asthma is relieved by producing a cough to bring up some of the thick mucus. These remedies are still in use in some parts of the country. Some of the better known are Brater's Powder, Dr. Guild's Green Mountain Asthmatic compound, Dr. Whetzel's Powder, Himrod's Powder, Kellog's Relief, and Power's Relief, as listed in Table 8.

When a patient is in an asthmatic paroxysm he may understandably seek a sedative to give him rest and sleep. Many a doctor succumbs to a plea of this sort although he knows better, for an excess amount of sedatives is dangerous in bronchial asthma. Perhaps the newer tranquilizers are not as risky as those drugs that put a person into a deep sleep, but they, too, must be used with caution. The chief objection to the use of medication to induce sleep is their tendency to depress the respiratory center in the brain and slow the rate of breathing. In addition, they may depress the cough reflex.

Slowing of the respiration is harmful; it diminishes the amount of essential oxygen that is taken in. When the regulator of breathing is slowed down, life is at a low ebb. A loose cough helps evacuate sticky mucus which is causing airway obstruction. When the cough is suppressed, this means of getting rid of the mucus is eliminated. Still, there are times when some form of sedation is necessary. One of these is when the person has had difficulty in breathing and has been gasping for breath for a long time (rare these days), and rest is essential. For this purpose one of the less harmful sedatives may be prescribed by the attending physician. Of these, one is chloral hydrate, an unpleasant-tasting medicine. Fortunately, it is now marketed in capsule form and as a syrup, which disguises the taste to a considerable degree; it is also available as a rectal suppository.

Another sedative drug considered relatively safe is paraldehyde. Since this drug has a distinct quietening effect, it is often given to a bronchial asthmatic who is excited. It has a very disagreeable odor, and is usually administered by intramuscular injection, or by a retention enema. Another mixture that is prescribed in a retention enema to induce sleep is anesthetic ether diluted in olive oil. Sleep provides welcome relief for the exhausted asthmatic. It is, as a rule, not dangerous, and when the person awakens, the asthmatic attack is spent and breathing is normal. This method of inducing sleep and relieving an asthmatic attack is employed only in severe cases. Phenobarbital prescribed alone or in adequate doses to provide sleep may be harmful and is not advisable as a routine measure.

Morphine is especially dangerous and in the past has perhaps caused many deaths in bronchial asthma because its depressent effect on the respiratory center was not fully appreciated. It also tends to abolish the cough reflex and is habit-forming. Doctors do not prescribe it today. Meperidine, known best under the trade name of Demerol, is often considered a substitute for morphine, and although it is claimed to assist in dilating the bronchial tubes, it also depresses the respiratory center and cough reflex. It too is a habit-forming drug and in addition is likely to produce nausea and vomiting. For these reasons it is rarely prescribed.

Another narcotic, cocaine, once used in an asthma spray, is habit-forming, and since today other asthma sprays are as effective, or more so, it is not prescribed. Codeine is derived from morphine and is a common ingredient of many cough mixtures. These should be used with caution since they, too, are narcotic and have the same effect as morphine, although somewhat less severe. Codeine is placed in cough mixtures to suppress the cough. In asthma, coughing is useful and necessary to bring up the thick mucus, and codeine may be harmful. Only in instances where a hacking cough acts to set off an asthmatic paroxysm, or where it is debilitating, is suppression of the cough indicated. Even then, only small doses of this medicine are prescribed.

CORTISONE

This term denotes one type of product of the adrenal gland, but it has become a common term, or almost generic, for all newer derivatives. The more scientific terminology for this group is *adrenocorticosteroids*, often shortened to "steroids." Adrenocorticosteroids are derived from the cortex (outer layer) of the adrenal glands, the small glands located just above each kidney. These are important glands, and the hormones they secrete have a profound effect on many body functions. ACTH, an abbreviation for *Adrenocorticotrophic hormone*, is closely related to cortisone. It is derived from the pituitary gland, a very small gland situated deep in the brain tissue. In addition to other functions, it produces a hormone which in turn stimulates the adrenal gland to manufacture and produce more cortisone. Therefore, for practical purposes, the effects of ACTH and cortisone (or "cortisone derivatives") are the same. Either, if used in adequate dose, will relieve asthma almost dramatically.

Since the introduction of these new medicines around 1950, the symptomatic treatment of bronchial asthma has been greatly altered. They have eased suffering, eliminated many days of illness, prevented "status asthmaticus," and have to a great extent lessened or even eliminated the need for hospitalization. Yet these medicines have been a mixed blessing because, along with the benefits they bestow, they may produce side effects which can be severe. Their proper use by a doctor who is aware of these side effects and regulates the doses accordingly constitutes excellent treatment.

People read a good deal in popular articles about the dangers of cortisone. To prevent fear of this medicine some doctors inform their patients that they are taking a "steroid" or a "hormone" instead of bluntly saying "cortisone." This is done not to deceive the patient but to avoid producing prejudice in the patient. ACTH, although it has a similar or comparable effect, differs from cortisone in that it activates four classes of hormones, of which cortisone is only one. Several of the others are related to male and female sex hormones. The use of ACTH is therefore considered a stimulation type of treatment while cortisone, which has no stimulating effect, is pure replacement or substitution. Its use may be compared to that of insulin for a diabetic in whom insulin production is lacking.

Cortisone Derivatives: The original chemically manufactured product was cortisone. Soon after, an improved chemical, *hydrocortisone,* was synthesized. From cortisone a new drug, *prednisone,* effective in one-fifth the dose of cortisone, was developed. From hydrocortisone came still another drug, *prednisolone,* effective in the same small dose as prednisone. Then a series of derivatives was developed, each claiming an advantage, particularly with regard to fewer and less severe side effects as compared with the older preparations. Prednisone and prednisolone were different from their predecessors because there was less water retention in the body. The newer preparations caused retention of even less fluid, but as each new medicine was devised, eliminating one side effect, it had a tendency to introduce a new one. Doctors are aware of these different side effects.

Side effects: There are numerous possible side effects of this class of drugs, ranging from the relatively unimportant and easily controlled to the serious and dangerous. Only the major ones are discussed.

Diabetes is not usually produced by a steroid in one who has no predisposition to it, but if one has latent diabetes or a tendency toward diabetes, the steroids are very likely to promote its development. For this reason, if long-term treatment with steroids is contemplated the doctor may require urine or blood sugar tests from time to time. *Osteoporosis* is a condition in which there is loss of calcium and a consequent thinning of the bones, particularly those of the spine and the pelvis. Occasionally it occurs spontaneously in older people, especially women, who have passed their change of life. It has been known to occur in persons taking steroids in large quantities over a long period of time. *Ulcer* of the stomach or inflammation of the stomach may be a complication of cortisone usage, and those inclined toward or suffering from peptic ulcer may tolerate steroid treatment poorly. *Infections,* particularly *tuberculosis,* can be aggravated by steroids. Frequent X rays of the chest may be indicated during steroid therapy, particularly if there is a history of tubercular infection. An interesting observation is that the symptoms of an infection can be relieved completely while the bacteria continue to cause damage. A person with pneumonia, a cough, high fever, and sweating may be completely relieved of symptoms while under steroid therapy. Yet an X ray picture of his chest will indicate progression of the disease with damage to the lungs.

High blood pressure and *heart trouble,* although perhaps not produced by cortisone, are usually aggravated and often considered contraindications to its use, particularly when long-term. In high blood pressure, diuretics are commonly used to rid the body of excess sodium (salt). Many of the diuretics also rid the body of vital potassium salt. The combination of steroid treatment and potassium depletion may be dangerous to the body. Doctors who prescribe steroids in the presence of high blood pressure recognize this and usually prescribe additional medication.

Emotional reactions to steroids may range all the way from a mild feeling of well being, or a more pronounced euphoria to severe depression (melancholia). Fortunately, although euphoria is common, extreme depression is rare.

Possible complications of steroid therapy may be minimized. One step is the replacement of possible loss of potassium by supplementing the diet with fruits (particularly orange and banana), cranberry juice, and meat. Sometimes the doctor prescribes potassium as a medicine, preferably in liquid form. To avoid sodium retention, salt and salted foods are restricted. Antibiotics and antitubercular medicines may be necessary. The stomach may be protected from ulceration by avoiding irritating foods and eating frequent small meals. Sometimes antacids (but not baking soda or any other substance containing sodium) can be taken between meals to prevent stomach symptoms. Loss of calcium in the bones (osteoporosis) can be counteracted by drinking plenty of milk containing calcium and vitamin D. In women, both female and male hormones are exceedingly useful. If signs of diabetes such as excess thirst, hunger, and frequent urination occur, the doctor should be consulted at once.

The cortisones also called steroids or cortisone derivatives but most correctly adrenocorticosteroids, are listed in Table 9.

TABLE 9 COMMONLY PRESCRIBED CORTISONES FOR ORAL USE

GENERIC NAME	EQUIVALENT DOSE	TRADE NAME
Cortisone	25 mgs.	Cortone
Hydrocortisone	20 mgs.	Cortef
Prednisone	5 mgs.	Delta-Dome, Deltasmul, Deltasone, Meticorten, Sigmagen
Prednisolone	5 mgs.	Cordex, Delta Cortef, Predne-Dome Sterane, Meticortelone
Triamcinolone	4 mgs.	Aristocort, Kenacort
Methylprednisolone	4 mgs.	Medrol
Paramethasone	2 mgs.	Haldrone
Fludprednicolone	1.5 mgs.	Alphadrol
Betamethasone	0.6 mgs.	Celestone
Dexamethasone	0.75 mgs.	Decadron, Deronil, Dexameth, Gammacorten, Hexadrol

Several steroid derivatives are available as injectables, in both rapid and prolonged-action form. The action of the rapid-acting variety is not as immediate as one would anticipate but is much more rapid than the oral form. Long-lasting injectable preparations, if given in large enough doses, may retain their effect for two weeks or longer. One slight advantage of the injection is that it is thought to be less harmful to the stomach, but this is still questionable.

Cortisone preparations are usually prescribed for use in one of two ways: they are either given in short courses until the person has recovered from his acute attack or are used continuously as maintenance doses in the smallest amounts that will keep the asthmatic symptom-free. For some unexplainable reason the asthmatic on long-term steroid treatment does not develop complications as frequently as the arthritic or others who use steroids for long periods.

GENERAL MEASURES

There are several nonspecific forms of treatment which are very helpful for the asthmatic. Air pollution or any kind of increased irritants in the air aggravates the illness of patients with bronchial asthma. Cooking odors also affect persons with bronchial asthma, as does smoke inhaled from cigarettes being smoked.

Patients with bronchial asthma appear to do better when the air is humid rather than dry. Yet dampness, particularly when cold, may aggravate the symptoms. For that reason, room humidifiers may be helpful. Sudden changes in temperature may cause a reflex spasm of the bronchial muscles; therefore, such changes should be avoided. In Europe it has been the custom for many years to send asthmatics to "asthma resorts" in the mountains of Switzerland. But high altitude and "fresh clean air" have not proved helpful for bronchial asthma generally. Some asthmatics do better at the seashore; others in the desert. Some are better in windy regions; others in still air. But nearly all asthmatics do well in the pressurized cabins of jet aircrafts.

In the United States there are several asthma "homes" for asthmatic children. These children are treated with all the modalities available and a large percentage improves. Considerable counseling and psychiatric care is given to these children, and the term *parentectomy,* which indicates separation from or removal of the parents, has been improvised to characterize the good results obtained. But it is likely that the better care given to the children at the home, the more rigid supervision of play, diet, and sleep, and the regularity with which treatment is administered account for much of the improvement.

BREATHING EXERCISES

Exercising of the accessory muscles of respiration to help an asthmatic breathe properly during an asthmatic attack is very valuable for those whose bronchial asthma is severe and for those who have emphysema. The normal mechanism of inhaling (breathing in) requires the use of the muscles of the chest and abdomen, but expiration (breathing out) is normally performed automatically by the elastic recoil of the lungs and bronchial muscles. If one wants to check his breathing mechanism, he need only lie down and place one hand on his chest and the other on his abdomen. During the process of inhalation the hand on the chest will go up and during exhalation it will go down, while the hand on the abdomen will not move.

In the bronchial asthmatic, the movements are exaggerated. He has the feeling that he cannot get enough air normally so he increases the activity of the muscles of the chest. Since he cannot exhale properly because of the spasm of the muscles of the bronchial tract and other factors, the lower part of his lungs becomes overloaded and filled with stale air. The primary purpose of breathing exercises is to teach the asthmatic to exhale completely, letting this stagnant air out and allowing room for fresh air to enter and fill the lungs. This requires training and effort. Unfortunately, for two main reasons the exercises are not always utilized adequately: the average physician may not take the time to instruct the patient and the patient may not exercise as regularly as he should. First, the individual must learn to relax—to realize that his lungs have adequate capacity and that he will not suffocate. Then he must be convinced, by demonstrations and experience, that he can control his breathing, rather than allow his confused breathing pattern during an attack of severe asthma to control him. Following that, he must be taught how to use active muscles to exhale the air from his lungs. The muscles used are the diaphragm (the large muscle separating the chest cavity from the abdominal cavity) and, to some extent, the muscles of both the abdomen and the chest wall between the individual ribs.

Muscular exhalation can be practiced at odd moments during the day to gain control and ultimately to make the new habit an automatic one. The breathing exercises also tend to build up the muscles and to increase their power. In addition, they assist in loosening up muscles of the body that are not normally used. This includes the muscles of the shoulders, the upper chest, and the abdominal wall. There are many useful routines; the following includes several modifications of the one recommended by the Asthma Research Council of England. It has been in use for more than twenty years.

Elementary

1. Abdominal or diaphragmatic breathing:

(a) Lie on back with knees drawn up. Place hands on upper abdomen, and while exhaling let hands sink in and contract abdominal muscles. Then take a short breath, relax abdominal muscles, making sure that upper part of chest does not move during the process.

(b) Sit on a firm bed or a hard chair with back supported. Place hands over lower ribs and, while breathing out, contract abdominal muscles. At the end of expiration squeeze ribs to push out any air that might be left in the lower portions of the lungs. Relax abdomen and take a short breath while lower ribs move out. This exercises the abdominal muscles as well as the lower ribs and diaphragm.

2. Elbow circling to loosen shoulders: While sitting on a firm chair with feet apart, place both hands on shoulders. Then bring elbows up to shoulder level, carry them forward, upward, backward, and down in a circling motion. Repeat this six or eight times, then rest with arms down and shoulders relaxed.

3. Blowing exercises: Pursed lip breathing, or breathing against an obstruction such as the lips held close together, is a valuable exercise, since the greater effort necessary to let air out exercises the diaphragm, the abdominal muscles, and the lower rib muscles. There are many methods and variations such as:
   (a) blowing bits of paper or Ping-Pong balls across the table,
   (b) whistling or humming,
   (c) blowing out a candle,
   (d) blowing bubbles in water through a straw.

4. Forward bending: While sitting with feet apart and arms hanging down loosely, bend body forward until head is at level of knees—at the same time breathing out. While sitting up and raising body, breathe in. During exhalation and bending-down procedure abdominal muscles should be contracted. During inhalation procedure, back should be rounded and gradually pushed out.

5. Shoulder loosening exercises ("windmill"): While standing with feet apart, circle both arms so they cross each other in front of the face. The circles intersect each other as the exercise is repeated.

6. Relaxing exercise: Sit on chair, shrug shoulders quickly, then relax them. Let arms hang down adjacent to sides of body and press head back. Relax all muscles that had been shrugged and pressed back, allowing head, shoulders, and back to sag.

Advanced

7. Abdominal trunk exercises with breathing: Lie back on firm couch or bed with knees drawn up and arms limp at sides. Exhale while rising and bending forward, placing head well forward between knees. Inhale while slowly sinking back and resuming initial position. Rest for a

moment and at the same time breathe out quickly using abdominal muscles. Before resuming exercise, inhale. Rest, while breathing normally, allowing only upper part of abdomen and lower portion of rib cage to move.

8. Head and shoulders side bending (loosening exercise): Stand with feet apart and arms elevated almost to level of top of head; keep fists clenched, elbows well back. Bend shoulders and neck over to one side, with corresponding arm going down to side of body in direction of bend. Fist of opposite arm may be used to help push head down. Repeat in opposite direction, using other arm. Repeat this three times in each direction making sure that only head-and-shoulders portions of trunk are allowed to move.

9. Advanced trunk side bending with breathing: Sit with feet well apart. With right hand over ribs on right side, bend over to that side, breathing out simultaneously and pushing hand into ribs. Inhale while assuming an erect position. Bend in opposite direction while exhaling again, and push other hand into ribs. Repeat about six times. During exhalation the action of the hand pushing the ribs should be forceful, and during inhalation the hand should be felt going out.

10. Advanced trunk forward bending (for posture correction as well): Stand with entire body (back, shoulders, head) braced against doorjamb or corner of wall with feet about six inches in front of body. Bend down slowly while exhaling; first head, then shoulders and back, with arms hanging limply down. Breathe in while resuming erect position in reverse manner: first body, then shoulders, then head. Before continuing exercise breathe out, using muscles of abdomen, and push back to feel lower part of back against corner. Take in a small, short breath before bending down again and exercising while exhaling.

11. Side bending with rotation (combined breathing and loosening exercise): Stand with feet apart and lift arms above head while breathing in. Bend slowly over to right as far as possible, while exhaling. While bending twist body counterclockwise so that arms are eventually outside right foot. During bending, breath is exhaled slowly; same time, muscles of abdomen are contracted. Raise body, turn back to normal position while inhaling, and resume starting position with back straight and arms over head. Repeat in opposite direction with bending and rotation to the right and clockwise. Do this approximately four times in each direction

and complete exercise during slow exhalation, standing upright with arms down at sides and abdominal muscles drawn in.

TREATMENT OF A SEVERE ATTACK (INTRACTABLE: STATUS ASTHMATICUS)

When all of the measures which have been discussed are ineffective, bronchial asthma is called *intractable,* or *status asthmaticus,* and additional measures available only in a hospital may be required. These, in addition to continuation of the treatments previously mentioned and discussed, may include injection of fluid into the vein and inhalation treatment.

Injection of fluid into the vein, *intravenous therapy,* by drop method (a regulated number of drops per minute) may consist of a salt and glucose solution to combat the lack of water and salt (dehydration) which causes the bronchial tubes to clog up. As much as three to four quarts of solution is often administered in a twenty-four-hour period. Frequently, this procedure alone is adequate to terminate an attack. At times the intravenous solution must contain other chemicals to combat acidosis or lack of certain minerals. If necessary, adrenocorticosteroid and at times aminophylline are added to the intravenous infusion. When aminophylline is used in an infusion, it must be preceded by a more concentrated injection of the undiluted material in order to elevate the level in the blood immediately. An iodide, usually sodium iodide, is sometimes added to the infusion.

Contrary to common belief, oxygen is not the best treatment for severe asthma, unless there is actual decreased oxygen saturation in the blood (hypoxia). It is often useless if given by the usual mask or tent technique. The reason is that the difficulty in bronchial asthma is usually airway obstruction rather than lack of oxygen.

Oxygen has just as much trouble getting through constricted bronchial tubes as the ordinary atmospheric air. To get air containing oxygen into the lungs, an apparatus supplying air or oxygen under pressure must be used, an intermittent positive pressure breathing machine (IPPB). It can be adjusted to any flow rate and to several degrees of pressure. It can also be used as a method of introducing drugs that dilate the bronchial tubes as well as an agent to thin the mucus. If used properly, these mechanical breathing aids are very beneficial, not only in relieving severe asthma but also in relieving emphysema. Blood gasses, electrolytes, and acidity must be monitored at all times.

As a last resort a doctor can thoroughly investigate the entire upper bronchial tract with a bronchoscope, a lighted hollow viewing tube. During this procedure, he may be able to remove mechanically the thick plugs that are obstructing the upper part of the bronchial tract. Many physicians trained in bronchoscopy use this instrument in severe cases to "wash out" the lungs (bronchial lavage). They commonly employ a weak solution of salt water and cleanse one lobe of the lung at a time. This is best done under anesthesia. In extreme cases where the muscles of respiration are paralyzed, a tube is inserted as an airway, and artificial breathing is used with the IPPB or other mechanical ventilator.

SURGERY FOR RELIEF OF BRONCHIAL ASTHMA

Over the years many operations have been recommended for asthma, but they have been discarded. Recently a surgical procedure called a *glomectomy*, recommended by the Japanese doctor Nakayama, has become popular in some centers. The procedure is simple, consisting of removing the glomus, a small tumor-like body in the neck. Although the operation does not appear to be dangerous, the early-published favorable results seem unsubstantiated and the procedure is still very controversial.

DIFFERENTIAL DIAGNOSIS

Hundreds of conditions that can produce the characteristic symptoms of shortness of breath with cough, wheezing, and production of mucus may constitute the symptom complex *asthma*, rather than the disease state *bronchial asthma*. Among these are a foreign body in the bronchial tree, enlarged lymph glands pressing against the bronchial tree, certain types of heart failure, infections in the small bronchioles, whooping cough, an enlarged thyroid gland, and an enlarged thymus gland.

One condition that in several aspects may mimic the symptoms of bronchial asthma, producing an excess amount of mucus, fatigue, and attacks of shortness of breath with wheezing, is *cystic fibrosis of the pancreas*, also known as *fibrocystic disease of the pancreas* or *mucoviscidosis*. In rare instances some cystic fibrosis patients have an allergy associated with this illness and may have been treated for bronchial asthma due to allergy for years before the proper diagnosis was reached. Cystic fibrosis is a congenital disease affecting the secretions of such material as mucus; it obstructs the small tubes of various organs. There is an associated lack of absorption of vitamins A and D. The disease occurs primarily in children and young adults and is characterized by cough, shortness of breath sometimes accompanied by wheezing, bulky, very malodorous stools, increased appetite accompanied by failure to gain weight, abdominal cramps, and diarrhea. There is a marked tendency to secondary infection, especially with the staphylococcus bacteria, as well as to emphysema, heart failure, and cirrhosis of the liver. The diagnosis is made by a simple test that estimates the amount of salt, particularly the chloride portion, in the sweat.

EMOTIONAL ASPECTS OF BRONCHIAL ASTHMA

The late Dr. Franz Alexander and Dr. Thomas French psychoanalyzed a volunteer group of young people with bronchial asthma in Chicago and found that a common denominator in their makeup was a fear of the loss of the mother. Others verified this finding, one calling the feeling of suffocation "smother love." A related theory holds that the asthmatic child is not only rejected but even resented by the mother. The overprotective mother who hovers over the bed of a sick, asthmatic child, according to this theory, is merely acting out her guilt feelings. Each theory, of course, accepts the premise that allergy is an underlying cause. Nevertheless, a frequent question asked of allergists is, "Isn't asthma all emotional, anyway?"

As with all theories, there is some truth to the theory of emotional asthma. It is for this reason that the distinction between the *asthma disease* (bronchial asthma) and the *asthma attack* (gasping for breath) must be reemphasized. The disease bronchial asthma occurs as a result of an allergy reaction, a tendency which is probably hereditary. Nevertheless, the extremely raw and sensitive bronchial tubes may also be affected by emotional disturbances and other nonspecific factors. In addition, swelling of the lining of the bronchial tubes, spasms of the bronchial muscles, and increased activity of the bronchial mucus glands secreting mucus are all influenced by nerves. Chapter 18 provides a discussion of the role of emotions in allergy disease.

Another important psychological mechanism operates in the opposite way. In the frequently overlooked "allergic fatigue" or "allergic toxemia," asthma itself affects the psyche; the patient is constantly tired and depressed. Furthermore, always living in fear of an attack makes for profound changes in one's behavior and general health. For that, the term *somatopsychic* as opposed to *psychosomatic* has been suggested.

SUMMARY

Asthma is defined as shortness of breath with wheezing and coughing caused by some obstruction in the bronchial tubes leading to the lungs. Some consider it a symptom rather than a disease. As a disease it is caused by allergy, which may be intrinsic or extrinsic. If it is extrinsic it is due to allergy to some substance outside the body; intrinsic asthma is due to infection and emotional causes aggravating the true allergy. Asthma as a symptom can be attributed to numerous causes. Bronchial asthma, on the other hand, is caused by allergy; its symptoms consist of episodes of asthma.

The respiratory mechanism is made up of a series of hollow muscular tubes. These lead into small air sacs, which constitute the smallest unit of the lung. Asthma results from swelling of the lining of these tubes, increase of mucus or phlegm production, and spasms of the muscular walls of the bronchial tubes. In addition, the mucus tends to harden, producing obstruction of the free flow of air in and out of the lungs through the tubes with the characteristic asthmatic symptoms. The allergic mechanism in bronchial asthma is the same as that involved in other allergy diseases; in asthma the shock tissue is the bronchial tract.

The symptoms of bronchial asthma are implied in the definition but can vary from a mild degree of "heaviness on the chest" to profound unconsciousness with major metabolic and chemical changes in the body. It can be constant or periodic, with long periods of freedom between the attacks. Intractable asthma resists the ordinary simple forms of treatment. Status asthmaticus is a term best reserved to denote severe and persistent asthma symptoms; the patient is extremely ill, with changes in the blood gasses and acidity of the body.

The main complication of asthma is emphysema, a condition in which the air sacs that make up the lung are permanently inflated and do not empty as they normally should. In uncomplicated asthma there is also hyperinflation of the same type, but the process is reversible and transient. In true emphysema the small air sacs have lost their ability to rebound, and the walls have broken down so that each air sac is no longer individual but rather is joined with other equally diseased sacs. Infection, in the form of bronchitis, when present, is thought to contribute substantially to this complication.

The treatment of bronchial asthma is both prophylactic and symptomatic. Since allergy is the cause of the asthmatic attacks, prevention, naturally, involves anti-allergy measures as in other allergy diseases. Avoidance of the antigen which incites the asthma is most desirable. If an inhalant such as pollen is responsible and cannot be avoided, specific allergic desensitization is indicated, as discussed in Chapter 7.

Symptomatically, epinephrine by injection or by inhalation will often relieve an attack quickly. Isoproteronol by inhalation is also effective. Ephedrine taken orally is effective, as is theophylline, usually in the form of aminophylline. Aminophylline is effective when given rectally and when injected within the vein. There are numerous anti-asthmatic medicines available with a doctor's prescription or at the drugstore without a prescription. Most of them contain ephedrine, aminophylline, and a sedative to counteract the nervousness produced by ephedrine.

Other measures helpful for asthma are medicines to thin or loosen thick phlegm or mucus. One of the best is iodide of potassium; another is glycerol guiacolate. Drinking a great deal of water and inhaling steam have the effect of thinning the thick mucus.

Old remedies, on sale nationally, persist. One type burns a chemical, saltpeter. The smoke is inhaled to make the asthmatic person cough and bring up some of the thick, obstructive phlegm.

Newer remedies are cortisone or cortisone derivatives. These are very effective but should be used with caution because they may produce harmful side effects. They are best taken in short courses, but not infrequently some people must continue them for a long period of time. In such instances, doctors prescribe gradual reduction until a minimal dosage is reached which is effective but not harmful. Such a person must be under the continuous care of a physician.

The most prominent and serious effects that occur following prolonged use of these products are diabetes, ulcer of the stomach, infections, high blood pressure, heart trouble, and emotional difficulties. These are not absolute contraindications to the use of these medicines, but their presence must be recognized and considered by the doctor.

People who have bronchial asthma should not smoke and should avoid marked changes in the weather. As a rule, they do not tolerate high altitudes very well, but they can fly with no difficulty in pressurized airplanes. In long-standing cases where emphysema may be present, breathing exercises are helpful.

Various surgical operations have been advocated from time to time to relieve asthmatic symptoms, but they have been disappointing. The benefits of glomectomy, the most recent of these, appear to have been exaggerated and the procedure is still controversial.

Chapter Thirteen

Allergy of the Skin

Skin allergy is probably the most common type of allergy. The skin is the largest organ in the body — using "organ" in the sense of its true definition, a part or structure in an animal or plant adapted for the performance of some specific function. In an adult it is approximately two square yards, increased by numerous creases of the hair follicles. Obviously, it is exposed to all varieties of allergens, by direct contact as well as through the bloodstream.

The most important skin manifestations of allergy are *hives,* or *nettle rash, eczema,* and *contact dermatitis.* Less common are the *"id" reactions,* and several that are considered *auto immune diseases,* which are discussed in Chapter 17. Each type can be correctly considered allergic skin dermatitis, an inflammation of the skin (*derma* skin, *itis* inflammation). Yet each differs from the other in many respects—appearance, distribution, method of production, means of investigation, among others. Each, too, has many synonyms which are confusing to layman and physician alike; some are archaic holdovers based on the appearance, others bear the names of the doctors who discovered them *(eponym).*

URTICARIA

The characteristic lesion of this variously named disease (hives, nettle rash, giant hives, angioedema, angioneurotic edema) is the hive, a collection of fluid in a localized area appearing as an elevated white plaque (wheal), surrounded by a zone of redness (erythema). The hive with its blanched appearance is formed as a result of an escape of fluid from blood vessels; the redness surrounding the hive is caused by widening of the blood vessels just under the skin. A similar reaction can be produced by injecting histamine between the layers of the skin or by rubbing the skin with the prickly or stinging *nettle plant,* of the genus *urtica* of the botanical family Urticaceae. This explains the terms *hives, nettle rash,* and *urticaria.* When the lesions are large in size, sometimes involving an entire eyelid or lip, they are called *giant hives.* Since the underlying process has been described as a swelling (edema) due to widening of the blood vessels (angio), the term *angioedema* is apt when the lesions are deep. The term *angioneurotic edema,* implying that there is a nervous element involved in this condition, is unfortunate. As in other allergy (and other illnesses, for that matter), persons may be neurotic, but not all individuals with angioedema are neurotic.

Urticaria may consist of a single hive, or of several scattered over the body. The individual hives may be very large and several or many of them may come together to form one very large irregularly shaped swelling, and may cover extensive surfaces of the body. When the blood vessels are involved in the tissues below the skin, the swelling and redness may be sufficiently extensive to cause an enlarged lip or eyelid, or even to extend much deeper, producing enormously swollen joints. In some instances fever may occur. In any case, the mechanism is the same; only the location of the blood vessel pathology may differ.

The outstanding symptom of hives or urticaria is intense itching. This may be slow in onset and preceded by a tingling or burning sensation, or the onset of the itching and swelling may be acute and sudden; it may disappear just as quickly, or may persist for days, weeks, and even months. Not infrequently, hives clear up for some time and then inexplicably return. They seem to occur at no special site. *Acute urticaria* denotes hives which develop suddenly and disappear quickly; in *chronic urticaria* they persist, or intermittently come and go for a long period of time.

Acute urticaria of the type that is caused by a specific contact such as food is rarely a treatment problem. Once the cause is determined and removed, the lesions will eventually subside, although it may take several days to a week or so for the skin to be clear again. In chronic urticaria, when the lesions persist or are intermittent over months or years, discovery of the cause may constitute a major problem. Foods, particularly seafood and especially shellfish, are the most common causes. Other foods that have been incriminated are chocolate, nuts, fruits and vegetables with small seeds, spices, and pork products. In fact, any food to which the person is allergic can produce urticaria. Horse serum, as may be contained in an antitoxin, is a notable producer of hives and even of the more extensive angioedema. Even sunlight, heat, cold, and physical pressure can induce their formation.

Reactions to a variety of drugs often result in urticaria. These include among many others those taken habitually, such as cathartics and vitamins. Penicillin may produce severe hives. In many instances, a chronic variety results which may persist for months or years. Insect bites characteristically produce urticaria; the mosquito bite is typical of a classical hive. The cause of hives may be as varied as the cause of allergy.

When the lesions of urticaria persist and there is no apparent cause, there may be a strong underlying emotional component. The element of nervousness is often evident in such instances and adds to the problem of treatment. It is easy to mistake for the cause the nervousness and apprehension that occur as the result of the illness.

Treatment consists of relief of the immediate symptoms and prevention of further attacks. It is usually not difficult to effect relief of symptoms even when the lesions are deep and the swelling large. First, a brisk saline cathartic is recommended to remove possible allergenic food from the intestinal tract. The medicines used for hay fever and asthma are equally effective in urticarial conditions, namely the antihistamines and the so-called decongestants. In this case the decongestants are used not to relieve congestion of the nose, but to relieve congestion of the skin.

When these medicines are not adequate, it is often necessary for the doctor to prescribe cortisone products. Large doses may be required, particularly when there is deep angioedema with swelling of the joints and high fever. An Adrenalin (ephinephrine) injection will render quick relief but unfortunately its effect is of short duration. Often soothing lotions and creams on the skin are helpful. These include calamine lotion with phenol or antihistamine creams. Soothing baths using starch, baking soda, bran, oatmeal, and even tar, as in other skin irritations, are useful.

Many people with acute hives may never have to visit a doctor since they have learned what produces the skin condition and avoid it. Sometimes it may be caused by eating lobster; or wearing woolen sweaters. Avoidance of the cause is the most effective method of prevention.

When the condition persists or recurs and the cause is not obvious, the individual must seek skilled help. Even then it may be difficult to determine the cause. The medical history is taken by the doctor as in any other allergy condition but with a special interest placed on medicines, as well as foods. Of particular concern are medicines taken habitually. Cathartics, vitamins, and especially aspirin, which is sold in many forms for various conditions, may not be considered "medicines" by people who take them regularly. Allergy skin tests are helpful, but unfortunately, in many instances the skin is hypersensitive and will produce a swelling when pressed or scratched in scarification allergy tests, injected by a hypodermic needle or just stroked (dermagraphia). This interferes with proper interpretation, and for that reason the skin tests are not as helpful as they might otherwise be. In addition, allergy skin tests to foods in general are not as reliable as they are for inhaled substances. Unfortunately, there are no simple, efficient skin tests for drugs that can cause hives. Even the skin test for penicillin is not particularly diagnostic in evaluating it as a possible producer of hives once they have developed.

Every effort must be made to discover and exclude the underlying cause of the hives. In urticaria due to penicillin allergy there have been reports of instances in which the urticaria was kept active by the person eating foods from animals treated with penicillin, or by drinking milk obtained from cows which had been treated with penicillin injections into their udders for mastitis (although Federal laws regarding such injections have been enacted). Because there are so many causes of urticaria, a doctor must sometimes perform many laboratory tests, aside from skin allergy tests. One that is performed almost routinely in chronic persistent hives is designed to ascertain if there are any parasites in the gastrointestinal tract, since these are known to be one of the causes of urticaria. When emotional problems are suspected as an underlying factor, the aid of a psychiatrist may be necessary.

There are several types of treatment used that occasionally seem to "break up" a chronic attack. Whether this is due to a placebo effect (placebo is a harmless medicine used for its psychic effect) or whether the treatment really alters the defense mechanism in some way is not known. One such treatment, autohemotherapy (*auto,* self; *hemo,* blood; *therapy,* treatment), involves removal of a quantity of blood from the patient and its immediate reinjection deep into a muscle. Occasionally it is successful. Another method is the artificial induction of a high fever with a vaccine such as typhoid, injected intravenously. After the chills and fever have subsided the hives may also disappear. Much less orthodox treatments used now and then prove successful.

PAPULAR URTICARIA

The synonyms of papular urticaria are merely Latinized versions of a description of the lesion and/or the symptoms (lichen urticatus, urticaria papulosa, prurigo simplex, strophylus pruriginosa). The condition is related to simple urticaria or hives but instead of just a blanched swelling and a red area surrounding the hive there is actual inflammation of the tissues involved. As a result the lesions on the skin and the symptoms do not disappear as quickly as they do in simple urticaria. Allergy is not the only cause. Sometimes the underlying cause of the rash, particularly in children, is a series of insect bites in a contaminated home where the bedding has become infested. In many cases, mild achiness and a slight fever accompany the illness. It often appears recurrently in spring and summer months.

Characteristically the lesion resembles the ordinary hive, except that it looks angry: the central area is red and elevated, sometimes with a small bloody crust in the center, like an insect bite. On the other hand, lesions may be of a variety of shapes and sizes; some are even blisters (elevated areas of the skin containing fluid). The rash is usually located on the exposed surfaces of the arms and legs, the buttocks, and occasionally on the trunk and face. The principal symptom is intense itching. Deep marks of scratching (excoriation) by the child are often evident. Sometimes ordinary urticarial lesions may also appear, with swelling of the eyes, lips, and face.

Treatment consists of relief of the itching with the use of antihistamines internally, and soothing lotions and baths applied externally.

Since insect bites, particularly those of the flea and sometimes the bedbug, are a common cause of papular urticaria, the most important preventive treatment is their elimination. House pets often harbor fleas and transmit them to the carpets and upholstered furniture in the home. A method of verifying the existence of fleas, which are usually difficult to detect, is to walk slowly around the sides of the room with a white handkerchief just touching the floor near the baseboards. The fleas will be seen as dark specks against a white background as they jump or fly in front of the handkerchief.

Aside from freeing the animal from his fleas with pesticides, the use of an insect repellent is often helpful. Most consist of the smelly oils of citronella, thyme, cedar, wintergreen, cedarwood, eucalyptus, camphor, bergomot and such. It has been recommended that the susceptible child wear a small piece of gum camphor in a little bag around his neck. Repellents such as these seem much inferior to the chemicals used to exterminate the reproductive ova of the flea, even if the pets must receive "flea baths" several times a month. A "flea collar" or "flea bag," which may be worn by the pet, is available at pet shops. The flea collar contains an insecticide formulated, it is claimed, to dissolve slowly, discharging its flea-killing vapors over a period of three months. These vapors permeate the coat of the animal and destroy the fleas. Patients have told us that these are effective when worn on susceptible subject's ankles. But contact allergy to these has already been reported.

ATOPIC DERMATITIS

Many of the terms for this allergy are obsolete; though still used occasionally. They include prurigo besnier, disseminated neurodermatitis, infantile eczema, eczematoid dermatitis, allergic eczema; and flexural eczema. The best-known and most widely used terms are atopic dermatitis, eczema, and neurodermatitis; the latter, although incorporated in the official nomenclature, is an unfortunate term since it suggests an emotional cause. The term "atopic" indicates the type of allergy which is inherited and inborn. The term "eczema" simply designates a skin rash that has persisted; it is used synonymously with "dermatitis" (inflammation of the skin). "Prurigo" merely means a skin condition that itches. The fact that many more names have been given to this skin disease is apt to confuse one who, if he consults different doctors, is likely to receive what he considers several different diagnoses of what is in fact the same condition.

Atopic dermatitis is well known to everyone and easily recognizable. The characteristic locations for the rash are in the bends of the elbows, the backs of the knees, and on the neck and the face. The appearance varies somewhat with the age of the patient. In infants, it is mainly a moist type of rash limited to the face and the outer portions of the arms and legs. In older children the locations are in the bends (flexural surfaces) of the arms, legs, and neck. In older children the eczema is dry, the skin is often thickened and even leathery. The area involved is usually sharply outlined with distinct borders. In adults the rash tends to be still drier, but it assumes many shapes and sizes and is therefore not as well defined or localized as in juveniles. In very old people there is often a reversal of the pattern to that of the infant-type, with moist lesions occurring on the face and corners of the mouth.

In severe cases the rash is made up of many small raised lesions that eventually become small blisters. When these blisters rupture they discharge fluid, producing a weeping effect. These tiny blisters often blend together to form one large rash. After the weeping effect the serum eventually dries, leaving a thickened, scaly, dry skin. When the severely itching rash is scratched, it not only makes the rash worse, but also is likely to invite infection.

Practically all patients with this type of skin disease have associated asthma and hay fever. They also are likely to show markedly positive allergy skin tests to foods and inhalants. The sweat glands, instead of emptying their material onto the skin, retain it and, in effect, send it back into the body. This introduction of one's own sweat into his own body may initiate itching; it may even act as an antigen to produce an allergy. The sufferer is in fact allergic to his own sweat. Another characteristic is a white instead of red response to stroking the skin (white dermographia).

Atopic dermatitis has been variously described as 1) merely a disturbance of the normal mechanism of perspiration with collection of the sweat in the bends of the elbows and knees; 2) a nonallergic illness which happens to occur in people who have allergies such as hay fever and asthma; 3) an allergy to one's self or to one's own skin; 4) a purely allergic disease just as hay fever is; 5) an emotional disease with scratching as the cause of the rash; and 6) an inborn disease of enzyme metabolism. It has even been suggested that all six mechanisms may be the cause.

The infantile type of the disease responds very well to food avoidance as a rule. The foods that are most suspect are milk, cereals, especially wheat, and eggs, as these are the only foods that the very small infant eats. Later, such foods as other cereals and citrus fruits may be the cause. No specific foods are more likely to produce eczema than others. Like the "milk causes mucus" myth there must exist an allergy to the food, and the child is just as likely to be allergic to bland food as to more complex foods.

In addition to foods, eczema may be caused by inhalants such as pollen and environmental substances found in the home. Rolling in the grass will produce it in the susceptible child; contact with cats and dogs, sleeping on feather pillows or any substance to which one is allergic can produce it. Since the skin of the person with atopic dermatitis is extremely sensitive, irritating soaps and detergents can often irritate it.

There are two important complications; fortunately both are rare. One is cataracts of the eyes. These never occur in infants, but may appear in adults who have had atopic dermatitis for many years. The second complication occurs only when an individual with eczema is vaccinated for smallpox: the vaccination reaction spreads to the entire skin, with severe generalized symptoms. For that reason, vaccination of a person who has eczema is contraindicated. Members of the household coming in contact with the child who has eczema should not be vaccinated either. When a vaccination is necessary one should wait for a time until the skin is clear. If foreign travel is desired the physician may write an appropriate letter to the public health authorities stating the contraindication. Such a statement is usually accepted. A hyperimmune gamma globulin (VIG) prepared from the blood of recently vaccinated donors has been used for the prevention of the complications of smallpox vaccination in atopic children. A more common complication is secondary infection as a result of scratching with dirty fingernails. This can be treated successfully with antibiotics.

Treatment of atopic dermatitis may create a problem. Most important is prevention or elimination of the itching; if the person does not scratch he will have no rash. For this, soothing lotions and creams are very helpful. Soap is not recommended and excess washing is harmful since it further dries the skin. Some doctors advise their patients to refrain from washing entirely, with the exception of a shower lasting but a minute or two with the use of soap only where necessary. In place of soap, a propylene glycol, cetyl alcohol compound (Cetaphil) lotion is an excellent cleansing agent. It is applied gently and the skin is patted dry.

Soothing baths have been used for many years and are still valuable. These are frequently recommended.

Starch: Two cups or one pound of cornstarch are mixed with enough cold water to make a paste and then added to the bath. An alternate method is to add warm water to the paste; the mixture is then boiled until it is thick and this is added to the bath.

Oatmeal: A special colloidal oatmeal can be purchased in the pharmacy. One cupful is mixed with two cups of cold water and this mixture is poured into the bathtub. One popular technique is to use three cups of ordinary cooked oatmeal tied in a cheesecloth bag. This bag is used as a washcloth, gently rubbing it against the skin and at the same time squeezing the oatmeal out of the bag.

Bran: This is used in the same manner as the oatmeal. Two pounds of bran are put into a cotton bag and soaked in hot water for fifteen minutes. The bran-filled sack is used as a washcloth.

Baking Soda: A half pound of baking soda is added to the bath water. The patient soaks in this.

Tar: Three ounces of coal-tar solution are added to the usual amount of bath water. Less tar is used for the child's bath. (Tar may stain the bathtub.)

Potassium Permanganate: (This chemical also stains the tub). The proportions are four teaspoonfuls of the crystal to a tub of water. Since this is a dangerous poison it must be kept away from the mouth and used with caution.

Cortisone has proved most valuable in the management of eczema, but it may also complicate the treatment considerably. Cortisone products and their derivatives taken by mouth in sufficiently large doses will dramatically relieve the symptoms and heal the rash in most circumstances. Unfortunately, often excessively large doses are necessary and invariably the rash recurs when the cortisone product is discontinued. Many individuals with long-standing eczema learn to accept some constant itching, which becomes part of their life pattern. When such a person is given cortisone he may become completely free of all itching. After this, any slight amount of itching, even a great deal less than he had been able to tolerate before, becomes intolerable. As a result, he insists upon taking the cortisone to the detriment of his general health.

Cortisone and cortisone-like products and their derivatives in ointment or cream form are also effective. There are several on the market prepared in varying strengths. Usually the stronger is used for the severe stage of the rash and the weaker to maintain improvement.

The stronger dilutions are still expensive but the weaker ones are comparatively inexpensive. Fortunately the material is effective even when used sparingly. When the cortisone creams are placed over the rash in fairly thick layers, covered with an occlusive dressing such as Saran Wrap or Pliofilm, then sealed with cellophane tape and left in place for forty-eight hours or longer, the rash responds to treatment more dramatically. The danger of absorption of the cortisone through the skin is negligible unless large areas of the body are covered and the occlusive dressing is used. Nevertheless, the cortisone creams and ointments must not be used indiscriminately.

When external allergens are incriminated and cannot be eliminated or avoided, desensitization is frequently employed. Most allergists agree on the great value of this approach but caution against using strong concentrations of allergy extracts, and urge that hyposensitization be performed with great care and the doses increased in very small increments. When hay fever and asthma coexist with the dermatitis, there is no doubt that specific allergy desensitization treatment is necessary and can be expected to provide relief of the skin allergy as well as of the respiratory symptoms.

Allergists and skin specialists agree on the following principles as a necessary part of treatment: 1) avoidance of substances close to the skin that might be either irritating or allergic, such as wool, 2) avoidance of contact with animal hair, particularly that of dogs and cats, 3) removal of feather pillows, rug pads, stuffed toys, and rugs and carpets, especially from the bedroom. Some recommend covering the arms and legs with tightly fitting pajamas or even bandages made of cotton, nylon, or some other synthetic material to avoid contact with the allergen and to prevent injury to the skin from involuntary scratching.

Characteristic atopic dermatitis or eczema is readily diagnosed in a child, but there are several other types of rashes from which it must be differentiated. One is *seborrheic dermatitis,* a condition marked by dandruff and prominent rash where the hair joins the skin and in the hair lines. The rash may become severe and extend to the forehead and cheeks, to the chest, and even to the pubic area. Often seborrheic dermatitis coexists with allergic eczema; there is a theory that oily hair with its dandruff is the antigen that produces the allergy. A condition known as *lichen simplex chronicus* is often considered a localized form of allergic or atopic eczema and therefore is also termed *chronic circumscribed neurodermatitis.* The cause of this rash is unknown although it often occurs in allergic individuals. It may consist of only one or of several localized areas of thickened skin with scaling. Often the site is on the nape of the neck and on the back of the forearms.

PSORIASIS

Although not an allergic skin condition, psoriasis is often either mistaken for, or thought of as, an allergic disease. Perhaps the reason for this is that it runs in families and is somewhat responsive to treatment with cortisone.

Psoriasis can readily be recognized by the thick placques seen in the chronic stage often involving the scalp, the outer surfaces of the extremities, the back, and the buttocks. Indeed no part of the body is exempt.

CONTACT DERMATITIS

The terms for this disease (dermatitis venenata, eczematous contact-type dermatitis, contact eczema, eczematous dermatitis) indicate the type of rash one acquires when the antigen is in contact with the skin, as opposed to internal contact. The best examples are the rashes of poison ivy, poison oak, and poison sumac, or "skin poisoning." The rash occurs at the point of contact with the offending substance and begins with a raised red area which rapidly develops small blisters. The degree and amount of redness around these blisters depend upon the extent of contact and the skin surface involved.

From the academic point of view, contact dermatitis represents a somewhat different type of allergic reaction, called the *delayed type of hypersensitivity*. Allergists distinguish between the *delayed type of hypersensitivity* and the *immediate* or *anaphylactic type of reaction*. Bronchial asthma, hay fever, and hives are examples of the latter type. In these allergy diseases, skin tests (intradermal or scarification) are performed and results are apparent within ten to fifteen minutes. Contact allergy is an example of the *delayed type of hypersensitivity*. Poison ivy and poison oak are examples of this type of reaction.

In contact allergy the test is performed by placing the antigen on the surface of the skin, covering it with a bandage or some other small dressing, and leaving it in place for twenty-four to forty-eight or seventy-two hours. A reaction may occur during or after that period of time and is considered positive when a rash is produced that resembles the original one, in miniature. A detailed account of all allergy skin tests is to be found in Chapter 4.

The outstanding symptom of contact dermatitis is itching at the site of the rash. The rash may spread to other parts of the body by way of the bloodstream. Smoke of burning poison ivy and other such plants can produce a rash in susceptible persons as the smoke harbors the allergen which can be carried long distances by strong winds.

Poison ivy, poison oak, and poison sumac are examples of contact dermatitis readily suspected and recognized by people who have been in areas where these plants could have been touched. Unless the reaction is violent, treatment is usually simple because the condition is self-limiting. When the contact is discontinued, healing is almost spontaneous. Subtle, contact-type allergies of the skin are much more difficult to diagnose and to treat since there is usually continued contact with the substance. For example, a rash on the hands of a housewife may be a nonallergic dermatitis caused by the numerous materials she handles daily and the frequent dipping of her hands in water. Or it may be a true allergic contact-type dermatitis caused by furniture polish, soaps, dust from dustcloths, fruits and vegetables used in cooking, the handle of a paring knife, or fresh flowers; the list is practically endless. (Table 10 lists some common contacts.) "Housewive's eczema," characterized by severe itching and a rash on the hands is very common and is thought to be caused by detergents. There is some question as to whether this is a true allergy or a nonspecific skin irritation in which frequent exposure to both detergent and water is the exciting factor. Probably there are elements of both involved.

TABLE 10

COMMON ALLERGY CONTACTS

1. SCALP

Scalp lotions, scalp tonics, pomades, soaps, hair dyes and rinses, wave sets, shampoos, patent dandruff removers, bristles of hair brushes, plastic combs, bathing caps, massage brushes, hair nets, hair pins and curlers, toupees, wigs. (The scalp is often remarkably resistant to external irritants and allergens. Thus, dermatitis caused by substances used on the scalp often appears not primarily on the scalp but predominantly or exclusively on other more sensitive skin areas such as the eyelids, ears, and retroauricular areas, nape and other parts of the neck, the face in general, and even the hands.)

2. FOREHEAD

Hat bands, hat linings, and other materials of hats, massage creams, sun-tan lotions and other cosmetics, material from bandanas, hair nets, celluloid visors, helmets, dye, and material from veils.

3. EYELIDS *(one of the most sensitive areas)*

Numerous substances used on scalp, face, and hands (cosmetics, soaps, hand lotions, creams, face powders, nail polishes and lacquers). Mascara, eyebrow pencil, eyelash curlers, etc., air-borne volatile agents and dusts (insect sprays, gaseous substances, nasal sprays, cleaning fluids, antimoth preparations, perfumes, benzine; dusts from clothing, furniture; air-borne pollen, etc.; materials of dyed clothing, fabrics, furs, gloves, handbags).

4. FACE
Cosmetics (face powders, creams, rouges, lotions): all possible materials transferred by hands or air-borne. All substances used on face, scalp, or hands. Shaving soaps and creams, after-shaving lotions, sun protectives.

5. EARS
Earrings, bakelite, other plastics, nickel, white gold, other metals; perfumes, hair dye, shampoo, lacquers, eyeglass frames, plastic ear phones, rubber ear plugs, bathing caps.

6. BACK OF EARS AND BRIDGE OF NOSE
Spectacle frames, hearing aids, earring materials as mentioned above.

7. NOSE AND AREA BETWEEN NOSE AND LIPS
Nose drops, nasal ointments, sprays, etc., perfumes, handkerchiefs, paper tissues, etc.

8. LIPS AND MOUTH
Lipsticks, their dyes, or other constituents. Mouthwashes, toothpastes, powders, throat lozenges and patent medicines, toothpicks, cigarettes, cigars, pipes. Sometimes certain foods and candies. (Many people have a habit of sucking on such things as pencils, erasers.) Acrylic denture material.

9. NECK
Collars, scarves, neckties, dress labels, furs, fur dyes, substances used on scalp, necklaces, perfumes, wave-sets, hair cosmetics and dyes, hairpins, nail lacquers, cosmetics and other substances used on face.

10. UPPER CHEST
Clothing contacts, materials and dyes (black, dark blue, and dark brown are considered the most common offenders). Rubber breast pads (falsies), brassieres.

11. ARM PITS AND SURROUNDING AREAS
Antiperspirants, deodorants, depilatories, dress shields, dyed materials, perfumes, shaving materials.

12. HANDS AND FOREARMS
Substances too numerous to list: Most occupational and industrial excitants; substances encountered in hobbies, games, professions; soaps, cleansers, plants, gloves, steering wheels, instruments, rings, bracelets; cosmetics, topical medicaments; all objects which may be touched, handled, held, or worn.

13. TRUNK
Clothing, material and dyes, girdles, sanitary belts, trusses, suspensory underwear, nightclothes, sweaters, bathing materials, bath salts, soaps, perfumes, massage creams.

14. ANAL AREA AND BUTTOCKS
Rectal suppositories, douches, substances in enemas, intestinal parasites, ingested foods—especially fruits and oils, topical medicaments, underwear, sanitary napkins, toilet paper, toilet seats.

15. REGION AROUND VAGINA
Douches, anticonceptional jellies, suppositories, sanitary napkins. Substances carried by the hands: perfumes, deodorants, prophylactic agents, condoms, pessaries, topical medicaments.

16. REGION AROUND PENIS AND SCROTUM
Condoms, prophylactic agents, anticonceptional medicaments, douches (used by

partner); fabric finishes and dyes in underdrawers, pajamas; rubber and elastic supporters; substances carried by the hands.

17. LEGS

Dyed materials and materials of trousers, underdrawers, socks, etc.; matchboxes, cigarette lighters, coins and other metallic objects carried in trouser pockets; volatile and air-borne substances, dusts inside trousers, etc.; garters (rubber, elastic, dyes, metal clasps).

18. FEET

Shoes, socks, stockings (leather dyes, tanning agents, dyes, shoe polishes and finishes of materials); galoshes, fur lining, ankle bracelets, medication; rubbers, cements, and pastes.

Any allergic individual can be allergic to virtually any substance that comes in contact with his skin. When the hands are vulnerable, rubber gloves, preferably with cotton linings are recommended. Several silicone-base hand lotions and creams are available which will allegedly form an impenetrable surface of silicone to protect the skin. But they have not been very successful. Some substances like cosmetics are more likely sensitizers than others. The chemicals known as *paraben esters,* found in cosmetics as a preservative, have recently been incriminated as one cause of contact dermatitis. This has led to the development of hypoallergenic cosmetics which are less likely to be allergenic because known sensitizing ingredients are omitted. Nevertheless, some of the substances in the nonallergic products may still be allergenic for some people.

With the increasing use of resins and plastics in clothes and almost every type of manufacture, a new type of contact allergy or dermatitis is being seen. Cottons and other materials are being processed to resist wrinkles; fabrics are being processed to stay pressed and innumerable new applications are daily being found. Dermatitis from plastics is not common but occurs often enough to pose a problem. It is most prevalent in workers in plastics plants who come in contact with the raw materials, which are usually the responsible agents. Along with these basic raw materials many other chemicals are used, such as dyes, solvents, fillers, plasticizers, catalysts, and hardeners. These can also cause contact dermatitis or other types of allergy.

The oldest plastic is made from the chemical formaldehyde. When the formaldehyde (and carbolic acid) is chemically treated with a catalyst, it can produce a soluble resin or plastic like that used in lacquers and paints, or it can be made into a hard, insoluble material for use in the frames of eyeglasses. After heating, the hardened substance loses all the formaldehyde; dermatitis from this is rare, but in the soluble form some elements of formaldehyde remain and rashes are more common. More sophisticated plastic materials made from different substances by diverse processes and with different chemicals added can be recognized by the names on the label; urea-formaldehyde, polyethylene, vinyl, acrylic, polystyrene, and cellulose acetate. An example is the so-called spun glass which is used in curtains and numerous other products. Brand names vary from country to country.

Once contact has been discontinued, future avoidance and symptomatic relief are the therapeutic goals. When contact with an allergy-producing substance has occurred, there is a possibility of preventing the skin rash with immediate precautionary measures. This is particularly applicable to poison ivy and poison oak contact; an immediate bath with a strong alkaline soap may remove the oily allergenic portion of the plant. This must be done very soon after exposure, for once the dermatitis has begun, the preventive measures are worthless. There are many commercial lotions and creams containing the chemical zirconium, which can neutralize the irritating effects of the poison ivy and poison oak allergen, but they must be used immediately.

An excess exposure to the poison-ivy variety of plants may produce severe generalized symptoms, including urticaria or angioedema rather than a minor localized rash. Extreme swelling of the eyes, extremities, and joints has occurred. Involvement of the deeper organs such as the kidneys has also resulted. Adequate amounts of cortisone products halt the spread of the disease, relieve the symptoms, and protect the body until the severe allergic reaction is terminated. Cortisone ointments, creams, and lotions are excellent as treatment for contact dermatitis.

"ID" REACTIONS

An "id" is a skin rash secondary to a primary infection elsewhere in or on the body; it is considered to be an allergic reaction to the circulating antigen. Thus, a person who has certain diseases may develop a rash as a result of allergy to that disease. *Tuberculids,* skin reactions to tuberculosis, and *syphilids,* skin reactions to syphilis, are no longer commonly encountered because the diseases are not as frequent. However, the skin reactions can also be to fungus infections such as ringworm or athlete's foot. These are called *trichophytids* and *epidermophytids;* the general term for all fungus infections on the skin is *dermatophytosis* and the general term for "id's" due to the entire group is *dermatophytid.*

The appearance of skin lesions which occur very often on the hands, is nondescript and similar to any other eczema type of eruption. The diagnosis can be made only by the appropriate skin test with antigen prepared from the fungus; the reaction is a delayed one, as in the tuerculin test. Further corroboration of the diagnosis can be made by identifying the cause of the original infection by culture and microscopic examination of the organism or fungus. Treatment is directed toward elimination of the primary infection.

SUMMARY

The skin covers the entire body and so is very vulnerable. The three most important types of skin allergy, and perhaps the only known ones, are hives (urticaria), eczema (atopic dermatitis), and contact dermatitis.

When the hives involve only the skin it is called simply hives or urticaria, although other names are in common use; when the lesions are deep and involve the tissues under the skin and perhaps even the joints, the condition is known as angioedema or angioneurotic edema. The term angioneurotic edema does not imply that the individual is neurotic.

The hives may be due to food, inhalants, and even absorption through the skin. The hive may be a severely itching, isolated, raised white area surrounded by a zone of redness; or may cover large parts of the body with large raised white areas, some of which may join each other to become extensive oddly shaped lesions. When the condition has reached the stage of angioedema, there is often swelling of the lips and eyes, swelling of some of the joints, and even fever. Severe reactions are often caused by medicines, notably penicillin.

When the urticaria is caused by food, inhalants, or something touched, it is self-limiting; the treatment is soothing lotions and creams to relieve the itching. Antihistamines are very effective. In angioedema, where symptoms are severe, cortisone-type drugs may be necessary.

When urticaria persists or recurs repeatedly, the problem is more difficult. It can be due to a food that is being eaten constantly, a drug, or emotional problems that keep aggravating the immune process. Many dermatologists feel that emotions alone are the cause of chronic, persistent, or recurring hives. But the allergist's concept is of a basic allergy which constantly flares up as a result of emotional problems. Only in this sense do they regard urticaria as psychosomatic.

A variation of urticaria is known as papular urticatus or lichen urticatus. This is usually caused by repeated insect bites. Unlike the usual hive which may disappear in hours, it is deep in the skin and persists for days or weeks. The treatment is identical to treatment of usual hives, but one must rid the house of the responsible insects. Sometimes these are fleas present on house pets.

The most common and intractable allergic skin lesion is commonly referred to as eczema but is well known as atopic dermatitis and by other names. Neurodermatitis incorrectly suggests a neurotic manifestation. The lesions of this skin allergy vary with the age of the individual, but the most commonly seen are the weepy or very dry scaly rash in the bends of the elbows and knees and on the neck and face.

Most people with atopic dermatitis have associated asthma and hay fever with positive allergy skin-test reactions. Despite this, many doctors feel that this type of eczema is not an allergic disease mainly because it has not been possible to reproduce it. In addition to the customarily positive allergy skin tests and the presence of other types of allergy, two important characteristic findings are present in this condition while absent in others. Sweating is markedly diminished, and when the skin is stroked with a blunt instrument, a white line develops (white dermographia) instead of a red one. The sweat retention syndrome has lead to the theory that sweat is absorbed back into the body and acts as an allergen.

There are two serious but fortunately rare complications to this dermatitis. One is the appearance of cataracts of the eyes in adults with severe lesions. Another is a serious generalized reaction of the entire skin and body to smallpox vaccination. People with active atopic dermatitis should not be vaccinated, nor should members of the household.

Treatment consists of relief of the itching to prevent scratching, which aggravates the rash. Oral antihistamines, soothing creams and lotions are useful. In severe instances cortisone-type skin creams and lotions are unusually valuable and effective. In exceedingly severe cases, cortisone drugs are administered orally. Although they are very effective they are usually prescribed only when absolutely necessary. The rash recurs when the medicine is discontinued. The side effects of cortisone are discussed in Chapter 7.

Contact dermatitis, a common allergy skin condition, is caused by contact with an offending material. The rash appears at the site of contact. The best-known examples of contact allergy are poison ivy, oak, and sumac dermatitis. But jewelry, the dye in fur collars, nylon-stocking dye, plastic spectacles, wrinkleproof clothing, cosmetics, medicines, and a host of others can be responsible for a rash.

To determine the cause of contact dermatitis the patch test is used. It consists of placing some of the suspected material on the skin, covering it and leaving it in place for twenty-four to forty-eight and sometimes seventy-two hours. A positive reaction is indicated by a small itching rash which develops at the site of the test. Because contact dermatitis from hair dyes is common, most hair dyes come with a card giving instructions for the performance of a test. If the test indicates an allergy, the dye should not be used.

The treatment of contact dermatitis is removal of the cause. For relief the usual antihistamines and soothing creams and lotions are helpful. In some instances cortisone creams are invaluable. When the condition becomes very severe, as it may in poison ivy, cortisone products may be required.

An "id" is a skin rash secondary to a primary infection elsewhere in or on the body. It is regarded as an allergy to the original infection, the antigen or allergen circulating in the blood. The most common is the trichophytid, secondary to ringworm or athlete's foot. The diagnosis is made by an allergy skin test and by the demonstration of the original infection. Treatment is directed at curing the primary infection.

Chapter Fourteen

Physical Allergy

Although it was not until 1925 that a direct relationship was suggested between physical agents and allergy disease, the deleterious effects of heat, cold, light rays, pressure, and effort on some people have long been recognized. Many patients who have bronchial asthma or some other allergy illness will testify that their illness is affected by such conditions. But it is still a matter of controversy whether all the reactions to physical agents are evidence of truly allergic (antigen-antibody) activity.

Those who do not consider physical agents antigenic feel that the release of histamine or a histamine-like substance causing the allergy-like symptoms results entirely from injury to the body cells by the physical agents per se. Those who argue that the reaction is a definitive allergy reaction maintain that physical agents act on the patient's skin, mucous membrane, or muscle to produce a chemical or physical-plus-chemical alteration of the tissue proteins, and that these transformed tissue proteins act as antigens leading to the formation of antibodies (auto allergy). Unfortunately, the proof of this hypothesis is made difficult by the fact that in physical allergy, antibodies are difficult to demonstrate. Some physicians disregard both of these theories and suggest that the release of histamine or a histamine-like substance may be stimulated by the central nervous system (brain and spinal cord) and the nerves going to the muscles.

In favor of the concept of allergic responses as physical reactive symptoms are these facts: (1) In many instances a history of some form of related allergy is present. (2) A local reaction can, as a rule, be obtained when sought at the site of exposure by skin test. (3) Generalized reactions can occur. (4) Repeated exposure to the same physical agent often produces tolerance (natural desensitization). (5) Desensitization with

225

gradually increased exposures is frequently successful. (6) Allergy medicines such as the antihistamines, ephedrine, and the corticosteroids, are often effective. (7) A transferable antibody has occasionally been demonstrated (Prausnitz-Küstner reaction). (8) An increase in the number of eosinophiles in the bloodstream may be present. For these reasons, most allergists think of allergenic physical agents as producing the symptomatology of allergy, using the term "allergy" in its broadest sense as "altered reaction" with antigen-antibody reaction present, although not always demonstrable.

TYPES OF PHYSICAL REACTIONS

There are two types of reactions that may result from exposure to physical agents; one is the local type that appears at the site of exposure and the other is a generalized reaction that may cover the entire body, although only a small part may have been exposed.

ALLERGY TO HEAT

Local reactions to heat are less common than generalized reactions. A person exposed to heat may break out with large hives (urticaria) only where the skin is uncovered. A generalized type of heat reaction may occur in persons who are exposed to heat at a site distant from the area of exposure. An example of this is generalized urticaria or an attack of asthma as a result of local application of a heating pad to one isolated portion of the body. Some susceptible individuals are affected by direct exposure to the sun's rays, sitting in a hot room, eating hot foods on a very hot day, wearing an excess of heavy warm clothing, or taking a hot bath. Although urticaria and asthma are frequent symptoms of heat allergy, abdominal cramps, diarrhea, migraine headaches, disturbances in the heart rhythm, faintness, flushing, and salivation are often experienced. Even collapse has been reported. It has been stated that an increase in body temperature of from two-tenths of a degree to one degree Fahrenheit can activate heat allergy in adults. Other forms of allergy may be present, and often there are contributing factors such as a preexisting infectious disease or an emotional upset that has reduced the person's resistance or allergy threshold, making him more responsive to heat.

Doctors usually test for heat sensitivity by applying a test tube filled with hot water or any controllable source of heat to an area on the skin. If a definite hive (urticarial wheal) appears at the site and is surrounded by a red, inflamed, itchy area, it is considered a positive heat reaction. Another procedure is to allow hot water (100° F.) to run over the hand or to soak the hand in hot water for a few moments. Again, whealing is considered a positive reaction.

Treatment consists of desensitization by careful exposure to gradually increasing temperatures, beginning with an exposure that does not produce any local or general symptoms. This is most often accomplished with the use of a heat lamp. The intensity of the heat is controlled by varying the distance of the lamp from the body. When a reaction occurs as a result of the exposure, it indicates overdosage, and the heat intensity is decreased until tolerance is established. For more general desensitization, hot tub-baths are used, regulating the gradual daily increase in water temperature by means of a bath thermometer. Warm to hot showers are substitutes but they cannot be controlled as carefully. Antihistamines sometimes give relief; in severe cases, corticosteroids ("cortisone") may be required, but at best medicines are not very effective.

ALLERGY TO COLD

The local type of cold allergy involves swelling of the face, eyes, ears, and hands after exposure to cold. Heat allergy, according to published statistics, is more common in adults; cold allergy in children. Local reactions to cold are more common than general ones. Extreme cold is not essential to produce a reaction; sometimes it can be activated by merely leaving a warm area and entering a cold one. For example, allergic persons entering cool air-conditioned buildings on very hot summer days may break out in sneezing attacks, urticaria, or some other allergy symptoms. Those who work in extremely low temperatures for a long period of time where, for example, there are walk-in refrigerators that must repeatedly be entered, frequently develop a resistance to cold.

The following generalized symptoms of cold allergy have been reported: urticaria (hives), diarrhea, visual disturbances, bladder irritability, hemoglobinuria (red-colored urine), fever, nausea and vomiting, dizziness, swelling of the lining of the nose, swelling of the palate, joint pains, muscle pains, drop in blood pressure, increase in heart rate, and shock. It is entirely possible that many unexplained deaths of swimmers are caused by shock in allergic individuals who are extremely sensitive to cold. Persons who are cold-sensitive often break out in hives following a cold shower.

The common tests for cold allergy are applying to the skin a test tube filled with chopped ice or ice water, placing an ice cube on the skin, or immersing the hand in cold water at a temperature of 40° F. As in heat allergy, a positive test is indicated if local whealing and a surrounding red inflamed area develops. Occasionally a generalized reaction is instigated. The threshold to cold may be lowered by concomitant allergenic exposures, by emotional upsets, or by the presence of an intercurrent infection.

Desensitization is usually accomplished by daily baths, the first of which are tepid. Using a bath thermometer, the temperature is gradually decreased until a relatively cold bath can be tolerated. Another method prescribes rubbing the body daily with ice or very cold wet cloths, beginning with a few seconds' duration and gradually increasing the time.

Injections of histamine have been employed with varying results. The treatment consists of hypodermic injections of histamine twice daily for two or three weeks, beginning with a very small dose, and increasing gradually until beneficial results are obtained. Then, the intervals between doses are lengthened, initially once daily, then every second day, then every third day, etc. Since no positive results are assured and since this treatment requires many visits to the doctor's office it is understandably not very popular. Added to this, collapse after an overdose of histamine injections has been reported. The best but often not the simplest treatment is for a cold-sensitive person to move to a temperate climate where there is little fluctuation in temperature.

ALLERGY TO LIGHT

Allergy to light is much more common than was previously realized. Light is merely a small portion of a vast spectrum of electromagnetic radiation, which includes radio waves, X rays, infrared radiation (heat), ultraviolet radiation, and gamma rays. In the solar spectrum the ultraviolet rays fall between 2,900 and 3,900 Angstrom units (a measurement used in physics to express the length of light rays). Visible light is between 3,900 and 7,700 A and infrared rays are above 7,700 A. Sensitivity to the sun's rays in the solar spectrum occurs in the vicinity of 2,900 to 8,000 A, with most light sensitivity being in the ultraviolet range (2,900 to 3,900 A). These comprise the ultraviolet, indigo, and blue rays of the sun.

Local reactions to light are easily recognized but must be differentiated from ordinary sunburn. There is initial redness of the area exposed, followed by an edema that is limited to the site. Surrounding the swelling, a flare into the surrounding tissues (red inflammatory reaction) develops. This is *urticaria solaris* (hives due to sunlight). Frequently, several hours may elapse from exposure to the onset of these symptoms, although they may appear immediately or within a few minutes in some exquisitely sensitive persons. Women are far more frequently affected than men, and an attack may last for several days. The tendency toward urticaria solaris may persist for years. Spontaneous improvement may occur in those sensitive to the ultraviolet rays but seldom in those sensitive to the visible rays.

Polymorphic eruptions, rashes that appear in more than one form, may be produced by light sensitivity. The most common types are: (1) Plaquelike patches on the skin. (2) An eczematous rash consisting of pinhead-size swellings, similar to pimples, that accumulate fluid which may become infected and change to pus and when they rupture produce a scab; these areas may itch intensely. They have been given the name *eczema solare*. (3) Small solid elevations on the skin varying from the size of a pinhead to a pea; these may be very deep in the skin; they are pale and itch. (4) A generalized redness of the skin (an erythematous rash).

When a portion of the body has been exposed to plants or to some special kinds of skin lotions, creams, ointments, or soaps, the effect of the sun's rays on those who are susceptible may produce a local reaction. This specially mediated response, known as *photosensitivity reaction* is not at all uncommon. It may also occur after ingestion of some medicines, of which the "sulfa" drugs are examples.

All the sun's rays may be adequately filtered out by the newer and efficient sun-screening agents readily obtained at all drugstores. Most of these contain p-aminobenzoic acid and are marketed as "suntans" or antiburn medicines. They vary in their filtering capacity. Some prevent burning but permit tanning; others prevent both. Antihistamines taken by mouth prior to exposure to the sun occasionally prevent a local reaction from developing, but their effectiveness is not constant. There are other medicines which help prevent a light reaction, such as amodiaquin hydrochloride and chloroquine phosphate (antimalarial drugs), but these require a doctor's prescription.

The generalized reaction to light is usually urticaria. It is believed that an underlying process, such as some disturbance of the the ductless glands (e.g., thyroid, ovaries, or pituitary), or some physical or chemical change in the body (metabolic disturbance) may be a precipitating factor influencing their production. For their detection, a thorough physical examination must be performed by the physician. The elimination of all foci of infection (parts of the body that harbor germs, such as tonsils or appendix) is important, and the treatment of any current infection is mandatory. Any abnormalities in the ductless glands (endocrine system) are treated with appropriate hormones, and metabolic disturbances are corrected. But, of course, avoidance of exposure to sunlight is the simplest and most efficient form of therapy.

There are several conditions associated with light sensitivity and photosensitization that also involve marked metabolic changes based on genetic anomalies. The general term for these is porphyria. They are not all clearly defined or completely understood. The ones involving the skin may be mistaken for simple physical allergy.

General exposure to light rays in gradually lengthened doses, accomplished by increasing the periods of exposure to a source of ultraviolet rays, such as an ultraviolet sunlamp, is a universal method of treatment. Locally, creams, lotions, and ointments containing sun-screening chemicals like those described for local light sensitivity are helpful to relieve symptoms. Photosensitizers should be avoided. These include the essential oils from which many perfumes are manufactured, fluorescent substances such as eosin and fluorescein, acriflavine, and fabric dyes. Coal-tar ointments, petroleum products, green soap and other soaps containing dibromoclan, when applied locally and the person is exposed to the sun's rays, may result in general as well as local reactions. Certain drugs when taken internally appear to be activated by sunlight and cause general symptoms of urticaria; among these the most prominent are the barbiturates and the sulfonamides. These must be avoided.

ALLERGY TO PRESSURE

Superficial pressure or scratching of the skin with the fingernail or stroking the skin with an object that is pointed but not sharp will produce a raised welt in some allergic individuals within a few moments. This is commonly called *dermographia* or *urticaria factitia*. Where stronger pressure is applied to a specific area, urticarial wheals or local swelling of the part may develop after a lapse of several hours. These symptoms are disturbing, but the latter may be disabling when it involves the buttocks from sitting, the hands from the handling of tools, or the feet from the pressure of shoes. In persons sensitive to pressure, often the slight pressure of a belt around the waist produces a band of redness with hives (erythema and whealing). Pressure allergy differs from the whealing that results from a violent mechanical stimulus such as a whiplash. In whiplash a large amount of force is applied, and the sensation is painful rather than itchy. Although whealing occurs in both instances, the mechanism of histamine release is thought to be entirely different.

Some dermatologists believe that the thickening of the skin seen in chronic eczema results from the rubbing and scratching of the skin. It is thought by some that the mechanical irritation of the skin by scratching produces some substance to which the person reacts. One of the reasons for accepting an allergic hypothesis for pressure allergy such as dermographia is the observation that continued stroking of the skin with a stiff brush several times each day diminishes the reaction; also, specific antibodies have been demonstrated in the blood of persons suffering from pressure allergy.

One of the methods of testing for pressure allergy is the application of the cuff of a blood pressure machine and inflating it to varying pressures for one to three minutes. Another method employed is the suspension of a known weight in a halter over one of the shoulders for five to ten minutes, noting the length of time and the amount of pressure necessary to produce the typical urticarial response.

Infections, intoxications, and the excretion of certain animal and plant pigments in the urine probably play a predisposing role in the formation of pressure allergy. Therapy consists of stroking large areas of the body daily with a stiff brush or a rough Turkish towel. Treatments are usually started at six-hour intervals and the duration of the stroking increased by five minutes daily as the interval between the treatments is gradually decreased. The antihistamines may be of value, as well as the corticosteroids; the latter, because of their possible serious side effects, are reserved for very stubborn cases.

ALLERGY TO EFFORT

This is the rarest of all physical allergies. Urticaria develops after exertion, in most cases reported after strenuous exercise or athletics. The condition is said to be most common in people between the ages of twelve and fifty. Women are more likely to be affected than men.

Many observers have felt that the urticarial wheals produced on exercise were simply evidence of heat allergy. While there are on record a number of cases in which no increase in heat distribution is present, still it is evident that cold deters the reaction and heat augments it. As in other forms of physical allergy the release of histamine or a histamine-like substance is involved in the production of the hives. Whether this is a pure allergy (antigen-antibody) reaction is doubtful. The present feeling is that the chemicals are liberated from stimulation of the central nervous system. Treatment consists of mild exercises slowly progressing daily or every other day to more vigorous ones. Diathermy has been used with some success, and since there is a strong suspicion that effort allergy may be nothing more than heat allergy, the treatment advised for heat allergy is often employed.

SUMMARY

Physical allergy is thought to be a true allergy manifestation but the release of histamine or a histamine-like substance said to cause the reactions is considered by many to be caused by mechanical stimulation of the cells, or by some effect on the central nervous system. The common forms of physical allergy are allergy to heat, cold, light, pressure, and effort. Both local and generalized reactions can occur. Urticaria is the most frequent lesion produced.

There are specific tests for physical allergies and treatment depending upon the form present. The most useful drugs are the antihistamines. In severe cases, it is sometimes necessary to resort to corticosteroids ("cortisone"). The best and simplest form of treatment is avoidance of the physical agent responsible for the discomfort.

Chapter Fifteen

Less Frequent Manifestations of Allergy

Although it is true that the majority of symptoms of allergy diseases originate in the respiratory tract or the skin, the site of an allergy reaction, the shock tissue, is not limited to these areas. Theoretically, any part of the body, any organ or system, can be attacked, so that allergic reactions may occur in such unrelated anatomical structures as the central nervous system and the bony joints of the body. Some organs, such as the eyes, and some structures, such as the gastrointestinal tract, are more commonly affected than others. In many of the conditions to be described, it has not been conclusively proved that allergy is solely or partially responsible, but in all there is a suspicion that it may be implicated in some way not yet determined.

ALLERGY OF THE CENTRAL NERVOUS SYSTEM

Headaches

Since an aching head is purely a subjective symptom and each person's tolerance to pain varies, headache is a symptom that is difficult to delimit and categorize. In experiments on the opened skull during brain surgery, the late Dr. Harold Wolff of New York and his associates showed that there are few anatomical structures within the skull that can produce pain. And in those few limited areas, they demonstrated that there are relatively few mechanisms able to initiate or stimulate painful sensations. These are (1) pressure on certain nerves with pain-conducting fibers; (2) the closing and opening of arteries within the skull; (3) inflammation of some sensitive structures of the brain; (4) the stretching of major blood vessels within the skull; (5) tightening of the muscles of the scalp and neck; and (6) any type of stimulation in a disease of the eye, ear, nose, or paranasal sinuses that may spread into the usual headache areas. Thus, the cause of a headache may vary from brain tumor, hemorrhage within the brain, infection, a change in pressure within the skull, an aneurysm (dilatation of the wall of an artery forming a pulsating sac), widening and narrowing of the arteries of the brain, to the common headache caused by emotions, the mechanism of which is difficult to explain. This last type of headache is also called psychogenic pain or tension headache.

Since the causes of headaches are so numerous, it is often difficult to determine the exact causative factor. Further complicating the problem is the inevitably present emotional component. In order to simplify the concept of the headache of allergic origin, some liberties have been taken with terminology. The term *allergic headache* has been adopted to describe the type of headache that varies in location and intensity, is often caused by food, and is not necessarily associated with any other form of headache. It is very likely that this type of headache is caused by some spasm of the cerebral arteries. *Headache associated with allergic rhinitis* (hay fever of either the seasonal or the perennial type) refers to an ache that most commonly involves the face and forehead as a result of sinus involvement accompanying hay fever. *Migraine* is a headache of an intense character attributable to disturbances in the blood flow within the skull; in many cases it is believed to be a true manifestation of allergy. *Histamine cephalalgia,* or *cluster headache,* is not universally considered a true allergy in the sense of an antigen-antibody reaction, although recently a group of investigators found food sensitivities to be responsible for a large percentage of their cases. This type of headache is associated with watering of the eye and runny nose on the same side of the head affected by the headache.

Allergic Headaches

These may be vascular headaches; that is, the blood vessels of the head or face are involved. Frequently, it is described as a severe throbbing ache or pain originating in the frontal area (the forehead just above the eyes) but gradually spreading and becoming general over the entire head. Occasionally they assume other forms. For example, allergic headaches may appear in any part of the head, face, or neck and not have any characteristic distribution. Every person with this type of headache forms his own individual pattern.

The allergic headache, first described in 1931, differed entirely from the well-known migraine headache that had been described many, many years before in that there was no family history of headaches; the attacks developed without any warning; the pain was variable in location and the attack was not ordinarily accompanied by nausea or vomiting or by a warning as is typical of the classical migraine headache. They are believed to be due to some specific allergen or group of allergens, usually ingested or inhaled. Allergy skin tests are used to detect the cause but cannot always be relied upon.

Among inhalant allergens, house dust is most frequently implicated. Nevertheless, any environmental element to which the person is allergic may be the cause. Tobacco smoke has been blamed by many, particularly those whose headache is not otherwise explainable, but most allergists regard it as a nonspecific irritant rather than a true allergen. On the other hand, nicotine has been recognized as a potent constrictor of blood vessels and it may well be that the nicotine content of tobacco smoke is the important factor. Attempts to prepare an effective extract of tobacco smoke for desensitizing treatment has not yet been entirely successful, but antigens to desensitize against other ordinary inhalants are readily available and constitute the form of treatment that is usually employed.

There are numerous medical reports regarding the allergenicity of foods in the allergic headache. In each report the number of cases cited is large and the methods used to prove that foods are responsible vary. Some investigators, for example, used skin tests, others employed a simple restricted diet, and many used a series of "trial diets." When relief was obtained by any of these measures, the suspected foods were not eaten for several weeks. Ultimately, the patients were returned to their regular diets. Some were permitted one food at a time, with a week or more between trials. If the headache returned after a certain food was eaten, it was withdrawn again. By repeating this procedure several times it was possible to state with adequate conviction that a specific food produced the headache. The reported results and the experience of allergists vary greatly. On the whole, however, with careful supervision of one's diet, if foods are the cause of the allergic headache, they can be discovered.

With the emotions playing a role in all headaches, particularly allergic headaches, suggestion and a sense of security inspired by confidence in the physician cannot fail to play a part in successful treatment. Those who embark enthusiastically on a series of diets or a restricted one in any form and remain faithful to them are particularly prone to suggestion; their hope of detecting the causative food makes them prone to color their reports. The likelihood of patients who have taken an unlimited number of injections pretending to have secured relief when none was experienced probably is not very great. A case has been reported of a woman who believed that her headaches were due to milk. She was given milk masked as a nondairy product and no headache developed. When water was substituted in the mixture and she was told it was milk, she immediately complained of a severe headache. This type of a case report casts only a slim doubt upon the reliance of food as a causative factor of the allergic headache, for in the large majority of cases a person's reactions can be relied upon.

Headaches Associated With Allergic Rhinitis

When Dr. C. H. Eyermann first suggested the term allergic rhinitis, he included in his classification those who had pain resulting from swelling (edema) of the nasal membranes and sinuses. This group of headaches was later separated from the type just described because of the site of the reaction. In the allergic headache the blood vessels are implicated; in the headaches associated with allergic rhinitis, the lining membranes of the nose and sinuses are affected. Such headaches are common during hay fever seasons. As seen by the doctor, the lining of the nose is generally pale, grayish-white or bluish-gray in appearance; the turbinates (thin curved bones on the outside walls of the nasal passage) are frequently enlarged; and nasal polyps obstructing the breathing space of the nose may be present. X rays may show the swelling of the membranes or the presence of fluid or even pus in the sinuses. However, it is well known that sinus X rays are not always clear because of the overlay of bony structures. There are tests, however, to determine whether a headache stems from allergy rather than from an infection.

The severity of the pain of headache associated with allergic rhinitis varies more with the individual than with the amount of swelling of the membranes and the degree of nasal obstruction. Tolerance to pain is an individual matter. In addition, nasal obstruction without sinus involvement need not produce headache.

Treatment of this type of headache is essentially the same as treatment of the underlying allergic rhinitis and sinusitis. Antihistamines (described in Chapter 11) taken by mouth often give adequate relief. The local use of nose drops or sprays to constrict and shrink the tissues of the nose and clear the sinus openings may give help temporarily by promoting drainage of the sinuses. Definitive treatment requires investigation by the doctor, including a diagnostic medical history, examination, and invariably a number of pertinent allergy skin tests. When the cause is determined, removal or avoidance of the cause is indicated, if possible. When pollen or another ubiquitous inhalant such as house dust is responsible, desensitization must usually be resorted to. This often relieves the allergic rhinitis and sinusitis and prevents or relieves the accompanying headaches. (See Chapter 11 for a description of the investigation of allergic rhinitis and for a description of desensitization.)

The boggy membranes of the nose and sinuses lend themselves readily to infection and this may complicate the problem of treatment. When infection is present, antibiotics by mouth or by injection are notably effective. The local use of antibiotics in nasal sprays or nose drops carries the hazard of the person becoming allergic to them; sometimes the use of this type of nosedrop also produces a primary irritation. *Rhinitis medicamentosa* is used to describe nasal symptoms due to irritation of the lining of the nose by medication.

Migraine

Migraine is one of the oldest diseases described in medical literature. The classical attack consists of three distinct phases: (1) the prodrome, or warning of the approaching headache, (2) the pain itself, and (3) the aftereffect of the headache. The prodromal stage in the classical case usually consists of the sensation of flashes of lightning before the eyes (scintillating scotomata). However, there is no limit to the variety of prodromal symptoms. They have been described as numbness of the nose, canker sores, abdominal pain, constipation, craving for sweets, dryness of the mouth, dizziness, and many other conditions. Even when the eye symptoms predominate, they are not necessarily limited to streaks of lightning before the eyes but may take the form of blurred vision, intolerance to light (photophobia), and varying degrees of blindness. The symptoms of this stage of the illness are believed to be caused by temporary constriction (narrowing) of certain blood vessels that supply the cerebrum, and similar constriction of the retinal vessels (the retina being that part of the eye that receives images). The changes in the cerebrum caused by diminished blood supply (ischemia) have been recorded by electroencephalography (a procedure for recording the electrical activity of the brain).

The headache is usually described as unilateral (one side of the head), but in many cases it may be bilateral. Occasionally, it begins on one side and then travels to the other. There are patients whose headache is confined to the back of the neck or the midline of the forehead. The quality of the ache varies but most frequently it is a throbbing or pulsating pain in its early stages. Sufferers describe it as "the pressure of an iron band around my head," "a feeling as if a hammer is pounding on the top of my head," or "the feeling of needles being pushed through my eye." When the throbbing stops it is usually followed by a steady ache that may last for hours or days. The pain may spread to the face, neck, shoulders, and arms. Usually the victim is more comfortable in a dark quiet room, since the slightest sound or even a ray of light may accentuate the ache.

Nausea and vomiting, sometimes only one but often both, usually accompany an attack of migraine. This is responsible for the name "sick headache." Rarely does vomiting, if it occurs, relieve the headache until dry retching occurs. Then the retching and the headache may subside simultaneously. In this stage the patient perspires and an abnormal amount of saliva may be produced and drool from the mouth. There may be tearing of the eyes. Toward the end of the attack there is often some fever.

During the headache, widening, swelling, and enlargement of the arteries within the skull occur. Electrical and mechanical tracings of the arterial pulsations show a very high amplitude of pulsation or throbbing. Stimulation of pain-sensitive nerves by the pressure of the dilated vessels is presumed to cause the headaches. In prolonged headaches the areas in and around the swollen arteries, as well as the arteries themselves, may become swollen.

The third stage of the headache, when it occurs, consists of a feeling of exhaustion, weakness, and need for sleep, especially if the attack has been of long duration. Excretion of urine is accelerated. It is evident that with the headache there is widespread disturbance of the entire body.

Migraine may start in childhood, often unrecognized by parents and some doctors who misinterpret the complaint of head pain and stomach distress. The symptoms are the same as those in adults, except that the head pain may be overshadowed by the stomach symptoms. Cyclic vomiting (periodic attacks of vomiting) is a common illness in children considered to be "nervous." There seems to be a clear correlation between such vomiting spells in children and migraine. They may alternate, or the cyclic vomiting may appear at an early age and be followed by "sick headaches" when the child approaches puberty.

The majority of those with migraine give a family history of similar attacks, and it is not uncommon for several members of a family to have migraine. Many patients have, or have previously had, some definitive allergy illness. These facts have led many to state unequivocally that migraine is a true allergy disease. Although allergy may indeed be a cause of migraine it is not the only one.

In some cases there is undoubtedly a hormonal influence, since the headaches are often associated with puberty, menstruation, and menopause. But there is no evidence indicating in what way these events are associated with the production of the headache. During pregnancy many women are relieved of their headaches, but again there is no explanation of why the change in the hormone secretion is responsible. Contrarily, there are many women whose migraine attacks are worsened during pregnancy.

In susceptible allergic individuals, foods have been proved to cause migraine attacks, and avoidance of these foods has given relief. Some attacks are initiated following contact with a specific inhalant allergen. An association with other allergy diseases may be found; an increase in eosinophiles is further indication that the cause of the headache may be due to allergy. But definitive proof verified by laboratory procedures that migraine is a true allergy (antigen-antibody reaction) is still lacking. Empirically, however, since a large number of migraine sufferers have been relieved with allergy management, allergy investigation is warranted. Milk, wheat, eggs, chocolate, nuts, pork, peas, peanuts, and fish have often been cited as causes but it is more likely that if foods are responsible, they are those not eaten regularly. Therefore, for detection of this type of food sensitivity, the keeping of a food diary as described in Chapter 8 is essential. Allergy skin tests are of limited value.

At best the treatment of migraine is not always satisfactory. Nonetheless, there are some medicines that do give relief when used properly, particularly at the beginning of an attack. Many medicines used for migraine contaim ergot; this drug is taken only under a doctor's supervision and is cautiously employed in the presence of high blood pressure, evidence of heart disease, or a circulatory disorder. Aspirin gives some migraine sufferers relief, but usually a stronger pain-relieving medicine is necessary; even narcotics are used.

In all cases an evaluation has to be made about the stresses and strains of daily life. The attitude of a person toward the problems with which he may be confronted is perhaps more important in the treatment of migraine than in most other diseases. Severe emotional strain is an important cause of any headache. Psychotherapists help a person to recognize and "ventilate" his difficulties in order to relieve his inner conflicts and reorganize his personality. A person who has migraine should realize the difficulties and time-consuming nature of the treatment. Above all, in this difficult disease, a good patient-physician relationship is essential.

Histamine Cephalalgia

This condition was first described by Dr. B. T. Horton of the Mayo Clinic who made the distinction between histamine headache and histamine cephalalgia. *Histamine headache* is the normal, full feeling in the head which every person will experience after an injection of an adequate dose of the chemical histamine or after any medicine which dilates the arteries, such as nicotinic acid or nitroglycerine. *Histamine cephalalgia*, according to Horton, is a distinct feeling which occurs in some people without the administration of histamine. The attacks are of short duration and last from a few minutes to an hour, but may recur several times during the day. The excruciating headache is usually unilateral and is described as burning, boring, and pounding; it frequently occurs at night, often starting and stopping abruptly.

Typically, there is watering of the eye and running of the nose (rhinorrhea) on the same side where there is pain; often perspiration is present. In the susceptible person the characteristic attack can be precipitated by a provocative dose of histamine under the skin or intravenously. The injection first results in the usual dull ache in the head, characteristic of the simple histamine headache. A short time later severe histamine cephalalgia is produced.

Horton advised a course of treatment with histamine ("histamine desensitization") intravenously. A modification of this form of treatment is injections given subcutaneously. The treatments are begun with an extremely small dose of histamine in a very diluted form twice daily. The injections are continued up to the maximum tolerated dose and the headaches are relieved. The maximum dose is given daily thereafter for two weeks. A transient, throbbing headache and flushing of the face is considered a normal response to a histamine injection; if a severe and intolerable headache develops during the course of "building up the dose," the subsequent dose is either repeated or reduced before an attempt is made once again to raise the dose. Horton recommends that a person be instructed to give his own injections and continue the maintenance injection dose indefinitely, even for life. Most doctors do not concur and do not even find this type of treatment effective. However, many who do have modified the procedure so that the injections need be given only at intervals of three to fourteen days. Some doctors use the histamine in drops under the tongue as an alternative to the injections.

Recently a group of investigators reported that they found food allergy to be the cause of histamine cephalalgia in 98 percent of their cases. It is such a finding that suggests allergy may be a factor in the production of histamine cephalalgia and makes investigation of food allergy essential. A very restricted diet is the best manner of discovering whether foods are at fault. A diet of lamb, rice, maple sugar, pears, and salt has been suggested. After a week one food at a time is added at intervals of three days. Adhering to a diet such as this is trying, but if good results ensue, it is worthwhile.

Epilepsy

This is the term used for any convulsive disorder of the nervous system. Epilepsy may be caused by organic brain damage, but in most instances the cause in unknown. There are several types of "idiopathic" (cause unknown) epilepsy classified on the basis of severity of symptoms. The most severe is known as *grand mal,* the lesser is called *petit mal.* When a momentary lapse occurs it is spoken of as a *psychomotor* attack. Still another form is the *infantile spasm* which occurs during the first three years of life but usually becomes the more severe type of epilepsy.

The grand mal attack in its most characteristic form consists of (1) an aura or premonition of an oncoming seizure, (2) a cry, (3) loss of consciousness, (4) a fall, (5) a fit, consisting of convulsions, (6) urinary and fecal incontinence, and (7) a lapse into a deep sleep or exhaustion. The psychomotor attack consists of loss of consciousness, performance of movements which are purposeless and automatic, without any falling or convulsion. It usually lasts only one or two minutes.

It must not be implied that allergy is a common cause of epilepsy. Nevertheless, there are numerous documented reports by competent physicians indicating that some cases of epilepsy are caused by allergy.

All agree that when the following criteria are met, allergy must be very seriously considered:

1. A family or personal history of allergy.

2. Eosinophilia (increase in eosinophiles, a type of white blood cell) preceding and during attacks.

3. Positive allergy skin tests.

4. Absence of demonstrable organic brain disease.

5. A characteristic electroencephalographic pattern of the disease.

Allergy management has proved successful in controlling the convulsions in a certain number of cases. Antihistamines have been used with variable results. They are helpful in some children; in some adults they appear to aggravate the symptoms. For this reason, antihistamines are used carefully in adult epileptics.

Multiple Sclerosis

Multiple sclerosis is a disabling neurological disease in which there is a disturbance of sensation, gait, and certain reflexes. The first symptoms are those of numbness and tingling of the hands and feet. Later, difficulty in walking develops since the position sense is impaired; there are other characteristic symptoms. The fact that the cause is unknown and the disease is characterized by remissions (periods in which the symptoms disappear for a variable length of time) has led to one theory that the individual may be reacting to some undiscovered allergen. Unfortunately, this question has not yet been satisfactorily resolved.

ALLERGY OF THE CARDIOVASCULAR SYSTEM

Allergy involvement of the cardiovascular system is a rare and controversial aspect of the broad field of clinical allergy. Nevertheless, there are certain aspects of heart and blood vessel diseases that appear to have a distinct allergy background. Another aspect of allergy as related to heart disease, known as autoimmune disease, is discussed in Chapter 17. These discussions do not imply that allergy is a major cause.

Although considerable confirming evidence has been presented, there still remains some doubt, since to prove that an outside allergen is capable of producing a heart or blood vessel disorder, the same evidence is required as in any other disease; that is, when the offending allergen is eliminated, the heart or blood vessel disorder should return to normal. When contact with the allergen occurs again, the same symptoms as originally described should recur. These criteria have not always been met in the cases reported.

The tissues do not revert to normal as in hay fever or bronchial asthma after the allergenic factor or factors have been eliminated. Once an allergen has injured the heart or blood vessels, the damage has been done and the condition persists.

Changes In Cardiac Rhythm

Abnormalities in the heart rate and regularity (rhythm) due to allergy have been described; in some instances, but not all, they have not met the criteria mentioned above. *Extrasystoles* (premature beats) have been reported. They are not really "extra" beats of the heart as perceived by the patient. An extrasystole is actually a missed beat of the heart followed by a premature beat just before the next one is normally due, so that two beats come in rapid succession, giving the impression of the extra or double beat.

In other instances it has been shown that certain foods can induce *paroxysmal tachycardia* (recurrent periodic attacks of an abnormally rapid heartbeat), as well as *fibrillation* (rapid rate with irregular rhythm) and *flutter* of the heart. Similar reactions have occurred after the administration of certain drugs such as penicillin. In some persons, smoking will cause an increase in the heart rate but this may be due to the normal pharmacologic activity of the nicotine rather than to an allergic reaction to tobacco smoke. When the heartbeat is affected by external allergens, the other manifestations of allergy are usually present.

Angina Pectoris

The symptoms of *angina pectoris,* principally sudden viselike pain and pressure in the chest, are produced by spasm of the coronary artery which supplies the heart muscle with blood. Certainly, there are more likely causes of angina pectoris than allergy, usually ascertainable during a physical examination and by laboratory procedures. But in a certain number of cases, pollen, drugs, a serum administered, or foods have been shown to be the cause. Tobacco smoke and physical allergy to heat or cold, if not essential causes, are certainly contributing factors in coronary spasm.

Acute Coronary Insufficiency

This is merely an extended state of angina pectoris. In angina, the pain is short and often severe, quickly relieved by rest and the use of blood vessel dilating medicines, such as nitroglycerin. In *coronary insufficiency*, the pain is prolonged and is not relieved as rapidly. In *coronary occlusion* there is actual death of heart muscle fibers in certain segments, often leaving a residual scar. The differential diagnosis of these three conditions rests on measurements of the electrical impulses of the heart by the electrocardiograph. Laboratory tests also indicate the presence of heart muscle damage in the early stages. Allergy has been implicated in coronary spasm (angina and acute coronary insufficiency) but not in coronary occlusion, except as damage to the heart muscle may result from anaphylactic shock. In an allergic individual with coronary disease, allergy should be investigated and treated promptly but diet, drugs, proper exercise, rest, and blood thinners, when indicated, remain the basis of proper management.

Essential Hypertension

Essential hypertension, also known as *benign, idiopathic* or *primary hypertension* is blood pressure that is above normal for the given age and sex and for which no cause has been ascertained. Allergy has been suggested as being implicated but the frequency with which high blood pressure is caused by an allergic reaction is in doubt. There is much, however, to indicate that allergy has a definite effect on arterial tension. In some instances omission of certain foods may lower blood pressure and eating these foods causes an elevation. In many allergy conditions blood pressure may drop instead of rise. This is true in some cases of angioedema and bronchial asthma. On the other hand, the labored breathing in bronchial asthma and the administration of certain anti-asthmatic drugs may elevate the blood pressure. Kidney disease caused by allergy factors is also a cause of high blood pressure.

A sudden drop in blood pressure is characteristic of anaphylactic shock, as described in Chapter 2. Nevertheless, essential hypertension due to a proved allergic reaction is indeed rare.

Thromboangiitis Obliterans

This rather uncommon disease, also known as *Buerger's disease*, is a chronic recurring inflammation of the arteries and veins, chiefly those of the legs, resulting in obliteration of the blood vessels. The pain is excrutiating and is generally worse at night. There is diminished sensation of heat and cold. Gangrene of the toes often develops. Because it usually appears in men between the ages of fifteen and fifty who are heavy smokers, smoking has been considered to be the most important factor in its production. One view holds that thromboangiitis obliterans occurs only in smokers and that if this diagnosis is made in nonsmokers there has been a confusion with some other form of arterial disease such as hardening of the arteries. Because of the type of tissue alteration (fibrinoid), the edema (swelling), and the presence of eosinophiles, there has always existed some suspicion that an allergic reaction was the basis of the disease. Dr. Joseph Harkavy of New York was perhaps the first to demonstrate by skin tests that a sensitivity to tobacco existed in the majority of the sufferers. But many allergists still question the conclusions of Dr. Harkavy and the allergic etiology of this disorder. The question of tobacco allergy, particularly as related to cardiovascular disease, remains controversial.

Myocarditis, Pericarditis, and Endocarditis

Myocarditis is an inflammation of the heart muscle. *Pericarditis* is an inflammation of the membranous, cone-shaped sac that encloses the heart. *Endocarditis* is an inflammation of the lining of the heart, often confined to the lining of the heart valves. These conditions are most frequently caused by infection but in some cases of myocarditis occuring in pregnant women it has been thought that it might be due to hypersensitivity to the unborn child. Although a few cases caused by external allergens have been reported, they are not well documented. The most frequently attributed allergy cause is a reaction to drugs and biological products, such as tetanus antitoxin or diphtheria antitoxin. Pericarditis as an autoimmune disease following coronary occlusion has been mentioned.

Hematopoietic

Hematopoietic means "relating to blood-making processes." The disturbances ascribed as possibly due to allergy include *agranulocytosis* (a disease in which there is a marked reduction or absence of neutrophils, a particular type of white blood cell in the circulating blood), different types of *purpuras* (diseases which result in hemorrhages into the skin), and various *anemias,* hemolytic and hypoplastic (conditions in which there is a reduction in the number of circulating red blood cells or hemoglobin by destruction or otherwise). Most, if not all, of these pathological states, if allergic, are caused by a drug reaction, or some allergen formed within the body. These are discussed in Chapter 9 and to a lesser extent in Chapter 17.

ALLERGY OF THE EYE

Allergy of the eye is very common. In hay fever the conjunctiva (the covering of the eyeball and lining of the eyelids) becomes red, the eyelids become swollen and itchy and the eyes water. An allergic reaction of the eye, however, is not limited to merely the eyelids and conjunctivas. The cornea (the clear transparent front part of the eye), the sclera (white portion of the eye), the uveal tract (middle pigmented segment of the eye), the lens (the crystalline section of the eye), the optic nerve (which harbors the special sense of sight), and the retina (the innermost part of the eye which receives the image formed by the lens and is connected to the brain by the optic nerve) may all be involved.

Lids

An allergic rash on the eyelids is usually due to contact. It is most often observed in women, since the most common cause is contact with a cosmetic. When cosmetics are implicated the change from one brand of cosmetic to another may provide a solution. Currently many fine so-called hypo or nonallergic cosmetics are manufactured, including face powders and facial creams, eyebrow pencil, mascara, and virtually every other form of makeup. Eyeglass frames have also been incriminated. Plastics, gold, silver, and nickel in the frame are responsible for many of the reactions in and about the eye.

The list of substances capable of producing contact dermatitis of the eyelids will continue to grow as new materials which may come in contact with the eyes are manufactured and used. Frequently a cosmetic perhaps applied innocuously elsewhere on the body produces a dermatitis when in contact with the eyelids. Fingernail polish, for example, commonly does not injure the nail at all, but when a woman inadvertently runs her finger over her eyes and the polish comes in contact with the lids, a dermatitis may be produced. The nail has thicker protection which acts as a barrier to penetration, whereas the skin of the eyelids is thin and of fine texture, allowing absorption.

The symptoms of dermatitis of the eyelids are the same as dermatitis elsewhere and range from mild irritation to severe itching and burning. The appearance of the skin in the area varies from slight redness in acute cases to brownish discoloration and thickening as the condition becomes chronic. In the case of a contact dermatitis the rash should subside when the contact is removed. While this is taking place a mild boric acid ointment or wet application with boric acid or witch hazel may be soothing. The commercial nonprescription eyedrops can be used; they are ordinarily harmless and may provide comfort. Since there are causes of dermatitis of the eyelids other than allergy, a physician should be consulted about such a rash.

Conjunctiva

The most common evidence of allergic conjunctivitis is that which accompanies hay fever. Intense itching, watering of the eyes, unusual intolerance to light (photophobia), and a burning and annoying sensation simulating a foreign body in the eye are present in varying degrees. *Acute allergic conjunctivitis,* however, may occur in the absence of any symptoms of hay fever, as a primary symptom of allergy caused by local exposure to an allergen; occasionally it may be produced by a food, but in that case there are usually more generalized and additional evidences of allergy. Since there are other causes of acute conjunctivitis including virus infection, a doctor should always be consulted when the conjunctiva is affected. This is particularly true in the *chronic* form where, although the symptoms are similar to that of acute form, there is little visible evidence of inflammation, such as redness and swelling. Because of this, many persons who have chronic allergic conjunctivitis and complain of the symptoms—but show little evidence of eye trouble—are often accused of being neurotic. One of the methods of confirming the diagnosis is the microscopic examination of scrapings from the eyelids. The presence of a large number of eosinophiles is often indicative of allergy.

Vernal conjunctivitis, or *vernal catarrh,* is a particularly severe type of conjunctivitis that occurs in the warm months of the year. Since this is the time of the year when plants pollinate, it has long been thought that pollen may be the cause. Sometimes this is true, but usually it is not. Actually the cause is still unknown. In this condition there is severe itching of the eyes and marked photophobia. Both eyes are affected and the conjunctiva of the eyelids when inverted discloses small elevations, routinely called "cobblestones." As in other forms of conjunctivitis, acute and chronic, scrapings of the eyelids reveal a large number of eosinophiles, suggesting allergic etiology. A delayed reaction to molds (mildew) sometimes occurs and there have been reports of successful treatment by mold desensitization, but on the whole, treatment of vernal conjunctivitis has been notably difficult. In severe cases, the condition may become so progressive and the "cobblestones" so large that surgery must be resorted to.

Phlyctenular conjunctivitis is another form of conjunctivitis in which small red elevations appear at the edge of the cornea where it joins with the sclera. This area is called the *limbus corneae.* Since the cornea is involved, conjunctivitis is not a very accurate term; keratitis would be more accurate. Thin, debilitated children are subject to this condition and may respond to proper hygiene and a balanced diet. Dramatic results have been noted from local and general treatment with corticosteroids.

Cornea

Inflammation of the cornea, *keratitis,* is often seen as an extension of the more superficial conjunctivitis. One form may develop in congenitally syphilitic children; this is thought to be an allergy to the germ of syphilis, the *spirochete.* Small pinpoint *ulcers of the cornea* have been described, resulting from local use of eye medications such as local anesthetics, from circulating pollen and dusts, and from ingestants such as foods. *Recurrent dendritic (tree form) corneal ulcers* have been ascribed to food allergy. These ulcers, unlike other manifestations of allergy, do not respond to the local use of anti-allergy medications, such as the corticosteroids, and they are not employed, since perforation of the ulcers has been reported following their injudicious use. The more accepted cause is herpes simplex, a virus, and the use of IDU (idoxuridine) is so successful that allergy as a cause is seldom probed.

Keratoconus, literally *conical cornea*, is a disease in which there is an irregular protrusion of the cornea with thinning of the layers. It has been reported to be of allergic as well as metabolic origin. It may be associated with atopic dermatitis and other forms of allergy.

Sclera

Attacks of *episcleritis* (inflammation of the layers of the sclera just under the conjunctiva) have been explained on the basis of an allergy to tuberculoprotein.

Uveal Tract

The uveal tract comprises the iris (the colored membrane in the eye controlling the entrance of light by contraction and dilation), the choroid (the dark layer of blood vessels of the eye between the sclera and the retina), and the ciliary body (that portion of the eye extending from the base of the iris to the front part of the choroid). Inflammation of these portions of the eye has been ascribed to an allergic reaction; a bacterial reaction is cited as the most common type of allergy with the tubercle bacillus most prominent. Proof of bacterial allergy has not yet been substantiated and the finding of an infection with *Toxoplasma gondii* in many cases puts in further doubt the concept of allergy as the underlying cause of uveal tract inflammation.

Sympathetic ophthalmia is an involvement of an uninjured eye following injury to the other. It is considered an allergic reaction, the uninjured eye being sensitized to the uveal pigment of the injured one. This is discussed in Chapter 17.

Lens

Allergic cataracts, which may occur with severe allergy of the skin, have been considered a manifestation of atopic dermatitis. They are not common. *Endophthalmitis phacaoanaphylactica* designates inflammation of the eyeball. Considered an allergic reaction to lens protein substance, it follows rupture of the lens capsule and escape of lens substance into the capsule. As an autoimmune disease it is discussed in Chapter 17.

Retina, Choroid, Optic Nerve

Isolated cases of involvement of these structures may be caused by allergy. *Edema of the optic nerve head* has been described following serum sickness reaction to tetanus antitoxin. *Retinal detachment* caused by food allergy and *retinal hemorrhage* following antitoxin have been reported, but rarely has a responsible allergic mechanism been proved.

GASTROINTESTINAL ALLERGY

No part of the gastrointestinal tract is immune. Symptoms ranging from *aphthous stomatitis* (canker sores) in the mouth to *pruritis ani* (itching of the anus) occur frequently, often as the result of an allergic reaction and most commonly an allergy to a food. At times the symptoms are nonspecific, not seeming to involve any particular portion of the gastrointestinal tract; at other times the symptoms are quite specific, implicating a specific organ or area and sometimes mimicking various very serious diseases that may occur in that particular portion of the body. Thus the symptoms may range from mild nausea and vague stomach distress or unexplainable diarrhea to a severe pain such as occurs in appendicitis or gall bladder colic. Gastrointestinal allergy is never fatal. The possibility of graver illnesses must be excluded before the diagnosis of allergy is made.

When other diseases are ruled out, and particularly when there is a history of some other allergy or a family history of allergy, gastrointestinal allergy is then carefully considered. Sometimes the eosinophile count in the circulating blood may be found above the normal of 4 percent, or a stool examination may show many additional cells. If so, this aids in diagnosing gastrointestinal allergy. For the most part, the diagnosis is made by exclusion except when there are special conditions which may be caused by allergy and which are discernible by simple methods.

The Mouth

Aphthous stomatitis (canker sores) are small white sores or spots that appear on the mucous membrane of the mouth. They are usually considered a virus infection but may also result from ingestion of some food or drug to which the person is allergic. They may be due to a combination of virus infection, an allergy, and an irritant. In some instances the activity of the virus may be intensified by the allergy or the irritant. Skin tests are seldom helpful; more often a detailed account of what unusual foods are eaten or what drugs are being taken gives a clue to the cause. Among the foods, nuts appear to be most often implicated, but any food to which the person is allergic can produce the sores.

For combating the virus infection the local use of antibiotics, in the form of lozenges which can be dissolved in the mouth or as the ingredient of a mouthwash, has proved helpful. Many antihistamines have a local anesthetic action and relief from the pain from a canker sore can sometimes be dramatically relieved by merely pressing an antihistamine tablet against it. A cortisone derivative in a specially prepared dental cream is often effective (Kenalog in Orobase).

Stomach

Here allergy symptoms are variable. They may be acute or chronic. In the acute form, the pain may be sharp and severe, accompanied by nausea, vomiting, and abdominal distress—in simple terms, a "stomachache." Often stomach allergy is mistakenly diagnosed as peptic ulcer; the symptoms are frequently quite similar. A severe allergic reaction involving the stomach and the rest of the tract is manifested by diarrhea with watery stools which may become bloody.

Gastroscopic studies indicate that edema of the lining of the stomach or lower portion of the esophagus is a constant finding. Biopsy may show eosinophile infiltration. If allergic involvement of the stomach continues over a long period of time, irreversible damage may be done to the lining of the stomach, interfering with food entering and leaving (cardiospasm and pylorospasm). Milk is the most common allergen causing such a problem in infants.

Intestinal Tract

In the intestinal tract *chronic ulcerative colitis* and *regional enteritis* are the two most common conditions that may be caused by allergy. In ulcerative colitis, as the name suggests, the lesions are in the colon and consist primarily of ulcers accompanied by intestinal spasm, watery stools, and mucus and blood. This may be followed by constipation. The patient is usually thin or emaciated, and afraid to eat because the symptoms might recur. Spasm of the intestinal tract causes pain and discomfort; sometimes there is an intense "burning in the stomach," causing the patient to become nervous, apprehensive, and tense.

Physical examination usually reveals very little except generalized abdominal tenderness. However, if a proctoscopic and sigmoidoscopic examination (by which the physician can look into the lower portion of the colon) is performed, ulcers may be seen.

When allergy to foods is the cause and the offending foods are identified and eliminated, relief of the symptoms follows. A diet—especially one maintained while the search is going on for the allergenic factor—consisting mostly of cooked cereals without hulls or bran, soft-cooked eggs, lean meats, rice, bread or toast, pureed vegetables, creamed soups, cooked or canned fruits without seeds or skin, is frequently prescribed. Alcohol and condiments are especially to be avoided. Emotional problems are often present and must be resolved. Sometimes surgery is required; as a rule, it is resorted to only after all other measures have failed.

Regional enteritis, also known as *terminal ileitis* or *Crohn's disease,* has been attributed to allergy by some investigators. Most allergists do not believe it is a gastrointestinal allergy but rather a complex collagen or autoimmune disease.

Liver And Gall Bladder

There are many causes for liver disease and damage; one may be allergy, particularly a reaction to drugs or food. The assumption is that normally a foreign protein may reach the vein conveying the blood to the liver unaltered. In liver damage due to allergy, because of some changes in the lining of the gastrointestinal tract, a large amount of inadequately digested substances enters the liver circulation and acts as an allergen, with resulting damage to the liver substance. Bile pigments are discharged into the blood, causing a yellowish discoloration of the skin (jaundice). Recurrent headaches and mild stomach and intestinal upsets such as nausea, vomiting, and diarrhea are common complaints. The liver is often found to be enlarged on physical examination.

Laboratory tests (liver function tests) effectively ascertain the extent of liver damage. These procedures are not painful and are simple to perform. In addition to eliminating the offending food or drug, a diet is instituted in which carbohydrates and proteins are freely permitted, while fats, salt, spices, and alcohol are excluded. Any person with liver damage should be under the special care of a physician.

An underlying allergy to a food, drug, or serum may be responsible for some attacks of *biliary colic.* Gallstones may eventually form and typical symptoms of gallstone colic may result. This is a very severe cramplike pain in the upper right quarter of the abdomen. The pain travels, as a rule, to the small of the back and to the right shoulder. Belching, nausea, and vomiting commonly accompany the pain. Both the liver and the gall bladder become enlarged and tender on palpation. X ray examination confirms the diagnosis. A therapeutic test that is frequently used to help in the diagnosis is the injection of a very small amount of epinephrine hydrochloride, a drug which releases allergic spasm. This gives immediate but only temporary relief.

Allergic diseases of the upper intestinal tract may be difficult to distinguish from true gallbladder infection. Nevertheless, allergy must not be overlooked.

Colic

Colic is common in infants and has become almost expected and normal during the first three months of life. There are recurrent intense abdominal cramps for which there is no apparent cause. The infant calls for attention to his trouble by crying. Often, cuddling the crying infant so that its abdomen presses against the mother's warm body relieves the pain. Sometimes, there is accompanying diarrhea or constipation. Although attacks of colic generally subside when the infant reaches three months of age, the condition may last longer. Allergy has been suspected as a primary cause because so many colicky babies are born to allergic parents; in addition, babies are fed on a foreign protein such as cow's milk or mother's milk, as well as other new foods as the diet is increased.

As the child continues to eat the food, he usually becomes "desensitized" to it and the symptoms disappear. Ordinarily, however, an abrupt change of formula, or a change from cow's milk to a substitute immediately stops the attacks. The finding of eosinophiles in the stools establishes the allergic nature of the attacks, but their absence does not exclude it. Allergy skin tests to foods are of limited use and cannot be relied upon. Antihistamines may be administered in doses appropriate for the age and weight of the infant. Paregoric, an old standby of mothers, is a narcotic and must be used with caution. It is not nearly as often prescribed by physicians for colic as formerly, since most doctors are more anxious to find the cause rather than suggest medication that merely gives temporary relief.

Rectum

There are many more common and important causes of *pruritis ani* (itching of the anus) than allergy, including hemorrhoids, anal fissures or fistulas, polyps, irritating vaginal discharges, intestinal parasites, and changes in the acidity of rectal secretions. But allergy has been found to be a direct cause, particularly in those cases that have resisted the usual forms of treatment and when no other more obvious cause has been found. Among the allergens that can produce pruritis ani, food, drugs, and local sensitivity to cocoa butter in rectal suppositories lead the list.

ALLERGY OF THE EAR

One of the most common sites of an allergic rash (*atopic dermatitis*), especially in infants, is the area just behind the ear. In the acute stages of this form of dermatitis, the area is generally moist with much "weeping" and subsequent formation of crusts. The itching is frequently intense and the skin is often covered with signs of scratching. Local treatment is required to give symptomatic relief but an allergy investigation should be pursued. This is discussed more fully in Chapter 13.

Dermatitis venenata of the ear is a rash caused by medication often applied to give relief to ear trouble or a condition in an adjacent area. When the offending medication is removed, the skin immediately begins to heal. Sometimes this condition may be caused by contact with eyeglass frames or earrings.

Repeated *swelling of the parotid gland* in young people may result from allergic sensitivity, usually to foods. The parotid, the largest of the salivary glands, is located behind the upper part of the lower jawbone, which partly overlaps it. Because it is close to the ear, a swelling of the gland may sometimes be confused with actual ear disease. Chronic swelling of the parotid gland may be caused by prolonged use or contact with heavy metals. The swelling must not be mistaken for mumps, which is the contagious type of inflammation of the parotid gland.

Occasionally, the parotid or the submaxillary gland, another salivary gland, situated toward the middle and below the angle of the jaw, reacts to potassium iodide, a drug frequently prescribed for bronchial asthma. The glands swell, but on discontinuation of the drug, the swelling recedes.

The middle ear can be affected by allergy in several ways. The eustachian tube is a connection between the nose and the middle ear which otherwise is completely enclosed. Obstruction causes pressure changes in the middle ear. Many persons experience a full feeling in the head and ears and even become deaf when flying in an airplane, especially in an unpressurized cabin on rapid descent. Allergic patients have much more trouble than others since the eustachian tubes are closed as a result of allergic swelling.

Another disturbance of the middle ear associated with allergy is an inflammation in the middle ear, *chronic secretory otitis media*. Here there is pain, fullness, and deafness, with an occasional accumulation of fluid. The excess fluid is formed as a result of allergy with or without infection. On examination, the doctor can see the eardrum bulging as a result of the fluid pressure. Often it is necessary for an ear specialist to puncture the eardrum (paracentesis), drain the fluid, and insert a small plastic drain which may be left in for weeks or months.

Ménière's disease or *Ménière's syndrome* is characterized by attacks of dizziness, variable deafness, and ringing in the ear (tinnitus), especially on changing position. Often included in the definition of Ménière's syndrome are numerous nondescript symptoms of dizziness involving the semicircular canals in the inner ear. In some cases, deafness may not be present; in others, the dizziness may not be evident, but in all cases there is some degree of imbalance associated frequently with nausea and vomiting.

Some allergists and otologists regard Ménière's disease as limited to attacks of extreme dizziness, nausea, vomiting, and nystagmus (involuntary movements of the eyeball), followed by tinnitus and deafness. The condition is progressive. The term *Lermoyez' syndrome* is used to describe the symptomatology: attacks of tinnitus and deafness followed by dizziness, nausea, and vomiting. This condition is temporary. The differences relate to the sequence of symptoms and the fact that one is usually progressive (Ménière's disease) and the other is temporary (Lermoyez' syndrome). An otolaryngological examination is necessary to differentiate these syndromes from other diseases with similar symptoms, such as brain tumors and diseases of the central nervous system. Allergy can instigate both symptoms.

In addition to a complete allergy survey and elimination of all allergy factors, a salt-free diet is usually prescribed and fluids are limited. When dizziness and loss of equilibrium are marked, it is advisable not to walk on the street alone since a fall could be serious. These persons usually feel better in a darkened room. Stimulating baths and massages are comforting.

Histamine liberated during an allergic reaction is thought to be connected with the production of disorders in the semicircular canals of the inner ear, but treatment with histamine (or desensitization with histamine) has been less than completely satisfactory. In one technique the histamine in solution is administered by intravenous drip, one to two hours daily for three to six days or until good results are apparent; then it is replaced by subcutaneous (under the skin) injections. In the method more popularly employed, all treatments are given by hypodermic injection.

Nicotinic acid is used intravenously as well as orally, but here also the results are variable. Potassium iodide has been employed but is of doubtful value. The same may be said of ammonium chloride. Sedatives and tranquilizers help to calm the patient and allay apprehension. Diuretics are helpful, as are the motion sickness medicines.

ALLERGY OF THE GENITOURINARY TRACT

Allergy of the genitourinary tract is frequently unrecognized, but it may be responsible for many obscure cases of *enuresis* (bed wetting), *painful urination, tenesmus* (spasm causing a persistent desire to empty the bladder with involuntary, ineffectual straining efforts), *urinary retention, cramps,* and *vaginal itching.* Food is the common allergen associated with enuresis. *Cystourethritis,* an inflammation of the bladder and urethra (the tube which extends from the bladder to the surface), may also be caused by allergy. This is rather common and causes painful, frequent urination and tenesmus. When the disease is intractable, bladder allergy may be responsible, particularly when the patient is otherwise known to be allergic or when there is a family history of allergy. The usual treatments consist of bladder irrigations and instillations of appropriate urinary antiseptics; some are given orally. Very probably allergies of the balance of the urinary tract such as the kidney, the ureter (the tube between the kidney and the bladder), and the prostate gland (a gland in males in the vicinity of the neck of the bladder and the central portion of the urethra) are more common than generally thought.

Pruritis vulvae, itching of the external female genitalia, is a most annoying condition that has many causes, among which is allergy. Undergarments, sanitary napkins, or douches may be responsible. Condoms are not used as much as they were prior to "the pill," but allergy to the material of which they are composed can initiate pruritis vulvae. Diaphragms and contraceptive jellies are also causes. Unfortunately, it may be difficult to determine the cause, but once this is done the cure is simple—elimination. For temporary relief, a soothing ointment or cream is helpful. In women past menopause, hormone therapy may be required.

ALLERGY OF THE JOINTS

The frequent involvement of joints in serum sickness has been described in Chapter 2. Among the untoward reactions that penicillin may cause, swelling of the joints is one of the most common. The extent of involvement varies from a mild swelling to a very marked inflammatory reaction. Another possible manifestation of joint allergy is *intermittent hydroarthrosis,* an inflammation of the joint with a collection of fluid within. This occurs most commonly in the knees of girls and young women. Again, treatment consists of removal of the cause. Antihistamines, corticosteroids, and other anti-allergy medicines give some relief.

Rheumatoid arthritis is a chronic disease in which many joints are affected by an inflammatory process resulting in swelling and stiffness, pain and tenderness, and in the latter stages, deformity of the joints. The specific cause is unknown, but it is thought by many investigators that this is a collagen disease in which allergy (autoallergy) may be implicated. This disease is more fully discussed in Chapter 17.

SUMMARY

Theoretically, allergy can attack any part of the body. Some structures are more often involved than others. In many of the diseases described, the allergic component is questionable but in all there is at least a suspicion that allergy may be implicated.

Allergic headaches, in which the vessels of the head or face are involved, are frequently termed vascular headaches. They have no characteristic pattern, varying from individual to individual. Foods are a frequent cause. In the detection of responsible foods, a restricted diet is more often successful than food skin tests. When an inhalant is the cause, it is most frequently house dust. Tobacco, like perfume, is an irritant to some people, but there is some doubt that tobacco is an allergen. A headache associated with allergic rhinitis is clearly associated with the thickening of the lining membrane of the nose and sinuses and is commonly noted during the hay fever season. Since it is difficult for most patients to remove themselves from pollinating plants or to remove the pollen from the air, desensitization treatments are usually prescribed. Antihistamines and the local use of nose drops often give symptomatic relief.

Migraine headache is a severe, often one-sided headache usually associated with nausea and vomiting. Although there are probably other causes, allergy is thought to play an important role. This severe type of headache may occur in children as well as adults. Frequently in children it is associated with cyclic vomiting. In addition to allergy, there may well be some hormonal cause inasmuch as these headaches are related to puberty and menopause in many people. Histamine cephalalgia are excruciating headaches that fortunately are of short duration. They, like migraine, are usually one-sided. Characteristically there is watering of the eye and running of the nose on the side of the headache. There is little doubt that this headache is related in some way to histamine, but histamine desensitization has not proved universally successful.

Epilepsy is a convulsive disorder of the nervous system of unknown cause. However, in some cases, particularly where there is a history of allergy either in the patient or the family, an allergic investigation may be warranted. The same is true of multiple sclerosis, although there are very few proved instances of an allergic cause.

Allergy of the cardiovascular system is rare and even controversial, but some types of heart and blood vessel diseases appear to implicate allergy. Changes in cardiac rhythym may occur, particularly as a reaction to certain drugs. Smoking influences the rhythm of the heart in some people and it has been suggested that there may be an allergic reaction to tobacco smoke. Some cases of angina pectoris, a sudden and severe attack of pain and feeling of oppression about the heart, have been reported to be caused by allergy. Allergy has also been implicated in acute coronary insufficiency, an extended state of angina, but has never been shown to produce coronary occlusion.

The causes of essential hypertension (high blood pressure) have not yet been discovered, but some cases appear to be affected by foods in the diet. Thromboangiitis obliterans is a disease that may result in obliteration of the blood vessels of the leg causing gangrene of the toes. It occurs in those who smoke considerably and some investigators are convinced that this is a disease due to tobacco-smoke sensitivity. The heart muscle, the sac that encloses the heart, and the lining of the heart are subject to infection but instances of allergy producing myocarditis, pericarditis, and endocarditis have been reported, although not well documented. The blood diseases that are thought to be caused by an allergy response are primarily those related to a drug reaction. They are discussed in Chapter 9. Some may be due to autoallergy, a reaction to one's own tissue cells. These are discussed in Chapter 17.

Allergy of the eye is very common. The lids are often affected by contact with some allergenic substance producing a rash. Cosmetics are frequent offenders. Allergic conjunctivitis commonly accompanies hay fever. It may also be caused by allergens other than those in the air, such as foods, but in this case more general signs of allergy are present. Vernal conjunctivitis, appearing usually in the warm months of the year, is thought to be caused by pollen. Molds may be an important factor since they are also present seasonally in the circulating air in particular sections of the country. Phlyctenular conjunctivitis develops primarily in thin, debilitated children. Corticosteroids have produced dramatic results in some cases.

In a disease of the cornea of the eye such as keratitis, corneal ulcers are regarded as a reaction to local medication as well as to circulating pollen, molds, and foods. Recurrent dendritic (tree-form) corneal ulcers are caused by a virus. Keratoconus is an irregular protrusion of the cornea with thinning of the layers. It is considered allergic as well as metabolic in origin. Episcleritis, inflammation of the layers of the sclera just under the conjunctiva has been described as an allergy to tuberculoprotein. Inflammation of all portions of the uveal tract has been periodically reported to have an allergic basis. In sympathetic ophthalmia the uninjured eye reacts to the uveal pigment of the injured one. This is discussed in Chapter 17. Allergic cataract, although not common, may accompany atopic dermatitis. Isolated cases of involvement of the retina, choroid, and optic nerve may be allergic. Retinal detachment caused by food allergy has been reported. Retinal hemorrhage following antitoxin administration may occur but is extremely rare.

The gastrointestinal tract may be affected by allergy; foods are most commonly implicated. Aphthous stomatitis (canker sores) are common reactions. Foods may be the instigating agent, but many are undoubtedly due to a virus. Chronic ulcerative colitis may be a pure allergy disease and many have been relieved by allergy management, but most clinicians feel that there are causes other than allergy which must be investigated.

Liver and gallbladder disease may indicate an allergy, but it is difficult to make the diagnosis accurately. Colic in infants is often a true allergy. Pruritis ani (itching of the rectum) has been cleared under allergy management but there are probably other causes as well.

Allergy of the ear is usually manifested by a rash (atopic dermatitis). Sometimes the rash may be caused by contact with, for example, the frame of eyeglasses or by a drug applied topically (contact dermatitis). Swelling of the parotid gland and the maxillary gland (salivary glands) may be caused by the medicine potassium iodide. When the eustachian tube is blocked, a feeling of fullness, pain, and deafness may be experienced. The tube is occasionally blocked as a result of severe allergic rhinitis (hay fever). Fluid may collect in the inner ear as a result of allergy with or without infection. It may not be absorbed and thus have to be drained by paracentesis (puncture of the eardrum). Ménière's syndrome is characterized by dizziness, variable deafness, and some ringing in the ear (tinnitus) especially when changing position. Allergy may often be responsible. None of the treatments available are very successful.

Allergy of the genitourinary tract may often go unrecognized. Enuresis (bed wetting) has been relieved by elimination of foods to which the person has proved allergic. Other symptoms of the genitourinary tract which may have an allergic basis are painful urination, tenesmus, urinary retention, cramps, and vaginal itching. Cystourethritis may also be due to allergy. Pruritis vulvae may be caused by allergy to undergarments, sanitary napkins, douches, or contraceptive devices.

Swelling and painful joints may accompany serum sickness, as discussed in Chapter 2. Intermittent hydroarthrosis is an inflammation of the joints that occurs mainly in the knees of girls. Many of the medicines used to treat other allergic manifestations provide relief. The specific cause of rheumatoid arthritis is still unknown, but it is thought that there may be an immune mechanism involved.

Chapter Sixteen

Occupational Allergy

If the definition of allergy as an unusual reaction based on an antigen-antibody reaction is accepted, it is almost impossible to categorize occupational allergy exactly because in so many instances the antibody cannot be demonstrated. In occupational allergy there are many diseases that are obviously the result of one's work but cannot be completely included as allergic in the strict definition of the term. Nevertheless, to the worker who has a rash on his hands or develops a chronic cough or severe asthma, the problem of the existence of allergy is purely academic.

A true allergy theoretically cannot occur on first contact; if symptoms result, they are due to the fact that either the person unknowingly has been sensitized, or the substance is an irritant, in which case the reaction is not a true allergy reaction. For that reason, in this chapter there will be many examples of illnesses which do not clearly fit into the exact definition of an allergic reaction. Yet there is some evidence that eventually they may.

The expansion of industry in the last few decades with the manufacture and employment of new materials which expose workers to different dusts, fumes, vapors, gases, chemicals, and abnormal physical factors in the environment has caused much concern. The most important problem is how they may be prevented. Much depends on the inherent susceptibility of the individual and upon the extent of contact or exposure.

Of all the workers' diseases, those affecting the skin are the most common, as the skin is the most likely to be exposed to allergenic contactants. Next in order are those illnesses that are produced by inhalation of noxious substances, particularly over a long period of time. These may be very serious. There are rare instances of occupational allergy due to ingestion and injection. There are many infectious occupational diseases, such as anthrax among leather tanners, and many

261

physical diseases, such as sunstroke or heatstroke in workers exposed to excessively high temperatures, and many other diseases which are often serious. We will only discuss those that are generally considered to be due to an allergy.

OCCUPATIONAL ALLERGIC DERMATOSES

Dermatoses is the plural of dermatosis, any involvement of the skin. Occupational dermatosis is a disease of the skin caused primarily by one's work. Allergy represents the presence of the specific mechanism for the production of allergy disease. A gasoline station attendant whose hands are constantly in gasoline, oil, and grease may develop a rash on his hands as a result of irritation. Although this is an occupational dermatosis, it is not necessarily allergic. A gardener, on the other hand, who has a severe rash on his hands as a result of pulling out poison ivy plants or planting primrose is most likely to have an occupational allergic dermatosis.

Workmen's compensation laws were introduced in the United States in 1911. Today they are commonly invoked, and the management of various industries has helped to control or reduce the incidence of occupational allergic dermatoses by improving plant facilities and instructing employees in how to protect themselves. The current increase in the incidence of contact dermatitis is probably attributable to the increased number of industrial workers and the constant introduction of new, potentially allergenic materials such as the plastics (synthetic resins), coal tar, petroleum products, and the synthetic substances derived from them. Approximately one percent of industrial workers in the United States are affected with some form of occupational dermatosis at any given time, and occupational dermatoses comprise about two-thirds of all occupational diseases for which compensation is paid. Many of these are of allergic origin.

Several factors predispose to the production of an occupational allergic dermatosis. Contact dermatitis, for example, is more likely to occur in one whose sweat glands are very active. ("Dermatitis" means inflammation of the skin.) Some rashes develop only in the presence of moisture. Another factor is the state of the skin. If there is an abrasion, a cut, or if for any other reason the skin is not intact, an otherwise preventable penetration of an allergic substance is likely to occur. One of the most recently discovered factors influencing contact dermatitis is the amount of dark pigment (melanin) in the skin; hence black people are more likely to react to skin irritants and allergens than white people. These dark skins are even more subject to skin cancer. On the other hand, melanin evidently protects the skin against ultraviolet light and heat so that the white person is far more susceptible to a physical dermatitis. Melanin also has an effect on the sweat glands. When sweat is present, the moist skin tends to soften and macerate and there may be a change in the degree of acidity or alkalinity of the skin. In some instances pores may close. This facilitates bacterial and fungus infection, and destroys the normal resistance to many allergenic contactants. Sweat may change the structure of certain ordinarily innocuous chemicals to make them allergenic.

Except for the palms, soles, and ends of the fingers, the exposed skin is usually covered with a protective film of natural oils which keeps it supple and prevents chapping and fissuring. It also helps diminish and even prevent the absorption of certain foreign substances. The fissuring and itching of dry skin may lead to infection, complicate an existing contact dermatitis, and perhaps help a new one to develop.

The skin of a worker who has had atopic dermatitis (eczema) with manifestations of other allergies is likely to react more readily to some allergic contactant. Sex is not a factor. There are fewer women with occupational dermatoses than men, but there are fewer women in industry, and perhaps women are more scrupulous about cleanliness and protect themselves more satisfactorily by washing frequently. The garment trade seems to be an exception, but this is more apparent than real because of the overall different ratio of men to women in this industry.

Textile Industry

Although, understandably, allergic dermatoses can occur in any industry, it appears very often in the wool industry. The wool comes to the factory in bales, and is sorted and then scoured. In the United States, oil solvents such as benzene are frequently employed and may cause a dermatitis in a susceptible person. At this stage, wool is dyed in the raw form; later it may also be dyed as yarn and cloth. This dyed wool may be allergenic, and the worker may be extensively exposed to it.

The process of sorting the waste and rags and tailor clippings into their varying qualities to make "shoddy" is a dirty job; the rags may be contaminated with all kinds of foreign matter which may be allergenic. Another source of occupational danger is in the weaving of the cloth. The weaver must thread the loom, using perhaps as many as fifteen hundred threads for a single piece of cloth. To do this dexterously, he must dip his fingers from time to time into French chalk which has oil and grease solvent properties. This may produce a dermatitis on the index finger and thumb caused by sensitivity not only to the chalk but also to the dye of the threads which he handles, as well as the threads themselves. This skin rash may be a true sensitivity, but in some instances in eczema-prone individuals it is probably caused by irritation.

The dye may be the chief offender in the allergic dermatitis prevalent in wool workers. The variety of dyes is innumerable. Some dyes adhere to the material directly; others require a mordant, a metallic compound that "fixes" the dye as it saturates and adheres to the fibers. The most common mordants are potassium chromate and other salts of the chemical element chromium. *Chrome dermatitis* is common among those who work with such solutions. Many workers wear protective clothing and gloves or gauntlets, but some men find it difficult to do their work with their hands encumbered and prefer to wash their hands often to prevent the dermatitis from developing. Since the strength of the chrome solution affects the frequency and speed with which the rash appears, it would seem that the dermatitis might be due primarily to the irritating quality of the chemical. Some feel that chrome dermatitis is not a true allergy, but most experienced specialists are convinced that "chrome allergy" is a well-established syndrome.

Some dermatologists believe that the rash frequently ascribed to a dye is caused instead by the hypochlorite solution often used to remove the stain of the dye from the skin after work. In the finishing process, the risk of developing an allergic dermatitis is slight. This is also true in the final manufacture of clothing. The dermatitis seen among those who work with wool at this stage is more probably produced by the roughness of the cloth.

Special finishers such as urea-formaldehyde resin have been known to produce a rash. Khaki may produce a fine rash in those who wear this type of shirt or trouser material in uniforms or in work clothes. More recently, this type of plastic coating is being used in many "stay-pressed" garments.

Cosmetics

Contact dermatitis caused by applied cosmetics has been discussed in

Chapter 13, but besides affecting persons who use them, they may also be a cause of dermatitis in people who work in the cosmetic industry, in drugstores, and in other stores that sell cosmetics, and thus come in contact with rouge, powders made from orris root, henna, quince seed oil, gum tragacanth, and gum karaya, among many other possible allergenic substances. The manufacture, processing, and packaging of cosmetics on a large scale is today a highly automated procedure. But personal contact can still take place, particularly in the laboratory, and result in respiratory difficulties as well as skin lesions.

In addition to the cosmetic salesperson who must handle and inhale the cosmetics, the beautician must work with soaps, bleaches, dyes, "fixers," "strippers," creams, lotions, body oils, chemicals, and innumerable other materials capable of producing either a true allergic reaction or an irritating one. The red inflamed hands of a beauty operator are not an uncommon sight in an allergist's or dermatologist's office. Respiratory symptoms from the inhalation of the ingredients of some cosmetics are not rare. The obvious treatment is change of occupation, but this is difficult for one who has spent many years learning the trade.

Medicines

Pharmacists who compound prescriptions are subject to many allergens. Nurses may develop a contact sensitivity to some antibiotics such as penicillin and streptomycin, as well as to disinfectants, ointments, creams, lotions, or aerosols which contain allergenic chemicals.

A nurse may also be exposed to allergenic substances in many other ways: in making of patients' beds, arranging flowers in the sick room, frequent handling of rubber, plastics, and many complex chemicals. Although the contact with allergenic substances may be brief, it certainly is varied. A physiotherapist comes in contact with the chemicals contained in the creams, ointments, and lotions that are used. Eczema can be caused in medical personnel by the procaine derivatives used in local anesthesia and is seen for the most part on the thumb, index, or middle finger which may encounter the anesthetic when the syringe is being filled. This is a particular hazard for dentists and their assistants.

Although general medical practitioners infrequently handle drugs, a large number have been sensitized to antibiotics or antiseptics because of contact with aerosols containing these medications. A surgeon may become sensitive not only to the rubber gloves he must wear but to the talcum that he uses to put them on after "scrubbing up." Lengthy contact with the gloves undoubtedly abets the formation of the dermatitis; enclosure promotes sweat and in turn maceration of the skin, altering the skin's acidity. So-called hypoallergic gloves of latex or neoprene can be substituted for the rubber, but a patch test must be performed to determine whether these too are sensitizers. Housewives sensitive to rubber may wear a cotton or silk glove under the rubber one. Some rubber gloves are lined with cloth of this nature.

Eczema of the fingers may occur in dentists who use their thumb and middle finger to roll metals together to form a filling. American or "silver" fillings contain a considerable amount of mercury, which is a potent sensitizer. There are other sensitizers he must cope with in his profession. These include soap, iodine, grinding dust, plaster of paris, and wax for dental impressions, among many others. Characteristic lesions such as overgrowth of the horny layers of the skin of the finger with deep fissures and often breaking of the nail have so frequently followed the use of Formalin or formaldehyde that the condition has been named formalonyx. Dentists can also be sensitized by the resin or vulcanite in their equipment.

Woods

Although wood has to a great extent been replaced by plastics, it remains the common component of furniture, and occupational allergic dermatitis caused by contact with wood is not rare. Some people are sensitive to just one kind of wood. This has been partly explained by the presence of hardness in some wood products. Coral wood from New Guinea often produces a contact dermatitis. This was not an unusual cause of "jungle rot" in World War II, but any wood can cause a skin reaction if the person is susceptible. Most allergy symptoms caused by woods, however, result from inhalation of their dusts.

Detergents

A person employed in an industry that requires repeated washing of the hands with a detergent may frequently develop a contact dermatitis. A similar dermatitis occurs in housewives; the expression "housewives' hands" is commonly applied. It is debatable whether the commonly used detergents are allergenic or whether the rash they produce is caused by their irritating quality. Patch tests do not appear to prove much. They have been performed on persons who are known to be very intolerant to a detergent and the results have been completely negative. Some investigators believe the reaction to a detergent is attributable to the nickel or chromium it contains.

Metals

Nickel is one of the metals most often responsible for dermatitis in susceptible individuals. In the textile, galvanizing, and graphic industries and in metal mills and joinery works, chromium and nickel are usually employed. Masons come in contact with chromium, and the rash is sometimes observed in bricklayers, perhaps indicating chromate allergy. In the Army and Navy where nickel and chromium identification tags are provided, there are some servicemen who are so sensitive to one or both of the metals that they cannot wear them in close contact with their skin but must let them hang loosely or enclose them in a leather-protected pouch.

Material Used In Printing

In addition to contact metals which are necessary in the printing business, the worker is exposed to numerous other materials. We have discussed the dye of the ink; in addition there is gum arabic. This is a plant juice obtained from the bark of the *Acacia senegal* tree of North Africa, especially in the Sudan region. On exposure to the air the liquid stiffens and is marketed in colorless or yellowish-brown lumps. It is chemically related to the pectins and is probably the oldest-known commercial adhesive. It is also used in pigments and textile finishing, in shoe wax, as a binding agent, in match-making, in confections, and elsewhere. In many printing plants it is used as a spray-on paint to prevent freshly printed pages from sticking together. Exposure to gum arabic can result in a contact dermatitis, while inhalation of small particles of the gum is more likely to cause bronchial asthma or other respiratory allergies.

Tobacco

One can become allergic to the tobacco leaf, and dermatitis among those who work with tobacco leaves, though not common, is demonstrable. This usually occurs among those workers who strip the stem from the leaf. A stripper's hand and wrist are in direct contact with the leaf during the process, making it possible for a contact dermatitis to develop.

In a cigar factory the "cigar maker" who puts on the wrapper uses primarily the thumb and the index or middle fingers; if a dermatitis develops it is usually at these sites. The older "wrapper" still uses his tongue to seal the cigar and consequently his tongue may show signs of a sensitivity reaction. Eczema caused by tragacanth, also used in cigar manufacturing, has been reported. Some manufacturers employ flavoring agents to which the worker may be allergic. Pastes and other adhesives required for labeling cigar boxes may produce a dermatitis.

Plants

Contact dermatitis resulting from the handling of plants by gardeners and nurserymen who come in contact with poison ivy, poison oak, or poison sumac has been discussed in Chapter 13. These plants and perhaps primrose, are the most common offenders, but it is possible that other plants, perfectly innocuous to most people, can also produce a rash in susceptible individuals.

Miscellaneous Chemicals

Photographers are in contact with many chemicals which have been shown to cause allergic contact dermatitis. The chemicals most frequently involved are the developers and fixers: acetic acid, acetone, banana oil, aniline dye, butyl alcohol, mercury, benzine, formaldehyde, hyposulfite (sodium thiosulfate), silver, potassium, chromic acid, or chromate, in addition to the film and printing paper. Leather workers and shoemakers, aside from the common leathers and dyes, handle a great many chemicals which can be allergenic. These include ammonia, antimony, benzine, mercury, copper, carbon tetrachloride, iron, formaldehyde, nickel, potassium, chromic acid, alcohol, turpentine, and various glues and soaps.

OCCUPATIONAL ALLERGIC RESPIRATORY DISEASES

Although the skin because of its size and position is the organ most susceptible to industrial disease, the most incapacitating manifestations of true occupational allergy are the respiratory diseases, such as bronchial asthma and allergic rhinitis (hay fever). These lead the list. The nose (some call it the air conditioner) is the first line of defense. Since it is an extremely sensitive organ, it is not surprising that in certain occupations it is a vulnerable site for response to allergens as well as to irritants. Inhalant allergens after passing through the nose are inhaled into the lungs and may cause bronchial disturbance such as bronchial asthma.

Dusts

Dusts, pulverized or powdery bits of matter, are the most common allergens that produce occupational respiratory allergy. These range from those in factories associated with the making of plastics to those in the outdoor air that are inhaled by outside workers. They include plant and mold materials. Most dusts, if inhaled over a long period of time or in sufficiently high concentrations, are intrinsically irritating, but there are many that, because of their high degree of allergenicity, are especially important in causing true occupational respiratory allergy.

Plastics

In the manufacture of plastics a number of substances which produce dust are utilized; some of these are merely irritating but an ever-increasing number appear to be allergenic. Among these are the *organic isocyanates,* the most commonly used of which is *toluene diisocyanate.* This is a source of asthma for many who come in contact with it. Another isocyanate commonly employed is *hexamethylene diisocyanate;* it is more volatile and may ultimately come to be considered just as hazardous.

The U. S. Department of Labor lists more than a hundred substances from which asthma occurs. The symptoms of asthma produced by these substances are identical with those of bronchial asthma caused by other allergens: difficulty in breathing, cough, and wheezing. The medicines used for relief are also the same and include ephedrine preparations, epinephrine (Adrenalin), and in some cases the corticosteroids. This asthmatic condition is entirely different from lung disease caused by toxic gases used in the manufacture of plastics which sometimes causes bronchitis and inflammation of the lung but more often liver damage and brain intoxication.

Toluene, in a volatile form, commonly employed in the manufacture of *polyurethane foam* plastics, is only likely to be encountered during the manufacturing process. Once the plastic has been formed and set, there is no danger of the gas being released. Polyurethane foams are used very commonly in packaging goods. Some have feared that when it is cut or sawed the toluene that may be released may be harmful. However, it quickly combines with the water vapor and is destroyed. Polyurethane foam products are frequently used in conjunction with asbestos, which is in itself a highly allergenic substance and if inhaled can produce much respiratory difficulty. Other fibrous materials with which urethane plastics may be joined are rock wool and glass wool. These intrinsically create no great problem, but if these fibrous minerals are inhaled from the dust created by sawing or sanding the plastic, they may lodge in the alveoli (the small air pockets in the lung) and cause considerable breathing difficulty. The very small particles may be retained permanently and slowly become surrounded by tissue cells. When they become large enough, they can lodge in the bronchioles during a spasm of the bronchial muscles. There they may remain indefinitely. In an effort to protect the body, nature isolates foreign matter by producing excess scar tissue around the area, with *pulmonary fibrosis* ensuing. Since allergic people are inclined to develop bronchial muscle spasms, it is apparent that allergic individuals under these circumstances are particularly subject to pulmonary fibrosis, even though it is not an allergy disease per se.

Fortunately, many of the plastics in common use do not present any allergenic hazard. *Polyethylene*, for example, is commonly used as a food-packaging material and in garment bags but it has no known allergenicity; nor do the *polyesterene plastics* or *polyvinyl chloride plastics* which are used extensively as automobile and furniture upholstering. Only occasionally is sensitization to *dibutyl* and *diamyl phthalate* as a cause of bronchial asthma reported. These are chemicals used in plasticizing polyvinyl chloride. *Polyepsilon-caprolactam,* contained in varying amounts in nylons, has been an alleged cause of allergic respiratory difficulty but, since it is soluble in water, all risk is over once the nylon is washed.

The *polyacronitrilic* plastics which include Orlon Buna N Rubber are not allergenic to the users of these products nor has there ever been any allergenicity attributed to the *saturated polyester resin plastics* of which Dacron is perhaps the most popular product. Nevertheless, in the production of Dacron, nylon, Orlon, rayon, and Lycra, the lubrication required to prevent the disruption of the delicate fibers may be a potential allergenic hazard to the plant worker if the lubricating oils should be dispersed into the atmosphere. The oils used are known in the trade as "finishers," and their chief ingredient is mineral oil, but other substances (surface-acting agents) may be added by manufacturers. Because of secret processes it is virtually impossible to know the exact formula of each product; some of the additives may be allergenic. There is, for example, a condition known as "yarn plant disability," common among those who are employed in synthetic textile operations, that causes difficulty in breathing. It has been postulated that this disease may be caused by an allergic response to one of the chemicals used as a "finish."

Teflon is practically inert but it contains *fluorine* (monomeric tetrafluorethylene). When Teflon is heated, the tetrafluorethylene is liberated and if oxygen is present, it is broken down into *hydrogen fluoride, carbon tetrafluoride* and *perfluoro isobutylene*. In addition to these products there is an as yet unidentified agent which on inhalation causes so-called *polymer fume fever,* or "the shakes." This agent is believed to settle on a burning cigarette and thus be inhaled. Not everyone who smokes such a contaminated cigarette develops "the shakes," so it is likely that this is an allergic reaction and not one resulting from toxicity of the chemical. The resulting influenza-like symptoms are transient.

The *phenol formaldehyde-type* of plastics is well known under the trade name of Bakelite, a hard substance used extensively in the electrical industry. Similar products are of the *phenol furfural-type* and the *resorcinol-type.* These produce allergy symptoms only if they are sawed, sanded, or drilled, and the dust produced is inhaled; then they can produce a physical effect on the respiratory system which may be attributed to sensitivity. There may be greater allergenicity from the materials with which the plastics are filled than from the plastics themselves; these include wood flour, cotton flock, asbestos, mica, rag, sisal, pulp, minerals, and pigments. If a person is allergic to any of these, their inhalation can cause nasal congestion or asthma. *Hexamethylene-tetramine,* the hardener used in preparing the plastic, may be capable of producing asthmatic symptoms during the manufacturing process, but such reactions are not common.

The *melanine* plastics are used principally as dinner wear and in themselves are not allergenic, although formaldehyde may be produced during the baking process in their manufacture, and inhalation can cause asthma in a sensitive person. Another potential danger in the manufacture of this plastic is in the additives to the plastic which may be allergenic.

The epoxy resin plastics are formed by the chemical reaction of *bisphenol* and *epichlorohydrin* with a hardener, usually an amine. The amine, if allergenic, can cause allergic respiratory distress. In addition, as in other plastics, fillers may be added: glass and asbestos are two that are most commonly utilized. The epoxy resins are especially valuable in automobile body repair. They are applied to the damaged metal in their liquid state, allowed to harden, and then sanded and smoothed preparatory to painting. The dust produced in this process can effectively produce allergy respiratory disturbances in workers, particularly if the plant is not well ventilated.

Of the unsaturated polyester resin plastics, the most popular is the *fiber glass* plastic; very little, if any, true glass may be in the final product, although the fiber has a glassy appearance. Allergic nasal and pulmonary symptoms may develop from inhaling the *monomeric styrene* during the process of manufacture. The fillers, asbestos or quartz (silica flour), may be important allergens since they may be inhaled when the fiber glass is being sawed, sanded, or pulverized.

The question of whether or not plastic hair-setting and luster-imparting sprays used in hairdressing can be the cause of allergy symptoms of the nose or lungs is a matter of some dispute. Although many of the ingredients are kept secret, in general they contain natural and synthetic resins, of which *polyvinyl pyrrolidone* (PVP) is a chief ingredient. Other substances included are various alcohols, lanolins, perfumes, and a propellant such as one consisting of equal parts of "Freons 11 and 12." Of these, polyvinyl pyrrolidone, together with *carboxyl methyl cellulose* or *dextran,* has been accused of causing asthmatic symptoms. Although there is considerable animal and human evidence that this chemical is neither allergenic nor otherwise productive of unfavorable reactions, hair sprays continue to be suspect because symptoms of allergic rhinitis and bronchial asthma are frequently found among beauticians and among persons engaged in hairspray manufacture.

There are on the market a number of so-called *pseudoplastics* which contain a glue that may cause allergy disturbance of the nose or lungs. *Methacrylate,* for example, can produce all the symptoms of sensitivity to methyl methacrylate. When plastic wood containing such a glue is sawed, the resultant dust containing glue or wood may be allergenic.

Grains

Respiratory allergy symptoms of the nose, the bronchi, and the lungs caused by the inhalation of grains differ little from those produced by pollen and other dusts in the air. Both cause sneezing and running of the nose alternating with congestion, often accompanied by a postnasal drip. In some instances the nasal membrane reacts to very little exposure; in others it takes many months or even years before symptoms develop. In the United States, wheat is most commonly cultivated and most sensitivities are due to wheat flour; rye is also an offender. Occasionally, the so-called wheat sensitivity is not entirely due to the cereal grain but to molds and smut fungi (see Chapter 6). Flour-improving and flour-bleaching additives may be a complementary or even a primary allergenic factor. Corn, oats, and other cereal grains may also cause respiratory distress. Those who work in plants where beer and alcoholic beverages are produced come in contact with barley, malt, corn, and rye, as well as wheat.

Farmer's lung is a disease characterized by cough, difficulty in breathing, fever, chills, and expectoration of blood. For some time, the cause of this illness was obscure. Then it was realized that it occurred principally among farmers who were exposed to moldy hay, grain, silage, or straw. Farmers who worked with "good" hay were seldom affected. It has now been proved that the cause of the illness is the molds which are produced by the hay and sent into the circulating air to be breathed in by the worker.

A similar disease is *bagassosis*. The symptoms are alike but this disease is associated with the inhalation of molds which develop from the dust of the fibrous sugarcane. Although it is felt by many that this disease, like that of "farmer's lung," is purely an allergic phenomenon, there are some who are not yet convinced.

Chronic disease of the chest marked by thickening of the lung tissue (fibrosis) resulting from inhalation of mineral dusts such as sand, asbestos, and coal dust is often designated under the group *pneumoconiosis* and is frequently referred to as *miner's asthma*. The wheezing that accompanies these diseases differs from that which occurs in bronchial asthma inasmuch as it is always present; in bronchial asthma there are periods when the wheezing cannot be detected. Although there can be no doubt that inhalation of the mineral dusts in the air is the cause of these diseases, the proof that they are allergy diseases is still lacking.

Baker's asthma, or *miller's asthma*, may be difficult to diagnose; it may be linked with the inhalation of flour, but the asthma can also be caused in other ways. If the asthmatic attacks occur only when the worker is in the presence of the grains, allergy to finely ground meal of wheat, rye, barley, buckwheat, or bean is suspect. Skin tests can be performed with samples of the flour to help make the proper diagnosis, but they are not always reliable. Concurrent allergic rhinitis is usually present.

Transient pulmonary eosinophilia or *Loeffler's syndrome* is one of the rarer diseases suspected and is discussed in Chapter 17. It is characterized by a slight hacking cough and a low-grade fever, some chills, sweating, and fatigue. The symptoms are similar to very mild pneumonia. They are transient and last but a few days. Often this condition is disclosed only by an X ray which shows some infiltration in the lung. There is an increase in the number of eosinophiles in the circulating blood, often considered indicative of an allergy disease. Other causes of transient pulmonary eosinophilia may be more common but certainly one is the inhalation of cereal grains among bakers or millers, as well as those who work in grain silos.

Possibly some cases of respiratory disease ascribed to grains are in fact a reaction to fungi or molds, such as blight, rust, smut, and others frequently present in mills or silos. Another possibility is that the nose and lung symptoms may be produced not only by the grains or even the molds, but by such contaminants as particles from insects like flies, mosquitoes, and some flour parasites.

Animals

Hairworker's asthma is due to human hair. The hair and dander of animals produce symptoms most often among hunters, animal keepers, and zoo workers. Laboratory researchers are exposed since they come in contact with the hair and dander of pigs, rats, dogs, cats, rabbits, and many other animals in their experimental work. Stablemen and grooms may become allergic to the dander and hair of horses. Often skin contact produces an inflammation of the skin (dermatitis), while inhalation causes bronchial asthma ("horse asthma"). Hat-makers may come in contact with animal hairs, particularly rabbit hair, in the making of felt hats. In addition, they sometimes become sensitized to bleaching agents such as banana oil and oxalic acid that are part of the manufacturing process. In the manufacture of bedding and upholstered furniture, animal hairs, as well as feathers, cotton, flaxseed, kapok, glue, and wood dusts, may be employed for stuffing. Any or all of these can cause bronchial asthma in a person allergic to them.

Workers in pet shops frequently develop allergic rhinitis or bronchial asthma as a result of inhaling the feathers of birds; hence the names *featherworker's rhinitis* and *featherworker's asthma*. Most frequently affected by animal hairs are furriers who inhale the hairs from the skins with which they work; the dyes as well may cause respiratory trouble. *Furrier's asthma* is common. The furrier may also develop an occupational allergy, usually a skin rash from the chemical used in his trade *(furrier's rash)*. The chemicals include benzine, copper sulfate, lead chloride, nutgall, sumac leaves, tartar emetic, tannic acid, potassium dichromate, arsenic, and mercury. *Apiarist's asthma* caused by inhalation of the emanations from bees is relatively rare. It is often associated with a pollen carried by the bees.

Beans

Castor bean allergy occurs in those who work or live in the vicinity of a mill that manufactures castor oil, where the powder is allowed to enter the air. The asthma is produced by the resin in the castor bean powder. Since the remnants of the beans are ground to a powder and then commonly used as a fertilizer, respiratory allergy symptoms from the castor bean resin may be observed in susceptible agricultural workers.

Most coffee beans possess the same type of allergen (ricin). (Guatemala coffee is an exception.) Workers in coffee grinding and processing factories may develop asthma from ricin inhalation. The soybean also contains ricin. The soybean is used in some countries in the manufacture of glue and adhesives. It is also used in the manufacturing of synthetic rubber, and in the processing of automobile parts. Soybean flour is used in bakeries that prepare health foods. Workers in industries using soybeans and who are allergic to them may develop bronchial asthma.

Woods

Dermatitis due to wood contact has been described. More common is the asthma that develops from inhalation of the wood dusts. This may be observed in carpenters, cabinetmakers, foresters, and wood cutters. The exotic woods are primarily involved, although *Maple Bark Disease* from native maple trees appears in the Northern Hemisphere. This may in fact be an allergy reaction to the fungus *Coniosporium corticale*, which grows on the bark of the maple tree. Among the unusual woods whose dusts have been known to cause asthma are the *African Iroko teak*, derived from the Chlorophora excelsa tree, the *South African boxwood*, from Gonioma kamassi, the *Angolan boxwood* (Pterocarpus angolensis), the *Mansoma wood* (Sterculiacea altissima), and the *western star cedar* (Thlaspicate). People who work with any of these may develop an occupational respiratory allergy. Workers in areas where poison ivy, poison oak, and poison sumac are eradicated by burning can be affected by skin rashes or severe asthmatic seizures, resulting from inhalation of the allergenic substances of these plants.

Suberosis is caused by cork inhalation. It is characterized by an initial cold, cough, and mild fever. If dusts from the cork tree *(Quercus suber)*, are inhaled over a long period of time, the initial mild symptoms may progress to those of severe intractable bronchial asthma. This is not uncommon among cork workers, particularly in the Iberian Peninsula, where most cork is produced. In the United States, where laminated cork is rapidly becoming very popular, it is possible that similar cases will be found among those working with this material over a period of years.

The gums derived from certain trees, notably the acacia trees that flourish in Africa and Asia Minor, are well known causes of bronchial asthma. The gums are *gum acacia, gum arabic,* and *gum karaya.* Since these are used to a great extent in the color-printing trade, the asthma they produce has been termed *printer's asthma,* and is caused by inhalation of the alcoholic mist of the gum.

Metals

Metal fume fever is a name that has been given to a syndrome associated with the inhalation of fumes from molten metals, particularly zinc, copper, and magnesium; the same set of symptoms can be observed as a result of the fumes from aluminum, antimony, cadmium, iron, manganese, nickel, selenium, silver, and tin. It has been named from time to time for the metal which produced it, or the type of work in which it appeared; hence the terms *galvanizer's poisoning, founder's ague, smelter shakes,* and *smothers.* Currently it results primarily from the fumes of polytetrafluorethylene, and has earned the name of *polymer fume fever.*

Cobalt is used annually in vast quantities and has manifold uses. Exposure to large amounts of cobalt can produce stomach and intestinal symptoms, a consequence of the toxic properties of the metal. In the lung, allergenic reactivity may take place with resultant spasm of the bronchi, cough, and other signs of allergy, including blood eosinophilia.

This cannot be explained solely on the basis of an allergy reaction, but since not all persons exposed to cobalt develop these symptoms, the possible allergic factor involving individual susceptibility cannot be disregarded. It should be noted that cobalt in very small quantities is essential to life and is contained in the vitamin B_{12} molecule.

Nickel may sensitize the skin by contact. Inhalation can also produce symptoms related to allergy, such as tightness in the chest, difficulty in breathing, and cough. Prolonged exposure to nickel has resulted in grave consequences. Probably not all of the symptoms prevalent among those who work with nickel are allergic, but no doubt many are. Not all workers are affected. Therefore, it is presumed that some workers have a specific individual susceptibility to this metal. This cannot be demonstrated by laboratory techniques, but the history of the illness arouses suspicion. The same sporadic evidence of lung disturbance in those who work with *tungsten* hints that here, too, an allergic reaction is responsible.

Cadmium is a metal used in industry. Exposure in some people results in lung damage with collection of fluid in the lung which can be fatal (edema of the lung). The kidneys are readily affected in some persons, but whether the kidney or lung effects are caused by allergenicity has not yet been proved.

Berylliosis occurs in those who are exposed to *beryllium compounds*. Beryllium itself is not allergenic but beryllium compounds may produce inflammation of the lung (pneumonitis) in an acute, subacute, or chronic form. The symptoms have been explained on the basis of toxicology, but the fact that persons with this disease react to a patch test with the compound has led to the speculation that berylliosis may be an allergy disease.

The reactions in the nose and bronchi are definitely allergic in those who work with the soluble salts of *platinum*. These are used in the electroplating process, as photosensitizers in photography, in X ray fluorescent screens, in the production of acids, and elsewhere. Workers who come in contact with the soluble platinum salts may develop signs of allergic rhinitis. The lung symptoms — difficulty in breathing, sneezing, and cough — are practically identical with bronchial asthma caused by other illnesses. Anti-asthmatic medicines such as the ephedrine compounds, epinephrine (Adrenalin), and if these fail, the corticosteroids, give relief. This provides further indication of possible soluble platinum salt allergenicity.

The metal *vanadium* is widely used in industry, and that which is not used is directly converted into *vanadium pentoxide.* Factory workers who inhale the dusts of *cadmium pentoxide* and *calcium vandate* may react to them. Those most affected are employees who clean oil-fired furnaces and reline firebrick kilns. Asthma and bronchitis are the common complaints. It is not yet known whether this is a true allergy or simply an irritation of the bronchial tubes.

Although inhalation of *chromium* as *monochromate salts* such as *chromic acid* may produce lung cancer, asthma is a rare result. A reaction of the bronchi to *silica* occurs frequently but has never been proved to be allergic. It may merely be an irritant. When silica is inhaled as *silicon dioxide, quartz, tricymite* or *cristobalite,* a complicated chemical reaction takes place between the compound and the circulating blood cells suggesting to some an immunologic or allergic reaction. When a tuberculous infection occurs in a person who is "silicotic," the lung destruction proceeds very rapidly. This has been regarded by some as an allergic reaction, but proof is lacking.

Halogens are substances that combine with metals to form salts. Among the most common are *bromine, fluorine, chlorine,* and *iodine.* It is doubtful that compounds of bromine such as *methyl bromide,* used as insect fumigants and fire extinguishers, are allergenic and able to produce an allergic respiratory disease. This is true also of *ethyl bromide* or *allyl bromide* or *bromoform* which are widely used in the petroleum industry. All chlorinated compounds including chlorine are active respiratory irritants, but at present there is no evidence of their allergenicity.

Organic Compounds

Among the organic compounds, *turpentine* may infrequently produce asthma. *Halogenated hydrocarbons* only occasionally produce sensitization and nasal or lung difficulties. This is also true of the *lactate esters,* the *benzoates* or the *carbonates* used principally in the lacquer, rubber, flavoring, and perfume industries. Whether or not *triphenyl phosphate* is allergenic has not yet been determined. *Silicate esters* are not known to be allergens.

Among the *aldehydes,* formaldehyde has already been discussed. *Acetaldehyde,* used in factories that synthesize dyes and rubber goods and produce disinfectants and pharmaceutical products, may be a sensitizing agent. *Acrylaldehyde,* known as *acrolein,* is employed in the manufacture of resins, plastics, and colloidal metals. It is a very irritating gas, producing marked lung symptoms but is of very doubtful allergenicity. *Furfural,* a solvent for organic materials such as lubricating oil, is a lung irritant. Sensitization, if it occurs, is rare.

Some of the aromatic *nitro-* and *amino-compounds* may be allergenic. Pulmonary symptoms, primarily asthma, may be caused by *aminophenol* (alpha, para, or meta), the *chlorodinitrobenzenes,* and the *dinitrophenols.* These are all used in the dye industry. Another used in the dye industry as well as in the manufacture of rubber and plastics is *nitrosodimethylaniline.* Two of the most potent sensitizers of this group causing severe asthma as well as dermatitis are *phenylenediamine* (para) and *aminophenol* (para). The latter is still being used in the fur-dyeing industry. *Tetryl* (tetranitromonomethylaniline) is an explosive that on inhalation can cause symptoms of allergic rhinitis in susceptible persons.

The only phenols used in manufacturing plants that may at times produce sensitization and asthmatic symptoms are *phenol, hydroquinone, quinone,* and *creosote,* which is a mixture of guiacol, phenol, dresol, and other aromatic compounds.

Inorganic Chemicals

Among the inorganic chemicals, *sulfur dioxide* and other sulfur compounds *(sulfur hexafluoride, sulfur monochloride, sulfur trioxide,* etc.) are irritating to the bronchial tree, as are *ammonia* and *phosphorous.* In this way, they facilitate the allergic response to other true allergens. Alone, they are doubtfully allergenic. *Nitrogen compounds* can be irritating to the bronchi and lungs, but no true allergy to any of them has been demonstrated.

DIAGNOSIS OF OCCUPATIONAL ALLERGY DISEASES

Many of the inhaled gases produce symptoms that resemble an allergy disease such as allergic rhinitis or bronchial asthma, but actually the symptoms may be the result of the toxicity of the chemical or its irritating quality. Similarly, a skin rash may seem to be a contact dermatitis when in reality it results from another — non-occupational — cause.

The diagnosis is aided and often made by the chronological history. The onset of symptoms after working in a factory a sufficient length of time to allow sensitization to take place is suggestive. Symptoms should in most instances disappear on weekends, or on holidays, when contact with the suspected noxious substance is interrupted. In contact dermatitis the closer and more often the skin makes contact with the suspected allergenic material, the more profuse the rash should be. When inhaled substances are the cause of an allergy disease, the nose is usually affected before the bronchi or the lungs.

Allergy tests may or may not be of value. One of the problems is in determining the proper strength of the testing material to be used. If it is too weak, no reaction may appear; if it is too strong, it may produce a reaction caused by chemical irritation rather than allergy. Each person has an individual threshold. Furthermore, patch tests (see Chapter 4) may be negative, when in reality the material is producing the skin condition complained of. With patch tests some people require more exposure time than others to develop the rash. In many, the skin of the forearm where the patch test is being made is not as sensitive as the skin of the face, for example, where the actual reaction is occurring.

A similar difficulty arises in the matter of the scratch or intradermal test where the suspected material is rubbed into the skin or injected within the layers. The strength of the testing material is difficult to determine reliably and with chemicals, such a test is hazardous. Chemicals are incomplete antigens (haptens) and do not react diagnostically.

Danger is augmented when inhalation or so-called provocative tests are used in which the person is asked to inhale the suspected vaporized chemical. Too high a concentration can aggravate the original condition and if the chemical is toxic, can result in grave consequences. There is no way one can positively predict a safe test concentration of any substance for a particular person. Usually the doctor begins with a weak concentration and increases the strength gradually in succeeding tests, if necessary.

When skin tests are performed, the doctor usually tests for other allergens as well as the suspected one. Positive responses to others indicate that the affected person is intrinsically allergic. Often persons who do not come in contact with the suspected allergen are also tested. If they show positive skin reactions, this indicates that the substance is probably irritating rather than allergenic. Allergy skin tests for sensitivity to grains are not uniformly considered reliable, but symptoms produced are accepted as reliable, and when any doubt exists a carefully performed inhalation test may sometimes be employed. If, after snuffing up a small amount there is no response (aside from the normal irritating feeling which can be verified by repeating on normal people), then a small amount is actually blown into the windpipe with an atomizer. Marked respiratory difficulty similar to an asthmatic attack is considered positive evidence of allergenicity. The asthma is promptly relieved with epinephrine (Adrenalin).

TREATMENT

The most effective treatment of all occupational allergy diseases is prevention. Factory owners should be aware of the allergenicity of the materials that they employ and limit their use, or substitute nonallergenic substances whenever this is possible. Environmental control is essential. There should be proper ventilation, adequate exhausts, and ample washrooms conveniently located. In some cases the manufacturer may be unwilling or unable to bear the cost. Public health officials, including physicians, check on all industries from time to time. In the United States at least one medical journal devotes itself exclusively to problems of industrial medicine.

Individual precautions include the wearing of proper clothing and gloves, the use of barrier creams, masks, and nonirritating, inoffensive cleansing agents. These are essential, but to be effective their use must be enforced. Industrial physicians often find that workers carelessly neglect these indispensable deterrents to allergy.

Fortunately some workers with allergenic manifestations lose their sensitivity. This process, called hardening, is particularly noticeable when there is diminished contact or the concentration of the previously offending product has been decreased.

Aside from adequate clothing and masks there is little that one who works out-of-doors can do to protect himself from allergens in the outside air. Of course an allergic individual should avoid working in any job where his specific allergenic materials may be present. Allergic persons are very likely to become sensitive eventually to any new allergens encountered, particularly those that are potent.

In some instances therapeutic desensitization, as described in Chapter 7, is effective but in most cases it is not. Allergists know which diseases are responsive. They also have at their command certain medicines — some to be applied externally, and others to be taken internally — that give relief, but the avoidance of contact with the offending material is the cardinal principle of treatment.

In other respects the treatment of occupational allergy diseases is similar to that of any other allergy disease. Hives and swellings (angioedema) are treated with antihistamines. Asthma is treated with ephedrine compounds, iodides, and aminophylline. Skin rashes are soothed with bland creams, lotions, and ointments. Corticosteroids are employed in intractable cases. Violent reactions are given prompt treatment with epinephrine (Adrenalin) and the cortisone compounds or derivatives.

The results of specific desensitization in occupational allergy are difficult to predict. Some sensitizers (e.g., wheat, horse hair) have been much more successfully dealt with than others (e.g., castor bean dust). Despite the fact that the results of specific desensitization are unpredictable, it should, if possible, always be attempted. There is nothing to lose, and fundamentally allergists have nothing else to offer.

SUMMARY

Occupational allergy is difficult to delimit or to prove. In many instances of occupational disease, the initial contact required for sensitization is apparently absent and the disease seems to develop on the first contact. Most occupational diseases undoubtedly are not truly allergic but are caused by the irritating quality inherent in the substance with which the worker comes in contact. Proof of an antigen-antibody reaction is usually lacking. Nevertheless, there is a strong suspicion that a large number of occupational diseases may be allergic, and they may at some time in the future be shown to be.

Certain infectious diseases are likely to appear in people who are engaged in particular occupations, but these cannot be considered allergic. There are rare instances of occupational diseases due to ingestion and injection. Of course any factors predisposing to the production of allergic diseases also predispose to occupational allergic disease. Probably the most important factor in the production of an occupational allergic disease is the allergic capacity of the worker to react. Those who have other forms of allergy are more likely to develop a new allergenicity to the material with which they must work than those who have never shown an allergy previously.

In the textile industry various materials used can produce a contact allergic dermatitis. The yarn as well as finishers used in perfecting the garment can produce a rash. Dermatitis caused by handling various medicines is noted mostly in druggists, physicians, dentists, and nurses. The various woods used by furniture and cabinet workers are known to be sensitizers. "Housewives' hands" afflicts housewives who develop inflamed hands and industrial workers whose rash is caused by frequent exposure to detergents.

Workers in all trades can develop an occupational allergic dermatitis. In the graphic industries, textile, galvanizing, metal industries, a number of metals are used; among them is chrome, which may produce a skin allergy. Printers and furriers come in contact with dyes, which often produce a dermatitis. Allergy to tobacco leaf in persons who work in tobacco factories has been observed and confirmed. Contact with plants of any kind can produce an allergic dermatitis, the rash so produced resembling poison ivy, poison oak, or poison sumac dermatitis. The list of occupational allergic dermatitises is practically endless.

In the usually more serious allergic respiratory diseases, the nose is the first line of defense and is most often affected, but the bronchi and in fact any portion of the lungs may be attacked. Dusts of all kinds are most important. They may be by-products of a manufacturing process. Many volatile chemicals are used today and any one of them is suspect. Inhalation of plastics, the chemicals used in their manufacture, or factory dusts may cause occupational allergy disease of the respiratory tract. Each industry presents individual problems. Farmers, for example, may become sensitive to the products they cultivate or to the molds in the air. Bakers can be troubled with an allergic reaction to cereal grains. Furriers are notably allergic to animal hairs inhaled from the skins they handle, and to fur dyes as well. Asthma is a common symptom.

Castor oil factory workers often develop asthma from the ricin in the castor beans. People who live near a castor oil factory may be affected when the castor bean dust gets into the air. The same ricin is found in soybeans and in most coffees. Asthma caused by inhaling wood dust is common among carpenters, cabinet workers, foresters, and wood cutters. Allergy is often a result of work with the exotic woods. Metal workers can become sensitized by inhalation of the metals they use, and the name "metal fume fever" has been given to their symptomatology. Most often associated with respiratory disturbances are zinc, copper, and magnesium. Similar symptoms have been observed in those who work with aluminum, antimony, cadmium, iron, manganese, nickel, selenium, silver, and tin. In many occupational diseases of the respiratory tract caused by inhalation of metals, allergy is suspected but not yet proved as the underlying cause.

The diagnosis of an occupational allergy is difficult. It is based largely on a chronological history. Lapse of enough time after exposure to permit sensitization to take place, and relief of symptoms when the worker is away from allergenic contacts are suggestive but not conclusive diagnostic points with the doubt being greater in respiratory affections. Allergy skin tests do not give sufficient information. In contact dermatitis the use of the patch test is complicated by difficulty in determining what strength solution to use. The inhalation test is sometimes resorted to when an inhalant allergen encountered in one's occupation is suspect. This test must always be performed with extreme care by a physician.

An occupational disease suspected as allergic is treated exactly as any other allergic illness. Symptomatic treatment follows the usual course of managing various allergy symptoms as outlined in other chapters dealing with the allergy diseases of the skin or respiratory tract. Desensitization has produced variable and unpredictable results, but it should be employed whenever possible as the best therapy available. With increased industrial activity, occupational allergy diseases deserve and are receiving greater attention by public health officials.

Chapter Seventeen

Newer Aspects of Allergy

Much of the research now in progress at medical centers throughout the world is focused on attempts to classify and explain diseases and reactions of the body not previously understood. In many, the key factor appears to be the antigen-antibody reaction, generally considered the essential mechanism of allergy disease (see Chapter 2). Although these obscure diseases do not fit readily into "clinical allergy," which is comprised mainly of hay fever, bronchial asthma, hives, and eczema, there is nonetheless a distinct connection between these and more recently observed conditions on the periphery of clinical allergy. Either these diseases have as their underlying cause a demonstrable basic antigen-antibody reaction, or when this reaction is not evident, the tissues of the organs affected show changes similar to or suggestive of allergy disease when microscopically examined on biopsy or autopsy. Some of the most important and medically interesting are known as *autoimmune diseases* (illnesses caused by allergy to one's normal tissue components).

Homograft rejection (inability of one's body to accept transplants or grafts from someone else) is a phenomenon that is equally intriguing. In addition to these are the *collagen diseases* (diseases involving fibrous or connective tissue found in the body between body cells. Yet another aspect of allergy is furnished by *hypersensitivity vasculitis* (allergic inflammation of the smaller blood vessels). This is often classified as a collagen disease.

AUTOIMMUNE DISEASE

A better and more accurately descriptive term would be *autoallergy* or *autoallergic disease,* since an allergic response to the tissue and

285

cells of one's own body is involved. This is incompatible with the original definition of allergy which stated that the substance to which one is allergic must be foreign to the body, such as one that is inhaled, ingested, or injected.

The realization that this is not always true began to come about when a very serious eye disease was explained on the basis of "self-allergy." *Sympathetic ophthalmia* is an inflammation of one eye which follows in a period ranging from weeks to years after injury to, or surgery on, the other eye. This is explained as caused by an allergy to the pigment of the injured or surgically repaired eye, the pigment having entered the general circulation. *Endophthalmitis phacoanaphlactica,* another eye disease, is similarly explained. This disease occurs following surgery for cataract or after a severe injury in which the lens material in the front portion of the eye escapes from its capsule and enters the chamber of the eyeball. The reaction is thought to be caused by allergy to the protein material of the lens which developed while remaining encapsulated and was not part of the general eye tissue itself.

Recently more and more diseases have come to be regarded as possibly caused by "self-allergy." An obvious reason for reluctance in accepting this theory is that if our bodies do in fact injure themselves we would all be ridden with frequent and violent allergy diseases directed against our various tissues and organs. And it is evident that our predominant allergy is to material outside our bodies such as pollen, animal hair, dusts, and foods. The explanation becomes reasonable with the concept of *immunologic tolerance.* This asserts that the body does indeed have a tolerance for itself and in fact does recognize "self" from "nonself" by not reacting to its own tissues as if they were antigens, but the tolerance is not absolute and under certain circumstances this tolerance can break down; the body can fail to "recognize itself" with resulting allergic reactions or diseases.

Practically every organ of the body is now being investigated as a cause or potential generator of an autoimmune disease. Various theories attempt to explain obesity, hardening of the arteries, infertility, kidney disease, the aging process, and many other problems on the basis of autoimmune disease. Many of these theories have been clinically verified, and some proved in the laboratory. The remainder and many not yet described will no doubt eventually fit into the autoimmune pattern. Among the diseases often classified as autoimmune are *Hashimoto's thyroiditis* (inflammation of the thyroid gland), *Sjögren's syndrome* (a disease characterized by excess drying of the membranes of the nose, throat, and eyes together with inactivity of the glands that produce mucus), *rheumatoid arthritis* (a form of rheumatism with inflammation of the joints, stiffness, and swelling), *ulcerative colitis* (an ulcerative disease of the large intestine), certain types of *nephritis* (kidney inflammation) and some red-blood-cell-destroying *anemias* (blood diseases in which there is a reduction of the number of red blood cells, hemoglobin, or both). Some collagen diseases such as *disseminated lupus* are also included, indicating overlapping in the classification of these diseases.

Post-myocardial infarction syndrome can be regarded as an autoimmune disease. This occurs not infrequently when a patient is convalescing from a coronary heart attack. He develops what appears to be another similar heart attack, but it is accompanied by inflammation of the sac surrounding the heart (pericarditis) and of the covering of the lungs (pleurisy). Despite the similarity of symptoms and even the electrocardiographic findings, this is not a new coronary occlusion but rather an allergic reaction to the structures adjacent to the cells of the heart muscle that had died in the original attack due to lack of blood supply. Nonvital cells are foreign and act as allergens, producing antibodies capable of instigating allergic reactions. This is an illustration of the way in which immunological tolerance can be overcome.

One manner in which autoimmune disease occurs is by alteration of the body tissues or cells, in order for them to become foreign or not part of "self," and thus capable of entering the antigen-antibody reaction. This is true of *Hashimoto's goitre* in which it is believed several cells become diseased or altered in some fashion and thus unrecognizable to the immunizing process of the body. There have been other mechanisms suggested for the production of autoimmune disease, most of which are extremely complicated. All are being studied.

The several types of autoimmune disease are classified by their symptoms as well as by their cause. One is "organ-specific" because the disease is limited to one organ for which there has been found an excess of antibodies. In another type, many parts of the body and many tissues and organs are involved. The thyroid disturbance just discussed exemplifies "organ-specific disease"; an example of the second type is *lupus erythematosus*, a skin disease with widespread involvement of other organs. These are the extremes. Some diseases, such as ulcerative colitis and Sjögren's syndrome, are thought to be mixtures of both.

HOMOGRAFT REACTIONS (REJECTIONS)

A *homograft* is a graft or other transplant from one animal to another of the same species. A *heterograft* is a graft from one species of an animal to another. An *autograft* is a tissue transplant from one part of the body to another in the same person. Autografts are invariably successful, and skin grafts and bone grafts from one portion of a person's body to another part have been a routine surgical procedure for many years. Heterografts have almost invariably been rejected. The cause of the nonacceptance or of rejection is an allergic or antigen-antibody reaction. Homografts from identical twins (from the same fertilized ovum) have been successful. Immunologic tolerance plays a key role here as it does in autoimmune diseases. We can tolerate transplanted parts of our own body but we tend to slough off the tissue of someone else's because we react to it as we would to any foreign body. Homografts from persons who are not identical twins tend to be rejected but are being used with increasing success. This is accomplished by altering the immunologic mechanism so that it becomes relatively indifferent toward a material that would normally produce an allergic reaction.

The fact that immunologic tolerance or the recognition of "self" from "nonself" is not absolute and can be influenced was indicated when twin cattle, though not identical twins, could in some instances accept transfusions and even skin grafts from each other. This has led to the idea that during early embryo life in the uterus of humans there is an interchange of tissue and cells between the mother and the unborn infant (fetus) sufficient to alter their immunologic tolerance to each other. Fetuses of chickens, mice, rabbits, and other animals were injected with antigens in order to produce artificially this tolerance to the antigen that was injected. The success of this procedure indicated that manipulation of the immune mechanism was possible, and other techniques were attempted. These have been called *immunosuppressive* measures, or measures to suppress the normal immune reaction. Drugs, surgical procedures, and general or total-body X rays have been tried.

The importance of the increasing success of homograft, or even of heterograft transplants, is evident. Skin grafts are a comparatively minor part of the problem because skin can practically always be secured from one's own body. But in the case of a person with a badly diseased heart or kidney when the prognosis is fatal, the possibility of securing a healthy organ as a substitute for the diseased one becomes exciting.

Though in an early stage of clinical development, the first procedures having been performed only in 1967, human heart transplants are being performed with increasing frequency. Kidney transplants have been performed for several years. Data published by Dr. Joseph Murray of Harvard University Medical School, based on work done in Boston, Massachusetts, indicates that a kidney obtained from a donor who is a sibling or a parent of the sick person has a 72 percent chance of functioning successfully for six months and a 67 percent chance of functioning successfully for one year. This operation is performed as a last resort and all the patients would have died within days, weeks, or months if they did not receive transplants or were not maintained by long-term dialysis. Dr. Murray's longest survival at the time of his report was ten years in a patient who received a kidney from an identical twin. The longest survival that he reported for a person not genetically related to the donor was seven years.

The most dramatic transplant, to be sure, is that of the heart. Since the first was performed in South Africa there have been numerous heart transplants performed all over the world. The basis of the drama is obvious. Nevertheless, though the surgical techniques have been perfected, the problem of reaction, with consequent possible rejection — allergy to the foreign heart — remains the major factor, as in all transplants of organs or tissue from others.

A transplanted organ is just as much an antigen as ragweed that produces an attack of hay fever. The difference, of course, is that the adverse homograft reaction eventually results in a sloughing of the transplanted organ and ultimate death. Aside from identical twins, who are the ideal donor-recipients, kidneys from close relatives seem to be most successful, but immunosuppressive measures still are required in an effort to prevent homograft reaction and perhaps ultimate rejection. In each instance, it is necessary for a healthy person to sacrifice a functioning kidney with the realization that the life of the recipient may not be saved. In addition, the donor must realize that if some unforeseen kidney accident should occur, or his remaining kidney should become diseased, it might mean death. A better source for a kidney transplant would be a young healthy person who died in an accident and whose kidney could be made available immediately. This is not often possible. A more practical source would be chimpanzees or similar animals, or homografts from other deceased donors. All of these have been attempted.

Not all patients with very severely diseased kidneys are suitable candidates for transplants. When the kidney disease is merely a manifestation of a generalized disease, or when there is a lower urinary tract infection, the operation is contraindicated. In these instances a new kidney cannot salvage the patient's health.

The surgical technique of kidney transplants has been perfected. The more difficult problem is that of the allergic reaction. Despite the fact that transplants have been successful and there are many people living and working with transplanted kidneys, it must be assumed that the kidney is nevertheless slowly being rejected; there is a constant allergic reaction in progress, suppressed as much as possible by medicines. Eventually, it is hoped, the body will take over; the immunologic tolerance will be altered sufficiently and permanently to accept the new organ. There is every evidence in the experimental laboratory that this is possible and will eventually occur. At the present time, however, immunologic tolerance is minimal and must be constantly influenced by medication.

Many medicines and procedures have been employed for suppression of the immune or allergic reaction (immunosuppressive drugs). Surgery of the thymus gland has been used. Greater success has been obtained with medicines and with X ray to the entire body (total radiation), but particularly to the organs that are believed to be the source of the antibodies that enter the antigen-antibody reaction. The medicines and drugs used are similar, often identical, to those used to treat cancer; for that reason they are called *antimetabolites,* or cytotoxic (cell-destroying) drugs. These drugs are intended to destroy the tissues that produce antibodies resulting from the newly introduced organ (foreign antigen) but also lower the body's resistance to infection. If the antibody is destroyed or even reduced, the antigen-antibody reaction is minimized.

Usually, a cell-killing medicine is given several days before the transplant operation. At the time of the operation large doses of cortisone are prescribed. Just as cortisone relieves attacks of bronchial asthma and hay fever, so it reduces the homograft reaction. Soon after the surgery, there is usually a period of marked allergic reaction. This is called the "rejection crisis"; at that time the dose of cortisone is further increased. The dose is reduced as tolerance increases and ultimately the smallest dose necessary to avoid reaction is maintained.

The technical problems of organ transplants are gradually being overcome. In addition to hearts and kidneys, transplants of lungs and livers have been performed. When transplanting is perfected and the rejection problem overcome, the possibility of substituting "spare parts" in the worn-out or diseased body, such as one substitutes parts of a motor, will become commonplace. How far away, then, will be the practice of storing the bodies of healthy young persons who die as a result of an accident, in order to provide (by "cannabalizing," some say) new hearts, kidneys, or other organs? There remain, however, many legal, moral, and philosophical problems.

COLLAGEN DISEASES: VASCULAR ALLERGY: HYPERSENSITIVITY ANGIITIS

The above terms are sometimes used synonymously. Although the diseases to which they refer, however, may have similar symptoms, run an almost identical course, display changes in the tissues or organs that resemble each other and have a suspected common cause, they are not all necessarily the same type of disease. Nevertheless, there seems to exist, although not entirely proved in all cases, an underlying antigen-antibody reaction of allergy.

In some the allergy is to one's self or autoallergy (autoimmune disease). In others the reaction is thought to be due to drugs and medicines. The list of the *collagen diseases* is becoming longer as more illnesses are found to fit into the pattern. The best known and the most intensely studied are *periarteritis nodosa* (or polyarteritis), *dermatomyositis, scleroderma, lupus erythematosus disseminatus* (disseminated lupus), *idiopathic thrombocytopenic purpura, rheumatoid arthritis,* and *rheumatic fever.* To this may be added some types of anemia, innumerable involvements of the kidneys, the heart, lungs, nervous system, joints, muscles, and nerves, all of which have been described at autopsy as showing specific evidence of inflammation of the small blood vessels, or special involvement of the connective tissue between the cells of the organs. Some show both and as a result many attempts have been made to connect all of the diseases and list them along one spectrum.

Polyarteritis

Polyarteritis is also known as *polyarteritis nodosa, periarteritis nodosa, Kussmaul-Maier disease, diffuse necrotizing arteritis, necrotizing angiitis,* and *essential polyangiitis.* Despite a multiplicity of synonyms, they are based on a common underlying pathology of widespread involvement of the medium- and small-sized blood vessels, usually in localized portions of the heart, nervous system, lungs, intestinal tract, skin, and liver. Although any organ may be involved, the kidney is most frequently affected. Lesions similar to these have been experimentally produced in animals by drugs used to produce a drug allergy reaction. Sulfa drugs, penicillin, and others have been used; this has caused investigators to feel that this is a disease due to allergy. But other causes have been described and some believe that infections and nervous disturbances are involved.

The symptoms vary; no organ or portion of the body is immune. There is usually an initial fever; the white blood cell count is elevated and there is often a large number of eosinophiles. The sudden onset of symptoms of kidney disease, heart disease, and asthma in males (usually stricken three times as frequently as females) in their thirties and forties arouses suspicion. The allergist may see him as a new asthmatic with no previous symptoms, the dermatologist as a patient with a bizarre rash accompanied by generalized constitutional symptoms, and the nerve specialist as a patient exhibiting peculiar nerve symptoms with weakness and numbness or tingling of the extremities.

The final diagnosis is made by a biopsy of the involved tissue or organ, but since the lesions are so dispersed they can be easily missed. Treatment is purely symptomatic as it is in all collagen diseases.

Dermatomyositis

Dermatomyositis is also known as *dermatomucomyositis* and *poikilomyositis*. This disease involves both the skin ("derma") and the muscles ("myositis"). Its connection to allergy is remote, based mainly on symptoms and findings similar to the other so-called collagen diseases which are more closely related to allergy (probably of the autoimmune type). The onset may be sudden, with chills, fever, intense redness of the skin, and muscle pain, or symptoms may appear slowly as vague feelings of tiredness and achiness of the muscles, with gradually increasing weakness.

The rash ranges from simple discoloration with swelling of the eyes, to scarring. In addition to lesions in the skin and the muscles there are also signs and symptoms indicating involvement of the internal organs, such as difficulty in swallowing, pain in the chest, enlarged spleen and lymph glands, changes in the eyes (retinal exudates). The resemblance to other skin and visceral diseases of the same group (collagen diseases), such as *scleroderma* and *systemic lupus erythematosus,* is often so striking that some believe all are merely variants of the same disease.

Scleroderma

Scleroderma is also known as *progressive systemic sclerosis, dermatosclerosis, sclerema adultorum,* and *hidebound disease.* The terms are descriptive of the disease which is characterized by progressive thickening of the skin and the tissues beneath the skin (connective tissue). Rigidity of the skin leads to relative immobility; less frequently it is localized: this is known as *morphea,* a benign manifestation. The disease occurs more frequently in women, and the intestinal tract is often eventually involved. Difficulty in swallowing caused by swellings in the esophagus is experienced and occasionally intestinal obstruction caused by paralysis of the bowel takes place. The kidneys may be affected with high blood pressure resulting as a late manifestation. Microscopic changes in the connective tissue link this disease to others definitely ascribed to allergy.

Lupus Erythematosus

Systemic or disseminated lupus erythematosus, sometimes also called *lupus erythematosus disseminatus,* must be differentiated from *discoid lupus erythematosus.* The discoid type is benign and localized to the skin, while the disseminated variety involves many organs and tissues of the body as well as the skin. Some physicians believe that discoid lupus may often eventually become the systemic or disseminated type. The localized variety is characterized by a rash across the bridge of the nose flaring to the flush portions of the cheeks known as the "butterfly" distribution.

Disseminated lupus is a wasting disease involving the skin and many other organs. It occurs most commonly in young women and there are pathologically the same connective tissue or collagen changes seen under the microscope as in others of the group. An antibody to the nucleus of the white blood cell can be demonstrated, distinctly suggesting that it is an autoimmune disease; this antibody is known as the *L. E. factor.* Other more sensitive tests are also diagnostic.

The symptoms are extremely variable and widespread. The butterfly rash formerly considered characteristic is but one of several types of skin rash that may appear. Among the others are redness of the skin, large blisters, ulcers, and sometimes patches of baldness. There are often symptoms of joint pain, attacks of pneumonia, heart trouble, enlargement of the spleen, liver, and glands, as well as kidney disease. The variability of the symptoms may make diagnosis difficult as in all collagen diseases.

Rheumatoid Arthritis

Rheumatoid arthritis is also known as *atrophic arthritis, arthritis derformans, proliferative arthritis,* and *chronic infectious arthritis.* This deforming type of arthritis occurs in young persons as opposed to *osteoarthritis,* which is not crippling and is common in those who are much older. There is no cogent evidence that rheumatoid arthritis is caused by an immune mechanism or is based on allergy, but because of its symptoms, occurrence, variability, and pathological findings, it is often classified as a collagen disease. There is a type of allergy test that seems to demonstrate what has been called a *rheumatoid factor* in this disease; when this is found, autoallergy is considered a possible definite cause. At present the rheumatoid factor is commonly demonstrated by the *latex fixation test.* Many claim that this test is not specific. Nevertheless, it directs attention to consideration of rheumatoid arthritis as one of the broad group of allergy diseases.

Rheumatic Fever

Rheumatic fever is a well-known disease occurring primarily in children and young adults. It begins with a fever, and the most pronounced symptoms are painful, swollen, often red, hot joints with symptoms which characteristically migrate from one joint to another. The disease is usually preceded by a streptococcal sore throat often so slight as to go unnoticed. One of the most serious sequelae of rheumatic fever may be permanent heart damage (termed rheumatic heart disease) which remains many years after the acute illness is gone. It has been estimated that one to two percent of all school children in the United States have rheumatic heart disease resulting from an attack of rheumatic fever so mild that it was overlooked.

The relationship of streptococcus infection to rheumatic fever and to rheumatic heart disease has been recognized for a long time. The question is whether the disease affecting the joints and the heart is caused directly by the streptococcus germ that has found its way into the tissue, or whether the symptoms of joint swelling and heart disease are an allergic reaction to the streptococcus organism. The consensus is that the heart disease, if not the joint symptoms, is certainly a reaction rather than direct invasion. As such, rheumatic fever and its complication, rheumatic heart disease, are examples of allergy of a distinct type due to an antigen which is the product of the streptococcus germ.

Hemolytic Anemia

Hemolytic anemia is a type of anemia in which red blood cells are constantly destroyed at a rate exceeding the ability of the body to replace them. There are many types of hemolytic anemia, some caused by infections, several due to hereditary absence of certain enzymes and others associated with the Rh type of blood such as seen in newborn infants. A specific type known as *hemolytic acquired autoimmune anemia* is believed to be caused by allergy to one's own body cells. There is a clumping of red blood cells when the blood is chilled, and several immunological tests performed on the blood yield characteristic results.

In addition to these questionably allergic diseases in which the antigen-antibody reaction is difficult to identify, there are several that can be considered hypersensitivity arteritis of a more clearly allergic origin. These include *serum sickness, drug reactions* and *Schönlein-Henoch purpura.*

Serum Sickness

Serum sickness is an allergic reaction manifested by swelling, hives, fever, and joint pains which may persist for days, weeks, and perhaps years after the initial use of foreign serums and even drugs. One explanation is that the antigen persists in the body, continuing to produce antibodies, perpetuating the antigen-antibody reaction. Another explanation which brings it into the realm of autoimmune disease is that the initial contact with the antigen produces changes in the cells and the changed cells act as an antigen. Hives produced after a reaction to penicillin may continue for many months, long after all the penicillin should have been eliminated from the body. Autoallergy is the most likely explanation. Drug reactions are in the same category and may indeed produce serum sickness.

Purpura

In *purpura* small hemorrhages are usually visible in the skin. They often appear as small discolored areas, like minute bruises. Purpura has several causes, some associated with a decrease in the number of platelets or thrombocytes (a type of blood cell that is active in producing clotting when a blood vessel is cut). In others, there is no reduction in the number of these cells. When there is a decrease in the number of the thrombocytes, the purpura is called *thrombocytopenic purpura;* when there is no decrease it is termed *nonthrombocytopenic purpura.* *Schönlein-Henoch purpura* is considered an allergic purpura and occurs mainly in children. In addition to the pinpoint hemorrhages in the skin there are associated pains in the joints and abdomen. There is also an *idiopathic thrombocytopenic purpura,* "idiopathic" meaning cause unknown. This is believed to be an autoimmune disease and thus related to vasculitis and the collagen diseases. Antibodies have been demonstrated which are directed against the platelets or thrombocytes, tending to destroy them, and in that way producing the thrombocytopenia or decrease in the number of thrombocytes. Very closely associated with this is *autoallergic hemolytic anemia* in which the antibody is directed against the red blood cell and attempts to destroy it (hemolysis).

There are many other disease conditions that may be classified as part of autoimmune disease, collagen disease, and hypersensitivity inflammation of the small blood vessels. One of these is *granulomas,* tumor-like masses made up of heaped-up scar tissue and cells.

Granulomas

Eosinophilic granuloma is found in the bones, occurring usually as a solitary mass with resorption and destruction of the bone tissue in its vicinity. A disease of young people, it must be differentiated from tumors of the bone which may be malignant. Cure is usually secured by surgical removal. Microscopic examination of the mass reveals many eosinophiles.

Loeffler's syndrome is a type of pneumonia seen on X ray in which the inflammation is due to many eosinophiles infiltrating the area involved. It is transient and often migrates to other parts of the lung. Eosinophiles are found on examination of the sputum.

Wegener's granulomatosis is a mass usually found in the lung; it produces ulceration and destruction of the lung tissue and involves other organs of the body including the kidneys; it is a progressive illness that may lead to death.

SUMMARY

A large group of allergic diseases is currently being investigated which, despite the fact that they do not demonstrate the antigen-antibody reaction, have many elements in common suggestive of allergy. Their pathology in some cases is similar or identical. Others in which the pathology is also identical appear to be definitely allergic; hence these diseases are often grouped in overlapping classifications.

One group of diseases is known as autoimmune diseases or autoallergy diseases. These are different from the usual allergy diseases in the sense that the allergy is to one's own body cells. True allergy had always been considered a result of a foreign substance, but today there is evidence that certain types of thyroid disease, intestinal diseases, heart diseases, eye diseases, and blood diseases, are caused by allergy to one's own body.

The explanation of this newly recognized ability of "self-allergy" is based on the theory of immunologic tolerance which states that the body can recognize itself and therefore ordinarily does not react to itself but that this tolerance is not absolute and can be altered.

Closely related to the problem of autoimmune disease is that of homograft and heterograft rejection, the inability of the body to accept transplants and grafts from others of the same or different species. This is caused by recognition of the homograft "nonself" in foreign material. However, with the recent knowledge of the mechanism of immunologic tolerance and of ways to alter it to prevent the body from recognizing the material as foreign, organ transplants are becoming increasingly successful.

Surgical removal of selected organs from one individual and transplantation into another's body has become a perfected technique. The main problem is in overcoming the allergic reaction to the foreign substance. Currently, most transplants are being done with kidneys, and X rays, cell-killing drugs, cortisone—all known as "immunosuppressive"—are being used to make the body accept the new organ. Although there are people who have been alive for years with newly transplanted organs, they still require constant medication. It is hoped that eventually they will develop an immunologic tolerance and that the medicines can be discontinued. When this problem is overcome the practice of using organs from deceased donors will become practical.

Another group of diseases connected with allergy and in some instances with autoimmune diseases are the collagen diseases; other terms of overlapping or similar diseases are hypersensitivity vasculitis, arteritis, or angiitis. Collagen refers to the connective tissue between the cells of the body. Angiitis, vasculitis, and arteritis refer to inflammation of various blood vessels. The most important diseases in this group are periarteritis nodosa (or polyarteritis), disseminated lupus erythematosus, and rheumatic fever. In addition there are various types of anemia, lung infiltrations, bone granulomas, blood clots and hemorrhages. The list is rapidly enlarging.

These diseases all have in common a peculiar type of involvement of the tissues between the cells and/or very distinct lesions around the small blood vessels. Some can be produced deliberately with allergy-producing drugs; most can be relieved temporarily with the use of cortisone. Some are definitely autoimmune since antibodies to the specific tissues and cells involved can be demonstrated in the laboratory.

Continued study of the collagen diseases and hypersensitivity vasculitis is making available more effective treatment of previously baffling illnesses.

Chapter Eighteen

The Emotional Factor in Allergy

The term "psychosomatic," meaning the effect of the emotions on the body and on the production of disease, has become part of everyday language. Allergy disease, by the very mechanism of symptom production, is particularly subject to the influence of changes in the nervous system. The physician specializing in allergy will invariably hear this question during the initial interview: "All allergies are emotional, aren't they, doctor?" Obviously the allergist does not think so; if he did he would have been a psychiatrist rather than an allergist. The layman's question is often precipitated by an inadequate knowledge of anatomy and physiology.

The relationship of emotional problems to organic symptoms is elementary. "Psychosomatic" means exactly what its foreign roots indicate: *psyche* refers to the emotional aspect, while *soma*, literally "the body," refers to the organic. We see examples of psychosomatic behavior in our normal, everyday life. The tears which come from the tear glands in the corners of the eyes are clearly organic, but the sorrow which produces the tears is emotional. A hearty laugh (activity of the vocal cords) and shaking of the body (moving of the diaphragm and chest muscles) is purely a "soma" effect of a "psyche"; the cause might be a funny story or a ludicrous sight. Other frequently encountered examples are blushing as a result of embarassment, pounding of the heart as a result of fear, and sighing as an indication of hopelessness.

All psychiatrists believe that emotional problems result from the interaction of the individual and his surroundings and from his experiences during the developmental period. The effect of heredity, although not denied, is minimized. Freud attributed special importance to the infant's sexual experiences; Adler made much of the individual striving for power or superiority, while Jung popularized the conception

299

of "extravert" and "introvert." The "eclectic" school prides itself on using all effective theories of each, depending on the patient who is being treated.

For our purposes the best explanation is the one that can fit into the framework of all the theoretical schools of thought, and will explain in a broad sense the cause, mechanism, and results of the psychosomatic problem. This has been called the adaptive or ecological theory.

We are constantly surrounded by challenging forces that make it somewhat difficult for us to maintain our equilibrium and even to exist. These include the forces of nature, such as earthquakes, floods, forest fires, and tornadoes or hurricanes; such simple rules and laws that prohibit us from driving an automobile faster than a given speed; bacteria and viruses that surround us all the time and make us vulnerable to disease; and the everyday problems of living in a complex society with its frustrations and competition for success. All of these and many more interfere with our everyday life, our equilibrium or balance in our environment, and our ability to cope with our surroundings. The medical term for this equilibrium is "homeostasis," defined in physiologic terms as "a tendency toward the maintenance of a relatively stable internal environment in the bodies of higher animals through a series of interacting physiological processes (as the maintenance of a fairly constant body heat in the face of widely varying external temperatures)." Disease prevention and allergen avoidance might also be included.

The definition of homeostasis in relation to psychological forces is "a tendency toward maintenance of a relatively stable psychological condition of the individual with respect to contending drives, motivations, and other psychological forces." The difference in the approach of the varying groups of psychiatrists involves "other psychological forces" and probably refers mainly to experiences during early developmental life. When socioeconomic and ecological factors are considered, the definition is "a tendency toward the maintenance of relatively social conditions among groups with respect to various factors (such as food supply and population among animals) and to competing tendencies and powers within the body politic, to society, or to culture among men."

These three definitions really constitute one definition involving all the external forces governing our good health and appropriate behavior. Whether this maintenance is the result of our infantile sexual experiences or is caused by other drives is a continuing point of argument. Of greater significance, in the view of most, is that there is probably a hormone involved in this mechanism, or perhaps several hormones, the most important of which is cortisone, secreted by the cortex (outer rim) of the adrenal glands, the small glands that are situated just above each kidney. Our response to stress of any sort is greatly influenced by the adrenal glands. Allergy, an abnormal response to a certain type of stress (food, inhaled material, drugs), is very responsive to cortisone. This is dramatically verified by people who take cortisone medicines for relief of asthma. Constant use of the hormone produces inactivity of the normal adrenal so that it cannot function. Cortisone or its derivatives, given as a medicine, act as a substitute, and the procedure is to administer only the amount necessary to maintain good health, or normal equilibrium. In some forms of stress such as surgery or automobile accidents there is a need for a greater quantity of the hormone to cope with the additional shock. Unless this additional amount of cortisone is prescribed, either aggravation of asthma or collapse ensues. Patients taking this hormone are urged to carry a card or other identifying information on their person. Unfortunately, cortical adrenal hormone does not always benefit psychological problems, although it does have a profound effect in many instances on the person's mood and behavior. It may cause depression or its opposite, euphoria.

A normal response to stress, whether it be a threat, an excess of pollen in the air, or a nagging wife, is to face it and fight it, or to escape from it. (The expression "fight or flight" has become an accepted scientific name for this.) The adrenal glands are instrumental in the escape or "flight" aspect and even perhaps in making the decision.

When the force or threat is purely an emotional one, there are two alternatives in facing the situation. In addition to fleeing and fighting there is the option of verbalizing, arguing, or objecting as one chooses. This is really a form of fighting but the fight is on a psychological rather than an organic basis. The other alternative is to withhold one's anger or frustration. When this happens, the theory is that the emotional charge must seek another means of expression, and this usually results in somatic (hence psychosomatic) symptoms.

Crying, laughing, pounding of the heart, and sighing are temporary, and once the cause is removed or forgotten the symptoms disappear. In many instances, however, the symptoms persist. A classical example is "conversion hysteria," a frankly organic symptom which has no evident organic explanation. Examples are a person who is paralyzed for years and suddenly begins to walk, and more commonly a form of blindness that has no apparent cause and may, after many years, be spontaneously cured.

Although the average "neurotic" may not exhibit these extreme conditions of hysterical paralysis or hysterical blindness, he may develop symptoms, which are minor in degree but qualitatively similar. Those who argue that allergy is a psychosomatic disease maintain that it is the manifestation of withheld emotional forces seeking a normal outlet. Allergists believe that while allergic symptoms result from an antigen-antibody reaction they may be subject to superimposed emotional influences because of failure of the normal mechanism of homeostasis, the normal response to stress. The body has difficulty in coping with the additional insult of the glands that maintain equilibrium. Such additional insult is frequently seen in infections, changes in weather, lowered resistance caused by fatigue, and many other factors, as well as psychological upsets.

All psychiatrists accept this thesis. To quote the late Dr. Franz Alexander, an exponent of the modified Freudian school of thought: "The recognition of emotional causes of asthma should not make one oblivious of the equally well-established influence of allergic factors. The latter are more conspicuous in seasonal attacks which appear simultaneously with the pollen to which the patient is sensitive. In cases where there is sensitivity to animal hair, kapok, etc., attacks can be produced in dramatic suddenness when the patient is exposed to the specific allergen in question. Desensitization is often effective in such cases." Often when the psychiatrist speaks of allergic disease he completely omits any reference to allergic factors. Perhaps he is speaking "in shorthand," omitting what to him is the obvious, the effect of allergy.

There is a tendency, however, to ascribe specific activity patterns, past experiences, responses to certain stimuli, desires, wishes, and many other forms of affective behavior to allergy symptoms. For example, hay fever has been explained as the result of the sexual factor or impulse of smell which has been insufficiently repressed. Another explanation of hay fever and even of the common cold is that they are "manifestations of frustrated passive receptive wishes with strong oral components." Dermatitis has been dismissed as a need to punish oneself by scratching the skin. Migraine headaches have been ascribed to hostility toward people who are loved or to frustration in intellectual sibling rivalry during childhood. Asthma, according to most psychiatrists and all psychoanalysts, is due to the fear of the loss of one's mother. The asthmatic wheeze has been vividly described as representing the suppressed cry of the child for its mother.

Perhaps most of the psychiatric investigation in allergy disease has had to do with asthma, since these are the sickest individuals. The results have been interesting. One group feels strongly that the cause is maternal rejection; that is, the mother does not really want the child and indicates it subconsciously with resulting asthma in the child. The overprotective mother who hovers over a sick asthmatic child during the night, according to some, has a feeling of guilt which she is trying to satisfy.

A distinction must be made between the allergy disease as a whole and the individual symptom which may be part of the disease. Asthma has been defined as a symptom or episode and bronchial asthma as the entire episodic disease. The disease state is a continuing series of individual symptoms, and in the case of allergy disease the underlying mechanism must be the allergic reaction. A favorite term for this among doctors is "continuum," indicating that it is a continuing series of individual symptoms making up a pattern. Although the allergy background must exist for the continuum or disease, each individual symptom can be produced by extraneous causes, among which is emotional trauma.

An individual attack of asthma, a fit of sneezing, or the sudden appearance of a rash can undoubtedly be caused by nonorganic causes. Some physicians have been able to relieve a severe attack of asthma by hypnosis. Many can initiate an attack of asthma at will in the doctor's office by discussing a subject particularly traumatic to the patient. In each instance, however, the patient must be predisposed to allergy disease. As in tuberculosis: "The soil must be fertile. When one spreads TB germs, some take hold and grow; others fall on barren ground."

Of course, the physician who concerns himself strictly with organic illnesses and the psychiatrist who deals with conflicts and frustrations are equally aware of the interdependence of their specialties. The enlightened internist, allergist, surgeon, and dermatologist realize that much of their treatment, aside from the complicated adjustments of the blood chemistries, blood enzymes, and electrolytes, is based on the rapport between patient and physician. Whether one chooses to call this "bedside manner," "interest," or "understanding," it is a form of psychotherapy.

An attempt has been made to correlate the purely psychological cause with an organic or physiological change in the body. Since an allergic reaction, which is the cause of the symptom, is assumed to be the result of the union of the antigen with the appropriate antibody in the chosen shock tissue, such terms as "emotional anaphylaxis," "psychoantigen," and "psychoallergy" have been devised to indicate that emotions can act as antigens. It is remotely possible that like other haptens (incomplete antigens which require union with a body protein to enter into the reaction), the emotional insult or injury alters some of the cells of the body or some fragments of the protein of the body sufficiently to make them antigenic. This is one of the theories used to explain allergy to light, heat and cold, pressure, and effort—the so-called physical allergies—and may very well be substantiated in the future. This suggests the problem of autoallergy or autoimmune disease, as discussed in Chapter 17.

Another explanation is that of the conditioned reflex. The experiment to indicate this type of response was carried out as follows: rabbits were sensitized with the cholera bacteria; then additional injections were administered to produce near-lethal reactions. Each injection was accompanied by the beating of a gong. Eventually it was possible to produce the severe allergic reactions merely by the beating of the gong. This experiment is in harmony with the feeling of many allergists that some of the symptoms of allergy, a severe attack of asthma, for example, is a "learned response." It has become a habit that follows certain incidents or procedures. Clearly, such symptoms are purely emotional. This might even explain the maternal dependency theory of asthma. A child learns that it can receive attention by crying, coughing, and ultimately wheezing. Eventually, the wheezing attack becomes a "conditioned reflex," or "learned reaction," as a request for the mother's extra attention. Again the symptom may be caused by a variety of stimuli, but the underlying disease or fertile ground for its development must be present.

Another theory of allergy based on response to psychological stimuli is that psychological disturbances make the blood vessels more susceptible to the absorption of material to which the person is allergic. In any case, it is felt that emotional problems never cause allergy disease; the disease must already exist although symptoms may temporarily be in remission.

One additional factor that must be considered is the possible effect of an organic illness on the emotions of a sick person. The term "psychosomatic" is popularly used to indicate the effect of the psyche on the soma, but why isn't the term "somatopsychic" employed to indicate the opposite effect? Attacks of asthma with their inherent fear of suffocation and death can easily affect one's emotional equilibrium. Even continuing mild attacks every night unaccompanied by fear can affect one's outlook on life. A constantly itchy skin with the impulse to scratch; a scaly, dry, unpleasant-looking rash on the skin; a runny nose or nasal speech—all symptoms of allergy—are certainly causes for unhappiness, self-consciousness, and alteration in behavior patterns. A common symptom of allergy disease is "allergic fatigue" or "allergic toxemia." Most allergists regard these as organic symptoms that coexist with allergy, but they may well be functional or psychological reactions to allergy, and many undoubtedly are.

SUMMARY

The effect of the emotions on allergy diseases must be considered in the treatment of all persons who have allergy symptoms. "Psychosomatic" indicates the effect of the mind, the "psyche," on the body, the "soma," and does not necessarily imply disease. Everyday examples of psychosomatic reactions are crying caused by sorrow and laughter caused by amusement.

Allergy symptoms, most of which are caused by changes in the caliber of the blood vessels and movement of involuntary muscles, are particularly subject to psychological influences.

Psychiatrists feel that psychological factors influence allergy disease, although most admit that the symptoms cannot be produced by emotional causes independently of an allergy background. The controversy among psychiatrists relates to mechanisms, particularly as they may involve infantile or childhood experience, behavior, the nature of conflicts and stresses that produce allergic rather than other types of organic symptoms. Allergists do not regard these controversial factors as important; most have concluded from the evidence that the psychological impetus is nonspecific.

In allergy, as in other organic diseases, psychological factors may be regarded as a force attempting to upset the normal equilibrium of the individual. The return to normal equilibrium, whether it involves treating allergy, fighting disease, or meeting the stresses of living is called "homeostasis." This adaptation to the normal is probably effected by the hormones; currently the adrenal gland seems most prominent.

The methods of fighting danger are to face it or run away from it. In emotional problems there are two alternative methods really in the "fight" category: these are to give expression to the problem by fighting or verbalizing or keep the problem within one's self. If the problem does not have an outlet the result is organic illness, the so-called psychosomatic disease or symptom.

In allergy a distinction must be made between the disease in general and the individual symptom. The disease is often referred to as a "continuum." Factors such as frustration, anger, fear, or desire may produce a symptom of the disease, but only in the person who has the disease pattern. Another factor that must be recognized is that of the effect of the "soma," the organic illness, on the "psyche," which might be termed "somatopsychic"—the opposite of "psychosomatic."

Important Hay-Fever Producing Plants

TREES

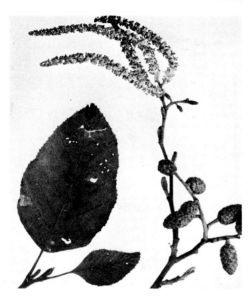

White Alder

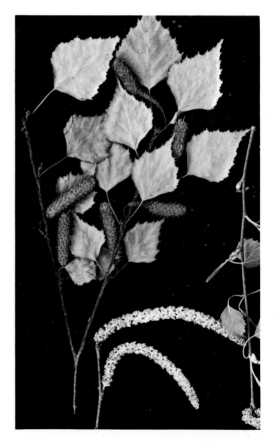

White Birch

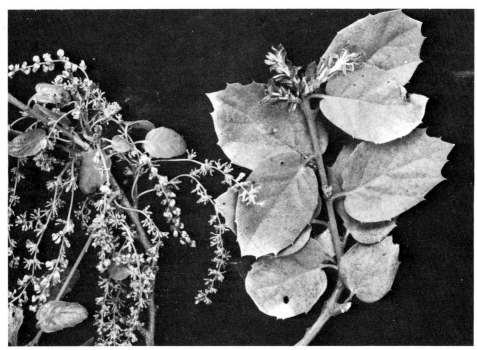

Coast Live Oak

Western Sycamore

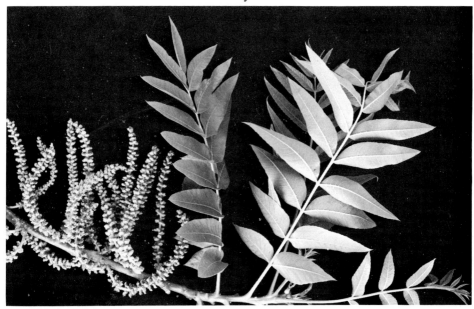

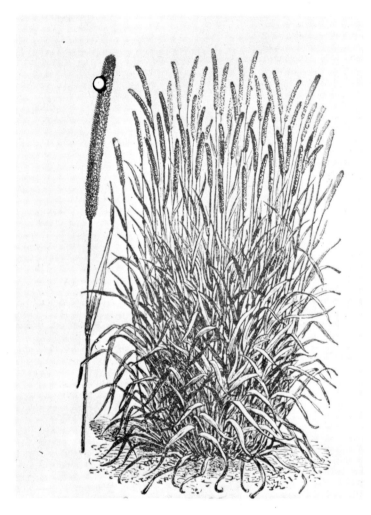

Timothy

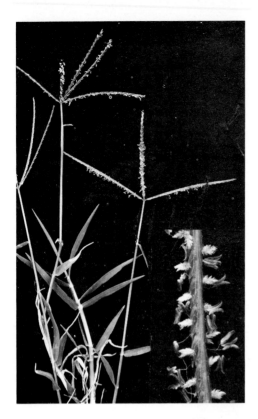

Bermuda grass. Left, stems with 3 to 5 terminal finger-like spikes. Right, enlarged portion of spikes with spikelets and protruding stamens.

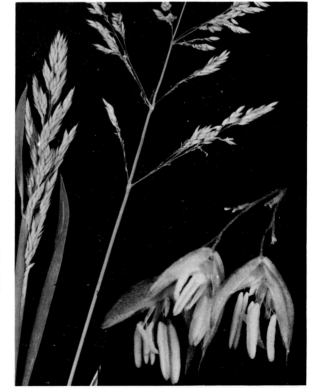

Velvet grass. Left, terminal panicles of spikelets. Right, enlarged view of spikelets with stamens.

Orchard grass. Left, few-branched panicles of spike-lets in one-sided clusters. Right, spikelets with protruding stamens.

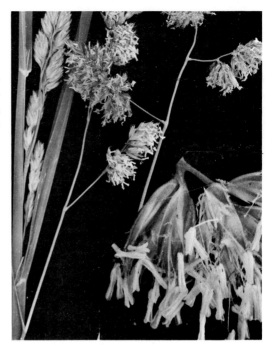

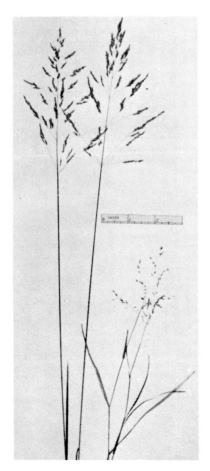

Annual bluegrass on right; Kentucky bluegrass on left.

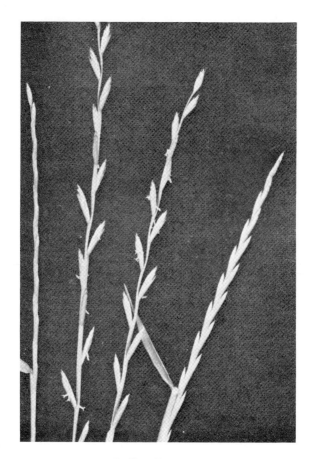

Italian Ryegrass

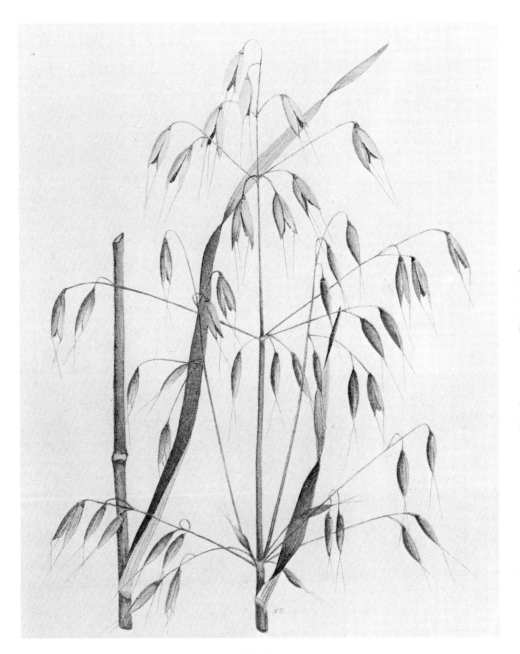

Wild Oats

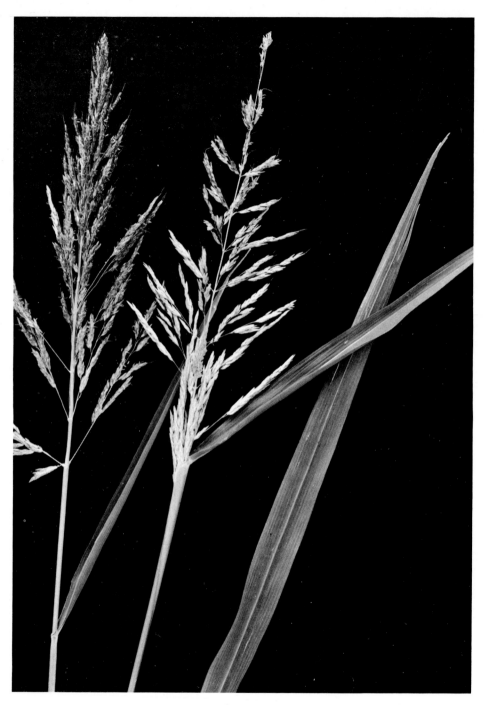

Johnson grass, open panicles of spikelets.

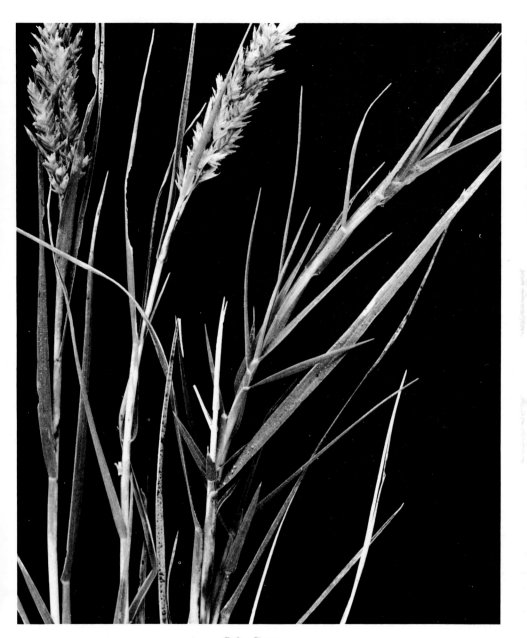

Salt Grass

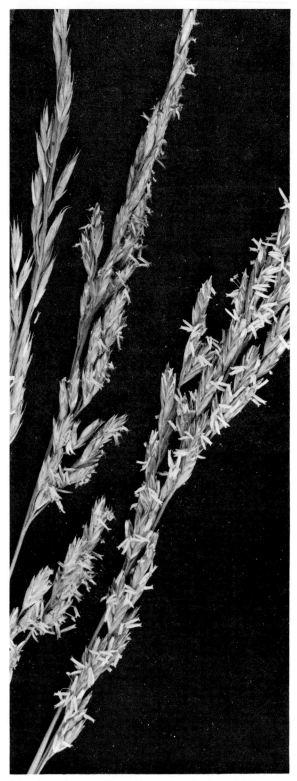

Meadow fescue. Panicles of spikelets with protruding anthers.

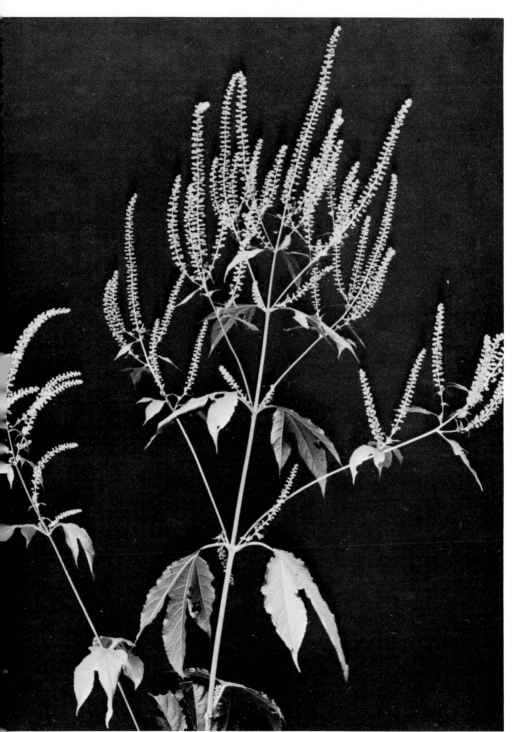

Giant ragweed. (*New York Botanical Garden*)

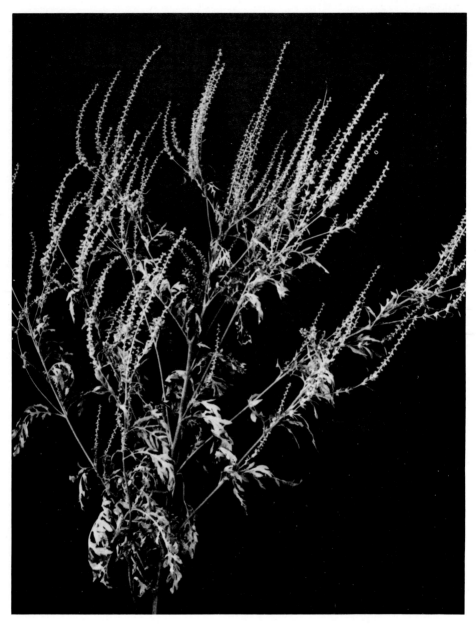

Dwarf ragweed. Note smaller leaves and spikes
than those of giant ragweed. (*New York Botanical Garden*)

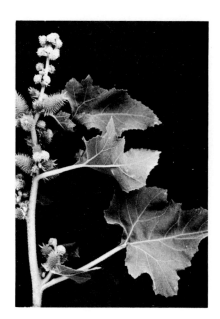

Cocklebur. Branchlet with leaves, small globular heads of staminate flowers (terminal), and pistillate floral clusters (axillary and basal).

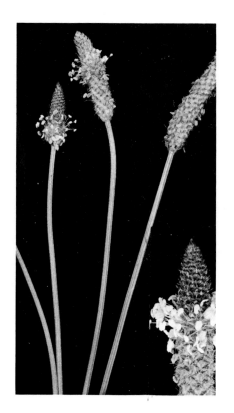

English Plantain

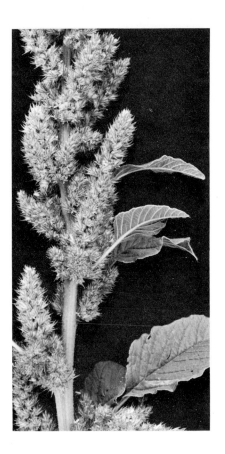

Rough Pigweed

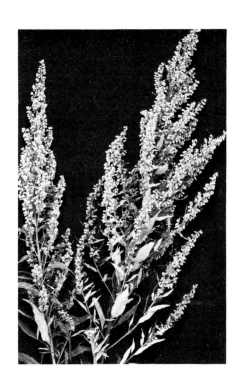

California Mugwort

Lamb's-quarters (White Pigweed)

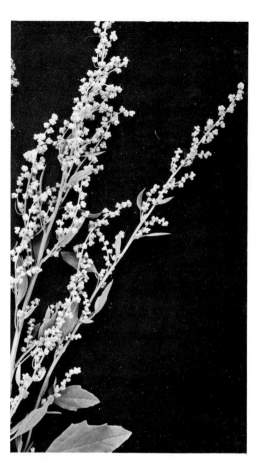

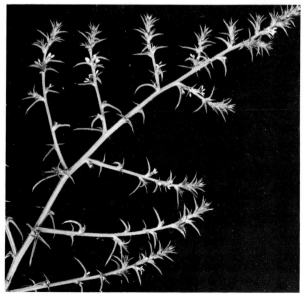

Russian thistle, branchlet
with small flowers.

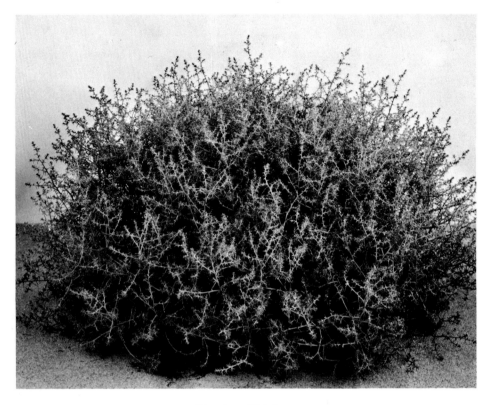

Russian Thistle

Chapter Nineteen

What To Do About Your Allergy

The information in this chapter should not be construed as suggesting self-diagnosis or self-treatment. This would be most unwise. In allergy, as in many other matters, an objective, specially trained individual should be chosen when help is required. When a person is emotionally upset, it is wise for him to visit a psychiatrist or psychologist; when business worries are present, he should call in a business consultant. An organic illness should be similarly approached.

The preceding chapters of this book do not imply that the diagnosis, or differential diagnosis, of allergy disease is simple. If this impression exists, it should be dispelled. Although some allergy diseases such as hay fever may be easy to identify, a well-trained physician may have difficulty in differentiating a case of allergic rhinitis from a coryza or cold caused by infection. In fact, both allergy and infection are very likely to be present at the same time. Laboratory tests, such as the microscopic examination of a nasal smear, may be required. Innumerable pathologic conditions can cause asthmatic breathing; many are very serious diseases, like tumors within the chest (which may be malignant), heart conditions, or whooping cough. Urticaria or hives may be easy to see, but the determination of their cause, particularly when they last for a long time, is one of the most perplexing problems in allergy. Eczema may be easily diagnosed by most doctors who are familiar with various skin diseases, but there are many variations of this illness which require differentiation and demand different forms of treatment.

There are instances where one may find it necessary to "treat himself." An allergist may not be available. Most physicians specializing in allergy are located in large cities and cannot be conveniently reached by all patients. Furthermore, allergy is a comparatively new specialty and until the past fifteen or twenty years was not taught in medical schools. Even today, it is often a neglected discipline. In addition, medicine is so highly specialized that doctors trained in other branches of medicine may have an insufficient knowledge of allergy. Therefore, if no allergist or other doctor equipped to handle allergy problems is readily available, a person who suspects he has an allergy may have to treat himself, at least for a time.

The symptoms of some forms of allergy are so distressing that immediate help to obtain temporary relief is required. In this connection, the individual suffering from allergy may wish to know how to evaluate the reliability of widely disseminated advertisements for proprietary allergy medicines. Such knowledge may be particularly useful in the event of minor sniffles or an occasional mild skin rash, which are unmistakably caused by allergy, but do not necessarily require the attention of a doctor. All people have some tendency toward allergy; in some it may be merely allergy to the poison ivy plant, which causes a reaction in up to 70 percent of the population, or to penicillin, an allergy which is becoming more and more prevalent. Or it may be asthma, hay fever, or eczema which affects 10 percent of the population. Only a fraction of the 10 percent seek formal medical care and the remaining 90 percent, who may have some mild allergy, usually try to help themselves. But one should remember that in the long run, self-diagnosis and self-treatment may be harmful. Treatment of symptoms without a definitive diagnosis is not recommended.

Finally, a person may wish to know how he can help his doctor. A person can assist his doctor by carefully studying his environment and neighborhood for possible allergens. By carefully scrutinizing the history form in Chapter 2 the patient may answer some of the questions and obtain some information about the possible diagnosis and cause of his allergy condition. A limited number of modified tests may even be performed on oneself. Despite these possible contributions of the patient to the alleviation of his own illness, this chapter is in no way intended to serve as a do-it-yourself kit nor to imply that one should circumvent a doctor's care.

Allergy skin tests may not always be essential in allergy diagnosis; when they are, they confirm the suspicion and the diagnosis derived from a careful history of the illness and the circumstances surrounding it. When the cause of the symptoms is an inhalant and cannot be avoided or eliminated, skin tests are necessary to determine which allergy material should be used for proper allergy treatment by desensitization.

This is particularly true of pollen that causes trouble only during certain months of the year and which requires that the use of pollen skin tests during the course of treatment be carefully calculated and adjusted.

Often the suspicion may be substantiated by an improvised self-administered "allergy test." There is hardly a need to perform an allergy skin test to cat hair, for example, when it is evident that asthma occurs each time one fondles a cat. In such cases, even a negative allergy skin test to cat hair and dander will not nullify a readily exhibited allergy to cats. If one performs a number of such informal tests frequently and they are properly interpreted, they are valid.

DIAGNOSIS OF ALLERGY SYMPTOMS

The allergist has three factors to consider in the management of a person with a suspected allergy disease. First, is the condition really an allergy? Second, what is the cause? What substance is the patient allergic to? Third, what is the proper treatment both to relieve the immediate symptoms and to prevent additional ones? The first question poses no problem if the allergy illness is a disease such as hay fever, the symptoms of which are well known and obvious. In a similar manner but less definitively bronchial asthma may be diagnosed. Here there are many causes of wheezing, cough, and difficulty in breathing other than allergy. A skin rash may be eczema but many skin rashes look very much alike, and a doctor must be consulted for an exact diagnosis. The numerous less common and/or rare conditions caused by allergy require diagnostic acumen. These include a variety of gastrointestinal symptoms ranging from mild abdominal cramps to severe diarrhea, frequency of urination, heart irregularities, and others. Some of these symptoms can be investigated by the sufferer just as he can investigate the cause of the more obvious allergy manifestations, but the final decision as to whether or not they are caused by allergy requires evaluation by a skilled physician. He must not neglect much needed medical care for a condition that may prove to be more serious. Sometimes, for example, being tired or lacking "pep" may be caused by allergy, but there are other serious causes of fatigue; therefore, it is important that all other causes of such a vague symptom should be thoroughly investigated before allergy is entertained as a diagnosis.

ALLERGY TREATMENT

Symptomatic treatment of allergy is usually not difficult. This encompasses relief of the current symptoms and preventive (prophylactic) treatment as well. Many medicines such as the usual "antihistamines" and "decongestants" can be purchased without a prescription. They are too numerous to list and many have a degree of local popularity. Most physicians are reluctant to approve patients' medicating themselves. As indicated earlier, this is a generally correct view. However, the U. S. Food and Drug Administration is particularly watchful of these over-the-counter medicines, restricting the dose sold to half that usually prescribed by a doctor. (See Chapter 12.) Addicting drugs, of course, are not available and others that can produce side effects in some people bear adequate warnings on the package. These may often be very frightening but are necessary primarily to protect a small minority of people who would react unfavorably. Individual state laws complement Federal law.

Many antihistamines and decongestants are popularly advertised and sold directly to the public. Some of them are identical with those the doctor would prescribe and several are even manufactured by the same pharmaceutical manufacturer. Those for asthma are listed in Chapter 12. The number of antihistamine preparations listed for sale directly to the consumer in the drug trade catalogue is currently more than two hundred. A partial list, along with prescription items, is listed in Chapter 12.

While many over-the-counter medicines are available for the relief of asthma and allergic rhinitis, it is difficult to treat one's skin allergy effectively without a doctor's help. However, a great deal can be done to prevent exacerbation and aggravation. Antihistamines and even the compounds used for asthma may be effective for the relief of hives, particularly those that contain antihistamines along with the other usual ingredients. Soothing baths with baking soda, starch, or oatmeal help to relieve skin rashes and allergy irritations. Strong salves and ointments, particularly those containing phenol (carbolic acid), menthol, and camphor are best avoided. Simple vaseline-type creams and boric acid (U. S. P. strength) ointment can be easily procured and are helpful. Soothing lotions such as calamine lotion and calamine lotion with an antihistamine are useful as antihistamine creams; they help relieve the itching. The most effective external medications for eczema contain a cortisone derivative and therefore cannot be purchased without a prescription.

Prophylactic treatment is more difficult than the relief of immediate symptoms. If symptoms result from allergy to a food, the treatment is avoidance of that food. If feathers in your pillow are the cause, synthetic or foam rubber pillows should be substituted. Avoidance of any implicated factor is always the best form of preventing future attacks. When the underlying cause cannot be avoided or eliminated, desensitization must be instituted by a physician.

ALLERGIC INVESTIGATION

In discovering which substances a person is allergic to there are several techniques of investigation that the sufferer can perform himself. Allergens entering by ingestion, inhalation, or contact can be explored by one's self; the other methods of allergenic entry are less feasible. Self-exploration does not mean the technically performed allergy skin tests described in Chapter 4, because these are dangerous procedures and must be performed under careful supervision by a physician. It refers to casual contact simulating common activities, such as washing clothes with a given detergent. Such a "contact test" may be invaluable.

Diet

The person who suspects that his difficulty is due to what he eats has a greater opportunity for self-investigation and self-help than in any other type of allergy. This is due in part to the fact that allergy skin tests for food sensitivity are not as reliable nor as diagnostic as the tests for what one inhales. So even while skin tests are being performed it is good practice for one to avoid suspected foods and then deliberately eat them one at a time in an attempt to induce symptoms and thus verify the existence of food allergy. One must be aware that there are several types of food allergy, as discussed in Chapter 8.

There are two main methods by which the exact nature of food allergy can be investigated: the use of a food diary and adherence to elimination diets. These methods are also discussed in detail in Chapter 8.

There are some misconceptions as to which foods are most important in the production of allergy symptoms. One is that "milk causes mucus." This is not true. Milk is an allergic factor only when a person is allergic to milk and has the type of allergy in which an overproduction of mucus is one of the symptoms. Merely to avoid milk for no logical reason is not warranted. On the other hand, in an infant whose diet consists only of cow's milk, it makes sense to change it to some other form of milk such as goat's milk, or to a substitute a nutriment such as soybean, if milk allergy is suspected as the cause of allergy symptoms. Although milk allergy may be caused by only one portion of the milk such as the casein (curd) or the protein (whey) fractions, it is simpler to avoid all milk products rather than to attempt to avoid the fraction to which the sensitivity exists.

Pollen

Most people are aware of pollen as a cause of allergy symptoms, particularly symptoms that are related to the respiratory tract, such as those of hay fever. The geographical plants and trees have been discussed in detail in Chapter 5. One must take into consideration not only the prevailing pollen but also one's habits. If you are an out-of-doors man or woman and play golf every weekend, you cannot be compared with an apartment dweller who lives in an air-conditioned apartment and stays at home during the weekend. Anyone can "investigate" his own living and recreational habits and form some sort of an idea of how likely he is to come in contact with the circulating pollen in the air. The next step must be to correlate these habits with his symptoms.

General Neighborhood

In addition to pollen prevalent in the area where a person lives and works there are often localized air pollutants that should be considered. A person with asthma who lives near a furniture factory may be dramatically relieved if he moves away. Although there is currently an attempt being made to control factory emissions, some get into the atmosphere and in the sensitive individual produce symptoms. If you look about, you may find sources of air pollution that were unsuspected. You can do this more easily than your doctor.

When one lives very near flower beds or works among them, they may produce allergy symptoms. This is particularly true when a person who is sick in a hospital has flowers in his room. If you are allergic, play it safe: do not keep cut flowers in your home, and if you must have a garden, plan it so that you will not have many allergy-producing plants.

House Structure

The age and state of repair of the house in which you live may be a cause of your allergy symptoms. If your house is old and damp, it may be subject to mold growth. The spores of the molds will often get into the air within the house, become part of the house dust, and produce symptoms. This is especially true in tropical and subtropical climates where there is much rain and dampness and where molds are very prevalent. They are also found in large numbers in the temperate zones where rain is frequent. In arid regions such as in Arizona, New Mexico, and southern California, molds are not so common but cannot be entirely disregarded because of the increased use of irrigation in these areas.

The type of heat that is used in a home may be important. Electric heat is practically innocuous. Forced-air heat depends on the use of a fan to blow the warmed air into the various rooms. If the source of the heat and ducts is dusty there is likely to be a considerable amount of dust blown into the house. Filters used in the furnaces are helpful but not completely efficient. You can investigate this if your home appears unusually dusty or if your symptoms are worse when the heat is turned on. A damp basement in which rotted wood is piled up, adjacent to a forced-air furnace, may be the source of molds in the house. Coal as the source of heat is probably not different from gas energy since stokers are used extensively. Often, change of filters, vacuuming air ducts, and use of mold-resisting chemicals may have to be resorted to.

Bedroom

More accurately than anyone else, you can go from room to room and examine the possible sources of allergy-producing materials. The bedroom is the most important room since one spends more consecutive hours in that room than in any other. Dust is the most common allergen, and it is essential to remove all dust catchers such as ornaments, pictures, books, knickknacks, and objects that may be used infrequently. The windows should be curtained with material that is easily laundered, and only throw rugs which can be frequently removed and cleaned should be used. Venetian blinds are very troublesome collectors of dust and should not be used anywhere in the house.

To eliminate dust from the bedroom as much as possible the following procedures are recommended:

1. The dust-sensitive person should be out of the house or room while all cleaning is being done.

2. Remove all the furniture, carpets, and drapes from the room; empty the closets.

3. Clean each piece of furniture, each article of clothing, and wash each curtain before replacing it.

4. Preferably, the floor should be bare wood—well-waxed—or tile. If carpet is necessary it should have a rubber underpad and should be of synthetic material rather than wool. Washable throw rugs, if kept washed, are acceptable.

5. If possible, beds should have wood or metal frames with metal springs, easily washable.

6. Pillows should be of foam rubber or synthetic, such as Dacron. However, some people find that when a rubber pillow becomes old, it tends to disintegrate, and the rubber dust that seeps out causes allergy symptoms, perhaps because of mold growth. If the pillows are stuffed with feathers, they should be covered with a special plastic zippered encasing.

7. Curtains should be washed frequently.

8. Avoid fuzzy wool blankets; if they must be used they should be enclosed in a tightly-woven percale blanket-cover encasing; or an extra sheet may be used to cover them.

9. Eliminate all excess furniture, especially upholstered furniture and dust catchers such as ornaments, stuffed toys, etc.

10. Do not allow any animals in the bedroom.

11. Clean the bedroom daily. For dusting use a damp or oily dust cloth. Vacuum at least once a week.

12. Keep the windows and doors of the bedroom closed as much as possible.

13. If there is a hot-air heating vent in the bedroom, have it sealed to prevent dust from being blown into the room with the hot air.

14. Avoid using insect sprays, particularly those containing pyrethrum and "pyrethrins."

15. Use the closet in the bedroom only for frequently used clothing; do not use it for storage.

16. For articles that cannot be properly cleaned or are suspected as being dust receptacles, the dust can be minimized and "sealed" by using a diluted solution of a liquid "antidust" preparation such as Dust-Seal or Allergex. Spray the solution at least annually on the curtains, drapes, rugs, carpets, furniture cushions, blankets, padded headboards, box springs, and mattresses.

Wool is another antigen of importance that is often found in the bedroom. It is of less consequence when it is used in polished form such as in men's or women's suits, but it may be a source of allergy when it is in the fuzzy form, such as blankets and coarse, bulky wool knit sweaters. Nor should one wear woolen stockings. Avoid wool in the form of fur, such as used for sheepskin linings for coats, gloves, and collars. Winter wear such as snowsuits and coats should preferably be made of cotton or some material other than wool. Electric blankets contain very little, if any, wool. Domestic rugs or carpeting were for years made only of wool, but there is an increasing tendency to use synthetic floor coverings. Chenille rugs contain cow hair, while Oriental rugs may be a combination of wool, cow hair, and sometimes dog hair.

Mattresses are made of cotton and, most often, raw cotton linters are used. Cottonseed may still be attached to the material and thus be allergy-producing. If, however, the mattress is adequately covered so that no fuzz leaks out and gets into the air of the bedroom, it is not likely to cause any trouble. The most expensive and softest feather pillows are those filled with goose feathers (down); others are mixtures of chicken and duck feathers. Dacron or other synthetic fiber pillows are being used more frequently today. They are not allergenic; nor are pillows made from foam rubber. A material commonly used for stuffing decorative pillows, less often bed pillows, and for sleeping bags, is kapok. Since kapok is a vegetable fiber it is an important allergen and should be avoided by those who are sensitive to it. To prevent stuffing from escaping, specially-made allergy casings for mattresses and pillows are now marketed. The spraying of a silicone or an oil-in-water emulsion, such as Dust-Seal or Allergex,* keeps the dust down in the bedroom or

---

* Dust-Seal is manufactured by L.S. Green Associates, 160 W. 59th St., New York, N.Y. Allergex is manufactured by Hollister-Stier Laboratories, 2030 Wilshire Blvd., Los Angeles, California.

elsewhere in the home. Either of these can be obtained or ordered from a drugstore. Directions for their use accompany them.

Living Room

All hidden residues of dust should be sought out and eliminated. Sometimes this creates a problem since certain dust-collecting structures may be part of the building. Fireplaces, for example, are very often major dust repositories. They should be enclosed with a screen that can be cleaned regularly and kept comparatively dust-free. As in the bedroom, the padding under the rugs and the furniture upholstery materials (both the coverings and the stuffings) must be considered. Furniture covering may be composed of any of a number of materials; the most important from the standpoint of allergy are wool and mohair. Mohair is derived from goat hair and is a common constituent of plushes, velvets, and velours. Silk may be a cause of allergy even when used as a furniture covering. Materials referred to as faille, satin, foulard, pongees, and taffeta are primarily silk. If you are sensitive to a particular covering or stuffing of your furniture, it may have to be replaced.

Federal law requires the manufacturer to attach a label to upholstered furniture designating the contents of the stuffing. A typical sofa label might read: "Concealed Materials Are New Materials. Contents: *Body:* Horse Hair 12½%, Hog Hair 87½%, together constituting 50% with Cotton Felt, 50%. *Cushions:* Duck Feathers 75% and Down 25%." Unfortunately some people remove these tags upon purchase of their new furniture. This later complicates the problem of finding out what the stuffing is composed of because it is not possible to guess the contents by touch. The upholstery must be ripped open.

Occasionally the wood burned in the fireplace may be a cause of allergy symptoms. Asthma caused by wood smoke is not uncommon and is sometimes caused by a specific variety of wood that is burned. Other factors in the living room which should be examined and considered include artificial leather substitutes and the heavy coating of furniture polishes and waxes. These can contain sufficient amounts of linseed (flaxseed) oil to produce symptoms in a very sensitive person.

Bathroom

To investigate allergy-producing articles in your bathroom it is necessary to list them inasmuch as each person keeps on hand medicines and toilet articles of his individual choice. The list should include all items including soaps, bath powders, after-shave lotions, and cosmetics. These are important from the standpoint of both ingestion (taking of medicines) and inhalation and contact (powders and scents).

Hairbrushes, shaving brushes, and toothbrushes must be considered in connection with animal hair sensitivity because some of the best bristles are made from the hair of such animals as the domestic hog and the boar. Orris root, which used to be a very common constituent of cosmetics and is a potent allergen, is rarely used today. But it may still be found as a carrier or a binder in some perfumes and scents, especially soaps, after-shave lotions, colognes, toilet waters, and other strongly scented toilet articles. The so-called hypoallergenic cosmetics, of which there are many readily procurable at drugstores, do not contain orris root, and although they seldom cause allergy symptoms, they are not completely allergy-free and can occasionally cause reactions in susceptible persons.

Linseed or flaxseed may be found in the bathroom in wave-set liquids, hair tonics, soaps, depilatories, and on tile floors. Denture adhesive powders may contain karaya gum which can act as an allergen. The gum is also found in some medicines, particularly cathartics, laxatives, toothpastes, wave-set lotions, certain diabetic foods, and hand lotions. Bathroom deodorants may contain sensitizers. If after using any of these products allergy symptoms develop, these products should be eliminated.

Kitchen

A list of all the foods, particularly those canned or packaged, should be made. The cleaning and scouring powders and the soap or detergent commonly used should also be noted, as well as brushes and brooms, starch, oilcloth, tile floor, twine, rope, candles, and any other nondescript items which may be kept about. Foods in the kitchen should be itemized on a food chart listing the hidden ingredients. The environmental status of the kitchen is similar to that of the other rooms but more extensive use is involved. If a person has symptoms aggravated only in the kitchen, food odors must be considered in addition to the contents. A woman spends much of her time during the day in the kitchen. If she is allergic to the items with which she comes in contact, they must be especially noted. Linoleum is a common kitchen floor covering. This is composed of linseed oil which has been treated with chemicals and then exposed to hot air to make it hard. Linseed oil is also a base for some of the widely used furniture polishes. It is also used in the preparation of oilcloth. There is some question about the allergenicity of many refined oils.

Brushes and brooms are made of wheat, rye, barley, and rice straw, and of animal hair, mainly that of the hog, horse, goat, sheep, and camel. Laundry starch is mainly corn but may be wheat or rice. Twine and rope are made of animal hair, cotton linters, straw, and flaxseed.

Closets

Closets are great repositories of dust. In some households they contain stored items of unworn clothing in addition to numerous miscellaneous materials, including old furniture. Fur coats and fur-trimmed coats should be identified because of possible allergy to the fur. The same consideration must be given to sweaters, particularly those made of goat hair, such as alpaca and Angora. Felt hats may be made of varieties of animal hair. Moths tend to propagate in dark closets and have been indicted as a cause of allergy, as have mothproofing materials like camphor and naphthalene. It is not possible to itemize all the possible allergens that may be found in the closet. A simple rule, if you are allergic, is not to allow the closet in daily use to contain anything but clothing in current and regular use. If storing is necessary, the storage closet should be as far away as possible from the area you live in regularly, and you should not enter the closet unless it is absolutely necessary.

Miscellaneous

Any room in the house may be a source of trouble for a person with allergy. It could be the den or "family room," the sun porch, the library, the nursery, a workshop, or a music room. Each should be carefully inventoried and the contents questioned as possibly allergenic if allergy symptoms are aggravated when the allergic person is in that room. A workshop with sawdust may be the culprit, or a sewing room with much lint in the air. Paints and varnishes contain linseed oil or corn oil, sometimes both, while animal hair is incorporated in plaster. They can cause severe allergy disease. Roofing tar has linseed oil, but it is usually the fresh plaster and the fresh paint and roofing that cause difficulty. Allergic individuals commonly react to the odor of fresh paint as well as to other strong odors. By carefully scrutinizing the materials in the home, one can often reach a diagnosis, or at least a suspicion of the cause of the trouble, and by elimination or avoidance effect a relief of symptoms. Allergy skin tests performed by an allergy specialist are invaluable in providing important clues.

CONTACT ALLERGY

On the surface it would appear that contact allergy would be the easiest for a person to diagnose by himself, since a rash on the skin, obviously in contact with some material, should present no difficulty. This is usually true but how often no one knows because the patients whom allergists and skin specialists see are most likely those who present perplexing problems and where the contact is obscure. Probably for every person with contact dermatitis who consults a doctor there are thousands who take care of the minor skin rash themselves. Several examples will illustrate this.

The most common type of contact allergy is the dermatitis caused by poison ivy, poison oak, or poison sumac. This is usually discovered and diagnosed by the victim; a physician is only called in if the person is very sick with a severe rash, generalized swelling, and intense itching. The doctor can diagnose but nature heals. The prevention of these rashes by desensitization is advocated by some doctors; others feel that it is not at all helpful.

Another example is that of the woman who finds a rash under her wedding ring, or under the metal necklace around her neck, or on her back where the zipper tab touches the skin. Other examples are rashes on the legs caused by synthetic stockings or dye, or rashes on the forehead resulting from hair rinses or dyes. There are many such varied examples. In practically all cases the diagnosis is made by the person who gets the rash without the help of a doctor. Sometimes there is merely suspicion, and verification is obtained from a doctor. A physician should always be consulted when any rash persists despite removal of the suspected contact.

Several commercial women's hair dyes include in their package a special small vial of the contents with instructions for the prospective user to perform a patch test on the skin to determine whether she is sensitive to the dye. This can be dangerous since a deliberate skin test with a suspected contactant may produce a severe reaction, if the individual is exquisitely sensitive.

SUMMARY

There are many things to do about an allergy even before consulting a doctor. One must first be "allergy conscious," reviewing all possible allergens that may be causing the symptoms, realizing that the most common allergy symptom-production is by ingestion, inhalation, or contact. The less common means of symptom-production are more difficult to ascertain by one's self, and in any event diagnosis should not be attempted, particularly if symptoms have existed for any length of time. There are many illnesses that resemble allergy diseases or coexist with them, so that the correct diagnosis is not readily or conclusively made in all instances.

Once the diagnosis of allergy is established beyond doubt, if relief of symptoms is all that is desired, there are many effective anti-allergy medicines available for purchase, even without a doctor's prescription. Many of these are almost identical with prescription products. It is never recommended that sick people medicate themselves indiscriminately without medical supervision. Although the medicines advertised may give relief, they do not remove the cause and they do not effect a "cure." There are many well-known hazards in self-medication, yet when a doctor is not available and immediate relief is needed, it may be necessary to resort to self-medication with the realization that this is not the best form of treatment.

The doctor is aided in his investigation of the cause of the allergy by an essential battery of skin tests. They are not infallible and the full complement may not always be required. The history of the illness can often give the allergic person as well as the doctor, an idea of the type of allergy and its possible causes. First, the foods that are eaten are considered, then the distribution of plant pollen, and finally the environment about and within the house. These skin contacts which may cause eczematous contact dermatitis are the most common causes of allergy.

The diet is investigated by food avoidance and food trial. For a further discussion of these techniques see Chapter 7.

Pollen is suspected as the cause of allergy symptoms when the trouble occurs during certain seasons of the year only. (See Chapter 5.) One must learn the geography and the plants of the region where he lives. The general neighborhood in which one works and lives may be important because it may have a particular tree or plant with a specific pollinating pattern. Also, the business and recreational habits of the individual are important since his exposure to the pollen varies in accordance with his activity.

The inhalant material within the house differs from room to room and it is recommended that an inventory be made of all the materials in each. Molds may be a factor in old, damp houses. The living room and bedroom as sources of inhalant allergy have also been discussed in Chapter 5. The type of heat is a consideration since forced-air heat may blow dust-laden air into a room. Fireplaces may be a source of allergy not only because they collect dust but because of the type of wood burned in them. In the bathroom, one must bear in mind not only the presence of medicines but also of toiletries. In the kitchen, there must be an inventory of all the food items as well as of the brushes, brooms, mops, cleaning supplies, twine, rope, laundry starch, and other items.

Contact allergy probably offers the best opportunity for diagnosis and treatment by oneself. Poison ivy, poison oak, and poison sumac dermatitis are easily recognized, and the history of exposure confirms the diagnosis without much question. Soothing creams, lotions, and washes are available for the relief of minor rashes at all drugstores; the more severe or persistent rashes require a physician's attention. The more potent medicines for the relief of severe rashes must be prescribed. Rashes caused by contact with a dye, metal, or other suspect substance can usually be identified simply by avoidance of the contact, which results in a clearing of the skin.

There is much that can be done by the person about his allergy if it is done intelligently and with understanding. Often, too much is done without proper insight. Self-diagnosis and treatment must be educated and reasonable, but they can be hazardous.

Chapter Twenty

Unconventional Treatment
of Allergy Diseases

The treatment of allergy diseases by a competent specialist is universal and quite well standardized. Patients who move from one section of the country to another, or even from a foreign country to another, can continue their treatment without interruption. All that is needed is a short report of the medication that they have been taking from the physician previously in charge and allowing for language and nomenclature with which every experienced allergist is familiar, the specific desensitization treatment as well as the treatment of symptoms need not be changed. One notable exception is Russia, where the symptomatic treatment is identical, but the concept of desensitization has not yet been generally accepted.

Nonetheless, as might be expected there have been developed over the years many unconventional and unorthodox forms of treatment. Their main appeal is simplicity or a purported shortcut to health. Some are based on folklore, some on misunderstood physiological principles; and some are utterly inexplicable. Many allergists regard most of these recommended medicines as placebos or as simply the products of quackery. Fortunately in this country strict laws now prohibit the marketing of any harmful or inappropriate medicine and have thus in large measure eliminated the sale of completely dishonest medicaments.

The history of frauds which have been perpetrated on the public under the guise of beneficial medicines makes interesting if somewhat pathetic reading. It includes not only medicines that had no medicinal properties but contraptions mechanically devised to fool the victim into believing that they had restorative powers. Those who suffered from asthma, for example, often as a result of misleading advertising, have purchased or employed these agents; in fact these products still appear from time to time. Once put out of business by the government, they may crop up elsewhere in another form. It is sad that the sick have been preyed upon in this way and succumb to promises which are not fulfilled. By doing so they neglect beneficial treatment from established sources.

Suggestion plays a prominent role in the treatment of all diseases, particularly those that are chronic. Many people will respond favorably to a placebo if they are under the impression that it is a potent medicine. Placebo literally means "I shall please," and is literally "a medicine, especially an inactive one given merely to satisfy a patient." Some may argue with this definiton since some placebos appear to benefit the person who has believed in it. The extent to which suggestion influences people has been demonstrated over and over again. In allergy, one interesting experiment was performed many years ago by an allergist who was in the habit of posting the current atmospheric pollen count in the local area on a blackboard in his office waiting room. During the hay fever season, of course, the more pollen in the air, the worse the symptoms would be. This allergist would occasionally falsify the figures, and in a substantial percentage of instances the hay fever sufferer's symptoms would be proportionate to the posted figures on the black-board rather than to the actual amount of pollen in the air.

Not all the unorthodox therapies being promulgated at present are outright frauds or placebos; many have beneficial effects but are not employed by the majority of allergists. Those discussed in this chapter are in that category. It is difficult to pass judgement on many of the methods that are unconventional. Despite the unscientific explanations of the manufacturers or promoters, the fact that they are still marketed indicates that surely some people have found them useful. At present, some may well have merit not clearly defined; others like the asthma powders and cigarettes possess asthma-relieving drugs in their formula.

ASTHMA POWDERS AND CIGARETTES

Most of the asthma powders and cigarettes contain stramonium leaves and potassium nitrate (saltpeter). In addition there may be leaves of lobelia, mullein, swamp cabbage, cubeb, chamomile, saw palmetto, eucalyptus, thyme, anise seed, and fennel seed. The action of the spices or herbs is probably nonspecific. The basic ingredient is the stramonium which contains atropine, a mild bronchial dilator. Ammonium nitrate is added to promote combustion. Burning produces pyridine and nitrate, which is also known to relax the bronchial muscles, so that the potassium nitrate probably is an important ingredient. The inhaled smoke irritates, as well as relaxes, the lining of the bronchial tubes inducing a cough. Some thick phlegm may thus be raised, relieving the airway obstruction. The continued use of asthma powders and cigarettes (*Schiffman's Asthmador formula* is said to have been available as far back as 1904) reflects some reliance of asthmatics on this form of medication. Among the powders similar to Schiffman's are *Kellog's Asthma Powder,* said to contain stramonium and potassium nitrate, *Himrod's,* a mixture of fennel seeds, stramonium, and niter, and *Power's Asthma Relief,* reported to consist of stramonium leaves, mullein leaves, anise seed, potassium nitrate, and inert matter. Some persons have ingested asthma powders that contain atropine and scopolamine for the purpose of "getting high." Deaths have been reported following such use.

URINE INJECTIONS

Some years ago it was proposed that allergies could be effectively treated with a series of urine injections. The procedure advocated was for the patient to collect his urine in a sterile container. Part of the collected urine was then injected into the buttocks of the patient weekly for eight consecutive weeks. It was asserted that 80 percent of those who took this treatment were "cured." It was claimed that the antigens responsible for the allergy are filtered through the glomeruli (the vascular portion) of the kidneys, rather than through the capillaries, into the tissue spaces (the usual route). By mechanically transferring the antigens to the tissue spaces, the allergy may be overcome. This did not accord with any well-founded immunological principle.

In 1933 Oriel described the presence of large amounts of a certain proteose in the urine. This protein-like substance, *Oriel's P Substance,* can be extracted with ether. Extensive experimental use yielded controversial results. Those who found the urine injections successful maintained that the proteose found in the urine enhanced the immune process.

AUTOHEMOTHERAPY

The reinjection of one's own blood into the body is not a completely unorthodox procedure, since it is still employed by many competent doctors under certain circumstances, one of which is chronic, severe, intractable hives. About ten cubic centimeters (one-third of an ounce) of blood is withdrawn from a patient's vein and immediately reinjected into the buttocks. This treatment is often given twice weekly. The concept is that in some way a nonspecific reaction to the immune mechanism "stirs things up," benefiting the patient. A more scientific explanation that has been offered is that blocking antibodies are formed.

ANERGEX (Poison Oak Extract)

Anergex is an extract of *Toxicodendron quercifolia,* which is related to the poison ivy plant. The claim is made that only several injections relieve any allergy condition, particularly asthma. The medicine is injected daily by a physician for six to eight days. This form of treatment is popular among some physicians who are not trained in allergy. The number of successfully treated cases as stated in the brochure of the pharmaceutical firm promoting the product is impressive. There is no need for allergy skin tests and each patient and each allergy disease are treated similarly. Severe local reactions at the site of the injection are common. The rationale of the treatment of an allergy disease with this material is not entirely clear. Perhaps it is to produce blocking antibodies against the plant *Toxicodendron quercifolia* and by so doing (hopefully) alter the immune mechanism so that other antibodies as well are blocked. In this way, it may be compared to the urinary proteose and the autohemotherapy methods of relieving allergies. The product was studied by a committee of the American Academy of Allergy. They reported in a double blind study using a placebo as a control that "eight daily injections of either Anergex or placebo into fifty-one patients did not reveal any difference between the two groups." It was the conclusion of the drug committee that "Anergex is without value in the treatment of ragweed pollinosis (hay fever due to ragweed)."

THE PRESENCE OF THE CHIHUAHUA DOG

The *Chihuahua* dog, since it has very short hair is thought by some to alleviate or cure asthma. This is not so, as it is the dander more than the hair that produces allergy. Yet the myth persists. Another type of a truly hairless Mexican dog known as the *Xoloitzcuintli,* almost extinct, is in great demand by physicians in Mexico for the treatment and prevention of asthma, but is virtually unavailable. It may be that this dog and the chihuahua are less likely to cause allergy in a person sensitive to dog hair, but there is no rationale for its being preventive or therapeutic. Yet the myth persists.

THE DIAGNOSIS OF ALLERGY FROM A BLOOD SAMPLE

For some years, at least one laboratory in the United States has been advertising that the diagnosis of allergies can be performed without skin tests merely by analyzing a sample of blood in the laboratory. The theory is that there are certain strains of *colon bacteria* which are individually specific to each food, pollen, dust, animal hair, and any other allergen. The diagnostic material is made by isolating the specific strains of colon bacteria from the substance and preparing a culture of it. The culture is then inactivated, standardized, and diluted. The test is performed in this way: One drop of the patient's blood serum is added to one drop of each specific culture, then this is incubated at a given temperature for twelve hours. The solution is then placed on a glass slide and examined under the microscope.

The technique has been tested by numerous allergists, bacteriologists, and other doctors over the years (it was first patented in Great Britain in 1931) without any correlation found between actual clinical allergy, skin tests, and the diagnosis as specified by the laboratory from the patient's serum. It is difficult to understand why there should be any correlation between the colon bacillus strain and allergy. Nevertheless, the method remains appealing.

HONEY

Eating honey is thought by some to be particularly good for sinusitis and for respiratory allergies. This notion is more common in the South, especially among the Cuban population of Tampa, Florida, where the honey, called *Cuban Honey,* was considered effective only if it came from Cuba. Whiskey is added to enhance its effectiveness. This form of treatment is probably based on the misconstrued idea of the effect of pollen as a cause of nasal allergy. Bees are known as carriers of pollen from one plant to another. Although the drab wind-pollinated plants are more frequent causes of respiratory allergy than the brilliantly colored, highly scented, insect-pollinated plants, it is true that if a sensitive person comes in direct contact with insect-carried pollen he can be similarly affected. Because bees carry pollen back to their hives along with the plant nectar, which eventually becomes honey, many allergists advise their pollen-sensitive patients not to eat honey except for the limited varieties such as those of orange flower and May grass. Either because it was assumed that eating honey would desensitize the hay fever sufferer, or because the proponents of the treatment were confused about the cause and effect of the bee-honey-pollen relationship to allergy symptoms, the use of honey as a treatment for allergy has become entrenched in certain localities. However, as far back as 1940, the *Journal of the American Medical Association* listed the "El Aquinaldo Cuban Wonder Honey," prepared in Lansing, Michigan, "misbranded as to claims for relief of bronchial asthma."

GOLD FOR ASTHMA

"Gold injections" have been used both here and abroad by some enthusiastic doctors since 1934 with reported results ranging from poor to good. But in this period of more than thirty years it has been discarded by practically all allergy experts in this country as of no value. The Japanese alternate the gold injections with injections of insulin to produce a hypoglycemia (lower than normal blood sugar level). Any possible benefit derived may be explained on the basis that perhaps the adrenal gland cortex is stimulated and an excess amount of cortisone is produced. This is pure conjecture.

IMMUNE MILK FOR HAY FEVER

There was a fairly well established practice some years ago, perhaps still in use in some localities, of injecting ragweed pollen into the udders of cows, and using the milk of those cows as an oral form of desensitization for ragweed pollen hay fever. The theory is that the cow builds up blocking antibodies as a result of the injection and these pass into the milk. By drinking the milk, the hay fever sufferer is thought to be "passively immunized" because it is postulated that the cow produces the antibodies instead of the person producing them. This method of treatment might be compared to the use of antitoxin derived from a horse that had built up immunity against lockjaw (tetanus). This form of treatment has not been found valuable.

ARGYROL NASAL PACKING FOR NASAL ALLERGY

For several decades, in cases of nasal allergy doctors often packed the nose with cotton saturated with *argyrol* (a silver proteinate solution). Argyrol was considered a valuable antiseptic and was used in all types of infections. The pack was left in the nose for five to ten minutes, then removed. Since argyrol is black this was a messy form of treatment, and with the advent of antibiotics, which specifically act against given organisms, it has been largely discarded. It is possible, however, that some nose and throat specialists still use this technique, which is also known as the *Hazeltine treatment,* after the name of its originator.

PROCAINE (H₃) TREATMENT FOR BRONCHIAL ASTHMA

In the late 1950's Dr. Anna Aslan, the head of an old people's home and hospital in Romania, reported miraculous success in the treatment of elderly people with chronic diseases including bronchial asthma. She simply employed *procaine* (a well-known local anesthetic, commercially marketed as Novocain). To be effective the procaine had to be extremely acid with a pH of 3.5 to 4.0. (Neutral is pH 7.0.) The treatment consisted of intramuscular injections (injections deep in the muscle) administered daily for two weeks, then once weekly and later less often.

In the United States, many doctors became interested in Dr. Aslan's reports, obtained the acidified procaine directly from Germany and added slight modifications of their own. Occasionally some physiological changes were produced by the procaine injections and there appeared to be a temporary improvement in the general health of the patient. One of the advantages of the treatment was that it was simple to give; no experience was necessary. Despite this, the general lack of asthmatic relief became quite evident and today few doctors are interested in this form of treatment.

INTRAVENOUS PROCAINE (NOVOCAIN) TREATMENT FOR ASTHMA

Quite a different form of treatment with procaine was introduced in the 1940's calling for a one percent solution diluted with equal parts of normal salt solution to be administered intravenously in 10.0 cc. (1/3 ounce) doses. Many physicians found it very effective, particularly in the treatment of hives and in the more severe manifestations of allergy such as angioedema with swelling of the eyes and joints accompanied by high fever and other very unpleasant symptoms. However, reactions to the drug itself were not at all uncommon, and today this therapy is seldom employed. Other procaine compounds such as *pronestyl* have been tried but have not gained much favor. Cocaine, with Adrenalin and ephedrine in a nasal spray, was once a classical remedy for hay fever. It shrank the nasal tissues and gave considerable relief but there was always the possibility of the person becoming sensitized to it. Habituation to cocaine also had to be considered, but in this form did not seem to pose much of a problem.

GLANDULAR TREATMENT OF ALLERGY AND THE HIGH PROTEIN LOW CARBOHYDRATE ALLERGY DIET

Females appear to have a change in their allergies during adolescence, the menopause, and pregnancy, suggesting to many that during these times the endocrine glands may play an important role in the production of allergy. Some allergies are made better and others are made worse during these phases of life of the female; one cannot predict which. Males also are likely to have allergy symptoms before adolescence and be relieved when their endocrine glandular systems become stabilized. All of this has led investigators to consider endocrine glandular therapy for allergy. *Ovarian substances, thyroid, insulin, pituitary,* and *testosterone* have all been employed but not with sufficiently satisfactory and uniform results to warrant general use.

An endocrinologist-allergist once enthusiastically recommended as a cure for all allergies *whole adrenal gland* injections combined with a diet high in protein, low in carbohydrates, and containing a medium amount of fat. This, he claimed, would cure all allergies. A grateful patient who had not responded to orthodox treatment hailed this form of therapy in a widely advertized testimonial book. There must have been many who purchased *Good-By Allergies* thinking that the cure-all for allergies was at hand. But despite the claims of the originator of the theory and the presumably honest author, allergy is still with us. Adrenal gland injections, whether of the whole gland or an extract, probably derive their benefits, if any, from the cortex of the gland which in effect is made up of cortisone and its product derivatives. These can be prescribed by a physician and taken orally at his direction.

DESENSITIZING NOSE DROPS FOR HAY FEVER

It would seem that if desensitizing injections in hay fever are valuable, it would be simpler and perhaps more effective if the material were administered directly into the nose. Accordingly, a nose spray was devised for this purpose. Pollen extracts could not be used, since it was quickly found that their instillation into the nose gave a marked hay fever reaction. But a number of chemicals were employed, most of which had very little use in medicine in the form recommended. The advised treatment was for the person to take increasing amounts of the nose drops daily until a certain maintenance number of drops were taken. For several years this material was available; then it appeared to lose favor and suddenly disappear only to reappear again with extensive advertising in late 1965 and early 1966. These nose drops have been tried by a number of allergists, but no benefits have been reported. The chemicals in the nose drops are guanine, uric acid, thymine, indole, glycerine, glutamic acid, alcohol, organic dye, liquid phenol (carbolic acid), acetylcholine, amino acid derivative, table salt, and water. This is what doctors commonly call a "shotgun mixture." No connection between these chemicals and allergy has been found by chemists or allergists.

THE SPA AND CLIMATIC TREATMENT

Some aspects of this form of therapy have been discussed in Chapter 13.

Spas (named after Spa in Belgium, world-famous for many years as a town where there were mineral springs of presumably medicinal properties) have sprung up in many parts of the world, but they are most popular in Europe, especially in France and Switzerland. One that is noted for "curing" asthma is the one at Mont Dore in central France. There, one must drink the medicated waters and inhale their hot steaming vapors as part of the treatment. At La Bourboule, also in the Pyrenees, is another spa often frequented by asthmatics. It has been suggested that the benefits derived are not so much from the spring waters as from the fact that people who go there experience a change of environment; they rest more than at home and live a more relaxed life.

In the Swiss resorts high in the Alps the air is pure and clean, free from dusts and pollen, and this may well be a reason for improvement. The nearest equivalents to European spas in the United States are those areas where there is little allergy-producing pollen. These have been named "allergy havens," many of which have been so advertised in the Great Lakes region and in the White Mountains of New England. These areas had at one time very little if any ragweed growing there, and for those who suffered from ragweed hay fever or asthma, it was indeed a haven during the fall months when ragweed flourished in their ordinary environments. However, the advent of golf courses and the desire to beautify the area with shrubbery, grass, and trees has also led to the introduction of many different types of plant pollen. This has rendered them far less acceptable to the hay fever sufferer.

The West Coast (and particularly California) has long been considered another haven for ragweed sufferers because none of the Eastern variety of ragweed grows there. However, there are many other pollinating plants which can cause allergy symptoms, and in an allergic person it is only a matter of time before a sensitivity to one or more of the newer pollen develops. Several years ago, there was an unfortunate article published in a popular magazine extolling the virtues of a suburb of Los Angeles (Sunland-Tujunga) as an ideal area for the asthmatic. As a result there was a large influx of asthmatics to this rustic, pollen-infested area whose only virtue was that it was at an altitude of 2500 feet and was protected from the ocean breezes. This area, despite its pollen count, is still popular for some asthmatics particularly because of its warm climate. However, many asthmatics do much better at the seashore where the prevailing winds from the ocean do not carry pollen. There is a children's asthmatic sanatorium in the Sunland-Tujunga area and others in Tucson, Atlantic City, Denver, Miami and elsewhere. The diverse pollen and atmospheric conditions of these locations refute the notion of an "ideal location" for all allergic persons.

THE GAY TREATMENT

Biloxi, Mississippi, became famous some years ago because of Dr. Gay and his clinic where many asthmatics flocked for relief. The asthma mixture he prescribed contained potassium iodide, a form of arsenic (Fowler's solution), tincture of digitalis, a sedative, and some red coloring. The dose was varied according to the need of the patient. In addition, bile salts with a cathartic were usually prescribed to keep the bowels open; included in the regimen was other medication that may have been necessary, following a complete physical examination. After two weeks patients usually returned home, continuing to take the medicines regularly. Many asthmatics reported relief with Dr. Gay's formula, at least for a period of time. Generally, the medical profession frowns upon the use of arsenic, especially when taken over several months or years. The value of the heart medicine, digitalis, was questioned, although for years it had been a constituent of many asthma mixtures. Potassium iodide is routinely used by most allergists, so that essentially there was not much new in this prescription aside from the arsenic. There have been very recent (1968) studies suggesting the merit of arsenic in asthma. The value of arsenic is therefore still moot, and the Gay treatment continues to be used.

NEGATIVE IONS

Negative ions in the air are particles of such gases as oxygen, nitrogen, and carbon dioxide which have acquired electrons and are therefore negatively charged. Positive ions are molecules of the same gases which have lost electrons and are positively charged. Normally we are surrounded by an equal amount of both positive and negative ions. It had long been believed by some that the general health of a person was benefited by the presence of negative ions. Those who considered the spas meritorious suggested that it might be due primarily to the negative ions in the mineral spring waters. A number of ionizing devices are manufactured to change the charge of ions in the circulating air from positive to negative in the hope that breathing in the negatively charged ions would be beneficial. Research by disinterested researchers produced results that were not in accord with those published by researchers associated with or endorsed by the manufacturing concerns. It is generally held at the present time that there is no value in the use of negative ion machines in the treatment of allergy diseases.

HAPAMINE TREATMENT

Hapamine (histamine-azo-protein) is a protein made by chemically combining histamine with despeciated horse serum protein (globulin). This drug was to produce antibodies to histamine which would neutralize any histamine liberated during the antigen-antibody union and in this manner prevent allergy symptoms. If all allergy symptoms were caused by histamine alone and this product was able to produce antibodies to neutralize the offending histamine, the treatment would be effective. But most allergists agree that although histamine is an important chemical liberated by the union of antigen and antibody it is not the only one and certainly is not responsible for all allergy symptoms. Although used extensively when first manufactured, very few physicians, if any, found it of value and it is not commonly administered today.

DESERT AIR LAMPS AND DEHUMIDIFYING INSTRUMENTS

A *desert air lamp* is designed to warm and dry the air in a room. Some allergy patients feel better in such an atmosphere; others feel worse. From the standpoint of allergy, damp or moist air—which represents microscopic droplets of circulating water in the atmosphere—often aids in holding dust of all kind in the atmosphere. Warming and drying the air effectively reduces the volume of dust particles suspended in the individual droplets. An infrared lamp accomplishes this purpose, so there is hardly any need for an expensive so-called desert air lamp, except perhaps for the sake of appearance.

Dehumidifiers are more complicated electrical devices, which dry the air. There are also humidifiers which add moisture to the air. Determination of which to use depends on whether dry or moist air is easier for the person to breathe. Most of these devices are indicated for infections such as infectious bronchitis where they are very useful. They are probably being overused for purely allergic conditions. Heat lamps and dehumidifiers are not actually unorthodox or unconventional modalities, but they should not be used unless prescribed by the attending doctor. It may be a waste of money.

STAPHYLOCOCCUS BACTERIOPHAGE

A bacteriophage is an agent that causes disintegration and dissolution of bacteria. Some years ago it was reported that unusually successful results were being obtained from the use of a specially prepared *staphylococcic bacteriophage* in treating bronchial asthma, sinusitis and nasal polyps. A number of competent allergists tried it on patients for a testing period but none obtained the hoped-for results. There is no valid scientific reason why this type of spray should be of any value in an allergy disease.

RESPIRATORY VACCINE THERAPY

Respiratory vaccine is used in the treatment of allergy disease by many thoroughly competent allergists who feel that it is definitely of value. It consists of bacteria usually found in the respiratory tract. These are killed, processed, and sterilized, then made into a vaccine that may be injected into a patient without producing an infection. The rationale is that allergy to bacteria is an important facet of allergy, and that desensitization to bacteria, just as one desensitizes to dust or pollen, is important and efficacious. The vaccine is sometimes made specifically for the person being treated, prepared from a culture of the bacteria found in his body—usually in the nose, throat, sinuses, or coughed-up sputum. Such a vaccine is called an *autogenous vaccine;* one consisting of the bacteria generally found in most people and prepared from several sources is a *stock vaccine.* Very small doses are claimed to help build up the blocking antibodies more rapidly by those who use it in addition to routine dust and pollen desensitization. Some allergists feel that good results can only be obtained with large doses of vaccine, either stock or specially prepared. The entire subject of vaccine therapy is controversial and confusing since the reported results vary widely.

TYPHOID VACCINE INJECTIONS

When an intercurrent infection occurs and a high fever is produced the asthmatic symptoms occasionally disappear. This interesting phenomenon noted also in certain other chronic diseases has led to the use of *typhoid vaccines* to induce a high fever in persons with intractable asthma. Malaria has also been induced for the same relief-giving fever in intractable asthma. These methods of stimulating the immune mechanism to help the allergy sufferer may be still used today in rare instances, although with the advent of the corticosteroid drugs such severe treatments are seldom required.

VITAMINS

Allergists uniformly recommend vitamins in a chronic illness such as bronchial asthma to keep up the body's nutrition. Whether per se they have curative or remedial value in allergy is open to question. Originally it was felt that vitamin C was valuable because it preserved cell membranes and bound the cells firmly together. Today this is in doubt. Yet vitamin C (ascorbic acid) is still advertised in the treatment of hay fever despite reports indicating no lack of ascorbic acid as a rule in hay fever or other allergy sufferers. In the experience of allergists, a saturation of vitamin C does not help. Vitamin D (viosterol) enjoyed popularity for awhile and some allergists prescribed it in addition to desensitizing injection treatment in the belief that it improved their results. Very large doses were administered often constituting overdoses followed by urinary frequency, gastrointestinal distress and vomiting. Because of the adverse reactions to the large doses and the fact that such doses are not free from danger this treatment is no longer used extensively. Vitamin E was also once in vogue, and may still be used by some.

CALCIUM TREATMENT

The argument in favor of calcium therapy in allergy diseases rests upon the observation that calcium deficit disturbs the metabolic balance of the tissue body salts; principally calcium, potassium, and sodium. This can play a role in allergy as well as other disease states. However, despite the occasional improvement noted with calcium therapy, laboratory studies show that in asthma there are normal blood values for calcium, phosphorus, potassium, and protein. Furthermore, the values of calcium, phosphorus, and potassium are similarly normal in the spinal fluids of asthmatic patients. In fact, all studies of ionized calcium are normal in allergy. Therefore, there is little scientific basis for calcium therapy despite its use by some physicians. Administration is usually by injection since it is absorbed poorly from the stomach. Intravenous calcium injections are used mostly for persistent hives to help relieve the itching. When calcium is injected into the blood stream there is an immediate feeling of intense heat all over the body. This so-called "hot shot," as patients describe it, may simply be a placebo.

INTRANASAL MANIPULATION

Manipulation within the nose occasionally produces relief of symptoms for varying periods of time. The techniques employed include (1) *cauterization* (chemical or electrical searing of the nose), (2) *turbinectomy* (removal of a turbinate bone of the side wall of the nostril), and (3) *injection of a cortisone* derivative into the turbinate bone. These treatments have been used primarily in perennial hay fever and are still employed by some nose and throat specialists, although allergists do not regard them with favor. The burning of the nasal membrane by whatever means gives only temporary relief, for when the new membrane forms it is just as allergic as the old. (A similar form of treatment is nasal ionization or *iontophoresis*). Removal of the turbinate bone may be followed by relief for months. The best explanation might seem to be that in the removal, more breathing space is obtained (such as also occurs after a straightening of the *septum*, the partition between the two nostrils). However, there is actually no real increase in breathing space following either cauterization or tubinectomy. Any temporary improvement has been attributed to increased cortisone production by the adrenal gland which usually follows an injury or surgical procedure.

Injection of cortisone into the turbinate bone was first attempted in 1951 and 1952 when hydrocortisone was first available. The results appeared promising but several alarming, unexplainable reactions occurred. Since the advent of the newer more soluble cortisone derivatives, there have been no reported reactions. Many nose and throat specialists still use the treatment, often in conjunction with more conventional therapy.

PIROMEN

Piromen is described by the manufacturer as a polysaccharide complex derived from a "pseudomonas species" (a certain type of bacillus; most of the pseudomonadoceae live in the soil and in decomposing organic matter). It is claimed that upon injection, preferably in the vein, the body's defense mechanism is activated by stimulation of the cortex of the adrenal gland. Advised for the treatment of allergies, Piromen was used quite extensively when first introduced. It continues to be marketed and may still be used, but certainly not as much by allergists as perhaps by dermatologists and ophthalmologists for non-specific treatment of skin and eye allergies. The published reports in medical journals of the allergy results obtained have not been very persuasive in recent years.

MISCELLANEOUS FORMS OF ALLERGY TREATMENT

Nosaki is a therapeutic mixture given by injection which is said to be similar or identical to the poison ivy (rhus toxicodendrum) extract. *Tyral* is a mixture of tyrosine with vitamins about which very little has been written. Allergists generally have paid little attention to either Nosaki or Tyral since there does not appear to be any scientific or justifiable explanation for their use.

Other treatments recommended and still used by some physicians in allergy diseases are *intravenous injection of hydrochloric acid* and the *intravenous injection of potassium iodide*. The explanation for the use of the acid is unknown. Iodides help thin the thickened phelgm which is usually present in the bronchial tubes of the severely asthmatic patient and therefore there is some reason for employing it, particularly when iodides cannot be taken by mouth. However, the sodium salt is the one regularly used along with fluids in severe asthma; there appears to be no valid reason for using the potassium salt intravenously.

Various body extracts have been used for the treatment of asthma and other diseases of allergy. One that was in vogue in 1949, and is still used by some, is an *extract of spleen* prepared in ampuls. Another is an extract prepared from the *white blood cells* (leucocytes). Their rationale has never been satisfactorily explained.

Some years ago Undecylinic acid, a drug currently used widely for the local treatment of ringworm of the feet, was reported as an excellent oral agent for the treatment of allergy. Several articles were published in the scientific journals and numerous allergists tested it; some found it efficacious at first. Nevertheless, like many other recommended medicines hailed enthusiastically in the beginning, it has now apparently disappeared. In 1947, there was a serious attempt to verify the value of a diet limited to *amino acids* (the chemical fractions that make up proteins) together with the necessary vitamins which would be lacking in such a diet. Several varieties of *protein hydrolysates* were tried both in adults with severe asthma not responding to the usual treatment, and in a number of institutionalized children with asthma. In both studies, although there appeared to be some evidence of improvement, it was insufficient to justify further trial. They are not generally prescribed at the present time.

Some time ago, a well known pathologist recommended a treatment for asthma that consisted of the use of an antihistamine drug combined with a chemical often used for the treatment of malaria. His theory was that this experimental compound eventually became localized in the respiratory tissues and caused alteration in the basic cellular structure (the reticuloendothelial system) which depressed antibody response. It therefore ameliorated or eliminated the allergic symptoms. The good results were not duplicated by many other physicians. However, investigation may still be continuing.

Sterilized milk has been injected into the buttocks of individuals for the treatment of allergy disease with the intent of stimulating the immune or allergic mechanism. In some instances it appears to help but the results are not consistent.

SUMMARY

Although the treatment of allergic disease is more or less standardized and universal so that doctors all over the world can continue both specific and symptomatic treatment started by another without much difficulty, there are many forms of treatment that can be considered non-standard or unconventional. Many have been used throughout the years and have been discarded; some persist. Their continued use indicates that they are beneficial in some way. Undoubtedly some are successful because of psychological suggestion; others are financially successful because of intense advertising or the influence of testimonials.

The injection of urine is an old technique tried by many and discarded. However, it is still being used by some. A highly advertised product is Anergex, a poison oak extract, which is given by injection once a day for six to eight days. This is not generally accepted by the allergy specialist. Blood removed from a patient and immediately reinjected into the muscles is an old procedure and is apparently still employed for some skin diseases. However, its use for other allergy diseases is certainly unconventional.

There is a myth that the presence of a Chihuahua dog will prevent one from having asthma. There is no basis in fact for this. It is true that this breed has very short hair and therefore is less likely to shed much dog hair and dander. There is one Mexican hairless dog, the Xoloitzcuintli, which is in great demand because of this, but this breed is almost extinct. Although the myth persists, asthma is not prevented by the ownership of such dogs.

One laboratory claims it can diagnose the allergy by examining a sample of blood removed from the patient, thus precluding the necessity of skin tests. This is based on the theory that a certain type of bacteria flourishes on each allergenic product.

For many years it has been felt that eating honey was beneficial for allergy and sinus trouble; this notion is particularly prevalent in the southern portion of the United States. The injection of gold into the bloodstream has been used for practically every disease and even at the present time it is a recognized form of treatment for arthritis. Although its value for treatment of allergic disease has been found wanting, it is still used by some. Another practice that persists is the use of Argyrol packs in the nose for the relief of nasal allergy. This was relatively successful in the days when Argyrol was a popular antiseptic, before antibiotics became known.

A vogue for several years was the use of an acidified solution of procaine for the treatment of chronic diseases of the aged, including chronic asthma. This was developed by a Romanian doctor and is still being exploited. Another treatment that has been popularized is the use of crude extracts of the adrenal glands in conjunction with a special diet high in protein and low in carbohydrates. This form of treatment was used more than thirty years ago and subsequently discarded by most allergists. However, there is a renaissance of this form of treatment among a small group of physicians.

A medicine administered in the form of nose drops and containing at least twelve chemical ingredients has been recommended as a cure for all allergies. One drop is initially instilled in each nostril and the number gradually increased to the maximum dose level. There is no known reason for its success, if there is any. Spas and climatic areas for mitigating allergic disease have been in vogue for many years. Certain resorts in Europe are particularly popular; in the United States, areas in California, Denver, Miami, and Tucson are the sites of children's asthmatic homes. There is also one in Atlantic City.

The Gay treatment originally practiced in a Mississippi clinic is apparently still used. The medicine developed by Dr. Gay is a simple mixture consisting primarily of potassium iodide and a form of arsenic, both of which had been used for asthma for centuries. Hapamine (histamine-azo-protein) devised to neutralize the effects of histamine is rarely used today. Devices to change the atmosphere in the room are still used. Those which filter the air are standard. There are contraptions that produce negative ions in the air to relieve respiratory allergy. Their value is questionable.

Staphylococcus bacteriophage is a vaccine produced from the staphylococcus organism and is used by some as a treatment for allergy. Mixed respiratory vaccine, a vaccine prepared from the bacteria usually found in the throat, sinuses, and bronchial tubes is used in varying doses for allergies. Although very small doses are most commonly employed, some doctors give very large doses. Despite case histories of benefits from vaccine therapy, this treatment is not universally accepted by all allergists. `

Other unconventional and unproven methods of treatment include various vitamins, milk injections, Piromen, calcium given intravenously, intranasal manipulation, and surgery. All of these are accepted by some but not all specialists.

Glossary of Allergy Terms

ACTH: Abbreviation for adrenocorticotropic hormone, a hormone secreted by the pituitary gland that stimulates the cortex (outer part) of the adrenal gland to produce cortical hormones (cortisone). ACTH is valuable in the treatment of intractable bronchial asthma as well as in other difficult or stubborn allergy diseases.

ADRENALIN: A proprietary name (Parke, Davis & Co.) for an extract of the adrenal gland (inner part) which is extremely helpful in the symptomatic treatment of most allergy diseases. The less familiar term is epinephrine. It is particularly effective in relieving attacks of bronchial asthma and in the treatment of constitutional (anaphylactic) reactions.

ALLERGEN: Any substance which produces allergy symptoms by joining with its specific antibody. Among the most common are inhalants such as pollen, molds, and dusts; ingestants such as foods and drugs; injectants such as drugs; infectants such as bacteria; and physical agents such as cold, heat, and pressure. There are many others. This term is synonymous with *antigen.* Another synonym not as frequently used is *atopen* but this has a slightly different connotation. (See Atopy, Antigen.)

ALLERGY: An acquired, specific capability to react on the basis of an antigen-antibody reaction; a mechanism explaining many diseases resulting from contact with something which in susceptible persons produces changes in the body leading to the production of symptoms. The sequence of events is (1) initial contact with the substance (antigen); (2) production of antibodies in the body (the person is then said to be allergic or sensitized); (3) union of the antigen with the antibody which had been formed; (4) subsequent release of certain chemicals. The effect of these chemicals on the body is manifested by allergy symptoms. The adjective *allergic* means "of," "relating to," "characterized," as well as "affected by" allergy.

341

ANAPHYLAXIS: A form of allergy occurring in certain animals. Anaphylaxis can be produced at will in animals but not in humans. The mechanism involving antigens and antibodies is, however, identical. The term anaphylaxis is also used by some physicians to describe violent allergy symptoms in humans with severe generalized manifestations, but most doctors prefer the qualifying adjective *anaphylactoid.* The antigen (or allergen) responsible for the anaphylactic reactions in animals has been termed the *anaphylactogen.*

ANERGY: This is the absence or lack of capacity to react. The term has been devised to indicate that allergy does not necessarily need to be an increased or a "hyper" sensitivity. The ability to react can be decreased or absent, as well. Anergy is a term used infrequently.

ANGIOEDEMA: A very severe form of urticaria or hives in which there are large, raised welts on the skin which involve the deeper structures of the skin. The lips, eyes, cheeks, and other portions of the body may become very much enlarged and even the joints may become affected. A more common but inaccurate term for this condition is *angioneurotic edema.* The swellings of angioedema are usually transient.

ANTIBODY: A specific substance derived from the protein material of the blood and formed in response to exposure to an antigen. This antibody can later join with the antigen on subsequent introduction into the body to produce an antigen-antibody reaction. There are numerous types of antibodies, some of which are named because of their specific antigen and the reaction that results. For example, a *hemolysin* is an antibody that affects the red blood cells; an *antitoxin* is one that neutralizes a specific type of foreign substance (a toxin); a *cytotoxin* is one that affects body cells. In clinical allergy the antibody that is produced is more properly called *reagin* or *skin-sensitizing antibody.*

ANTIGEN: A substance, usually protein, which when introduced into the body is capable of stimulating the production of antibodies and which on subsequent introduction can join with the specific antibody it has produced to cause an antigen-antibody reaction. The union of the antigen and the antibody with the release of certain chemicals to produce allergy symptoms is the hallmark of the allergic reaction. There are many types of antigens; some have specific names. The one involved in allergy is frequently designated as an *allergen* or an *atopen.*

ANTIHISTAMINE: A medicine that acts to block the action of histamine, one of the chemicals liberated during antigen-antibody union and which is thought to be the cause of many, if not most, allergy symptoms. The adjective is *antihistaminic.*

ASTHMA: A symptom or syndrome characterized by shortness of breath with coughing and wheezing. It can be caused by any interference with the free flow of air through the small bronchial tubes. It must not be confused with *bronchial asthma,* a disease state in which asthma is a symptom.

ASTHMATIC BRONCHITIS: Symptoms of asthma due to an infection of the bronchial tract. Some use this term to indicate bronchial asthma caused by allergy to the infecting organism.

ATOPY: This term was devised to indicate clinical allergy in which there were (1) a history of allergy in the family, (2) the presence of skin-sensitizing antibodies that could be demonstrated and (3) an immediate wheal and flare-like allergic response to a skin test. Today atopy is used primarily as another term for clinical allergy.

AUTOGENOUS: This means "originating from within" or "self-generated." The term is applied generally to bacteria which originate within the patient's body. A vaccine prepared from these bacteria is called an *autogenous vaccine.*

AUTOGRAFT: Tissue or organ taken from one part of the body of an animal or person and placed in another part of the same animal or person.

AUTOIMMUNE DISEASE: A disease that is thought to be due to allergy to one's own body tissues, often called *autoallergy.* As in other allergy diseases, the presence of a specific antibody is often demonstrable. This may be specific for one organ such as the thyroid, kidney, or colon, or the disease may be generalized; in that case the antibodies are not limited to only one organ.

BACTERIAL ALLERGY: Allergy to live or dead bacteria which may be demonstrated by skin testing. The *tuberculin test* is a demonstration of this form of allergy. In clinical allergy, it more precisely indicates an allergy reaction to living organisms or their products which may be present in the body. This is difficult to prove by skin testing or any other means and the actual existence of clinical bacterial allergy is controversial.

BLOCKING ANTIBODY: This is a particular type of antibody that is produced in the body as a result of hyposensitization treatment. This antibody can be demonstrated in laboratory tests and is differentiated from the one that joins with antigen (subsequently producing allergy symptoms) by the fact that it is heat stable and resists destruction at 56 degrees Centigrade. The theory of the relief of symptoms following hyposensitization treatment is based partly on the production of these antibodies. When they join with the antigen without releasing any harmful chemical that results in allergy symptoms, they give protection. The blocking antibody is sometimes called a *neutralizing antibody.*

BRONCHIAL ASTHMA: A continuing disease state characterized by repeated attacks of asthma. The basic cause of the disease is allergy, but there are some who feel that infection and emotional disturbances play a role in the causation. (Definitions of bronchial asthma given by the American Thoracic Society, the American Medical Association, and Webster's Dictionary differ on that point.) Allergists feel that the underlying cause is allergy but that infections and emotional difficulties can influence the symptoms by triggering, perpetuating, or aggravating them. It is customary to divide bronchial asthma into two types, *extrinsic,* produced by allergens from outside the body, and *intrinsic,* resulting from allergens within the body.

BRONCHIECTASIS: A condition in which segments of the bronchial tubes become dilated (pouched). Pus and mucus tend to accumulate in these areas of dilation. This condition may be present in bronchial asthma, but usually bronchiectasis is a complication of such infections of the lungs and bronchial tubes as bronchopneumonia, chronic bronchitis, tuberculosis, and whooping cough.

BRONCHIOLES: These are the smallest subdivisions of the bronchi. They do not have any cartilagenous (gristle) rings as the larger tubes do. Instead, they are surrounded by rubber-band-like muscles.

BRONCHOEDEMA: Swelling of the lining membrane of the bronchial tubes which diminishes their lumen (open area), hindering and obstructing the free flow of air through them. This is one of the main causes of the difficulty in breathing observed in bronchial asthma.

BRONCHOSPASM: Narrowing of the lumen of the bronchial tubes by contraction of the muscles that surround them.

CARDIAC ASTHMA: A condition marked by symptoms of coughing and shortness of breath, with wheezing, due to heart failure. The symptoms are relieved by medicine used for the treatment of the heart condition.

CLINICAL ALLERGY: This refers to the frequently encountered common allergic manifestations such as hay fever, eczema, hives, and bronchial asthma in contrast to the less common and experimental types of allergy.

CONJUNCTIVAL TEST: An allergy test performed by placing a small amount of suspected allergen (antigen) in the eye. A positive reaction is shown by redness and inflammation of the conjunctiva where the allergen was placed. Such a reaction occurs within minutes and is relieved by neutralizing it with a drop or two of Adrenalin. This test is used occasionally to verify a questionable positive skin test, or when allergy to an inhalant substance is suspected but the skin test is negative. It has also been advocated as a follow-up procedure to evaluate response to allergy treatment.

CONSTITUTIONAL REACTION: A generalized or systemic reaction following the administration of an allergen during treatment or in the course of performing skin tests. Instead of the expected reaction of itching and swelling at the site of the injection, symptoms develop which involve the entire body. These may be any one or a group of allergy syndromes such as itching, hives, angioedema, hay fever, or asthma. The most severe symptoms occur within minutes after the injection but occasionally they may appear as long as twenty-four hours later. Application of a tourniquet above the site of injection and immediate treatment with Adrenalin or some other brand of epinephrine is highly effective. Other drugs such as antihistamines and corticosteroids are sometimes employed. Rarely is the reaction severe enough to cause death. Similar violent symptoms following administration of tetanus antitoxin or penicillin are also called constitutional reactions, but the term is usually limited to the untoward reactions which may result in allergy testing or treatment.

CONTACTANT: Any substance which will produce an allergic reaction by mere contact with the skin or with the lining membrane of the body cavities.

CORTISONE: A hormone that has been isolated from the cortex (outer layer) of the adrenal gland. (It is also prepared in the laboratory synthetically.) Cortisone was the first adrenal cortex hormone used for the treatment of intractable asthma and status asthmaticus. Since then many other derivatives have been manufactured. Their names are Hydrocortisone, Prednisone, Prednisolone, Methylprednisolone, Paramethasone, Dexamethasone, Triamcinolone, Fluprednisolone and Betamethasone. These are very effective but must be used with caution because too large a dose, especially if taken over too long a period of time, may have serious effects. They must never be taken except while under a doctor's care and supervision.

CO-SEASONAL: This term means "during the season." It is commonly used in referring to allergy treatment given during the pollinating season of plants to which a person is allergic. It is distinguished from *pre-seasonal* and *post-seasonal* treatment. *Perennial* treatment is administered throughout the year, without reference to any pollinating season.

CUTANEOUS: Relating to the skin.

DANDER: Dander are the small, loose particles of dried skin attached to the hair or fur of animals, similar to dandruff in humans. They may act as allergens.

DELAYED REACTION: A positive allergy reaction, usually to a skin test, which, instead of appearing within minutes such as an immediate reaction does, may take twenty-four to forty-eight hours to become manifest. Delayed reactions are characteristic of bacterial allergy, the best example of which is the *tuberculin test,* which is not expected to show a reaction until twenty-four hours later. It is also characteristic of the *patch test,* which is performed to ascertain the cause of a contact dermatitis. In a patch test, the reaction may not appear for forty-eight or even seventy-two hours after it is performed.

DERMATITIS: Dermatitis refers to an inflammation of the skin. In allergy there are several: urticaria or hives, neurodermatitis, which has many synonyms but is perhaps best known as eczema, and contact dermatitis. Dermatitis must be distinguished from *dermatosis,* which signifies an involvement of the skin without actual inflammation.

DERMATOPHYTE: A microparasitic fungus, usually a mold or yeast, that can infect the human skin, grow, and set up local inflammation. It is also capable of producing an intensely itchy eruption at a distance from its original area of growth.

DERMATOSIS: Any skin involvement (as contrasted to dermatitis, which signifies inflammation of the skin).

DESENSITIZE: To build up a person's resistance to the material to which he is allergic and which is causing his allergy symptoms. The procedure is termed *desensitization* and usually refers to a series of hypodermic injections of the allergen to which the person is allergic with increasing doses until the optimum dose is reached. This reduces the symptoms without causing any severe reaction. Since the term suggests complete neutralization of the antigen, an objective not obtainable in allergy, the term *hyposensitization* is preferred by some allergists. Hyposensitization is a more exact but awkward term for the process; desensitization is more popularly used.

DISTANT REACTION: A positive reaction to an allergen that occurs at a site remote from that of its introduction or application.

DUSTPROOF: A term applied to certain fabrics, textiles, bedding, upholstery, etc., which are impermeable to dust particles. There are many such materials available—their use is particularly advisable for those who are highly sensitive to house dust.

ELIMINATION DIET: An elimination diet is used for the diagnosis and treatment of food allergy. It involves avoiding the foods which are either the suspected cause of the allergy symptoms or have been found to be positive on skin testing. If the person is relieved when these foods are eliminated from the diet, it is assumed that one of them is the cause of the symptoms. To determine which food is involved, the avoided foods are eaten one at a time, several days or a week apart, and the clinical reaction to them is noted.

EMANATION: In allergy this is considered to be any substance that is given off by a plant, a living creature, or other entity. It refers especially to the shedding particles of epidermis, dander, hair or feathers from animals and birds, or lint from bedding, furniture, or clothing.

EMPHYSEMA: A condition of the lungs in which the air cells are overdistended and ruptured. It usually results from prolonged interference with expiration such as occurs in bronchial asthma, where chronic infection is also present. It is not as frequent a complication of bronchial asthma as commonly thought.

ENDERMAL: This is a term infrequently used. It means "in" or "into the skin." It is a Greek derivative and corresponds to the Latin term, *intracutaneous.*

ENDOCRINE GLANDS: Glands that produce an internal secretion which is discharged into the blood and lymph and is circulated to all parts of the body. Common examples of endocrine glands are the thyroid, the pituitary, and the adrenal glands. Endocrine glands are differentiated from *exocrine* glands which discharge their secretion outside of the body as, for example, the sweat glands.

ENDOGENOUS: This means "generated from within." The term is applied to any allergen originating within the body, such as bacteria, which may exist in a so-called focus of infection.

ENVIRONMENTAL CONTROL: This alludes to the removal or control of those elements in the environment of an allergic person that are known or suspected of causing the allergic reaction. The term is usually employed in reference to inhaled substances to which one comes in contact in one's daily life (particularly indoors); it does not refer to control of food allergy.

EOSINOPHILE: A type of white blood cell which is found in the normal person and which can be seen microscopically during a blood count examination. In severe allergies and certain other disease states, there is an increase in these cells as compared with the other types of white blood cells. The increase is known as *eosinophilia.* Usually the eosinophiles are counted and eosinophilia is determined by their percentage to the other white blood cells. At times, they are actually counted and listed as so many per unit of blood.

EPHEDRINE: A medicine that can be taken by mouth and has an effect similar to that of Adrenalin or epinephrine, given by hypodermic injection. Ephedrine is an important drug in the treatment of allergy diseases and is a common constituent of practically every mixture of medicines prescribed for the relief of bronchial asthma. Originally an extract of the Ma Huang plant, it is now produced synthetically.

EPINEPHRINE: The active hormone from the medulla (inner or central portion) of the adrenal gland. It is probably the most important medication doctors have for the immediate relief of most allergy symptoms. Epinephrine is manufactured synthetically and no longer needs to be a true gland extract. There are several trade names for epinephrine. One of the best known is Adrenalin (Parke, Davis & Co.).

EXCITANT: A substance capable of producing allergy symptoms. Occasionally the term is used as a synonym for *allergen* or *antigen.*

EXOGENOUS: This means "having origin outside the body" and is used in discussing excitants such as pollen and house dust. A synonym is *extrinsic.*

EXTRACT: A term loosely used in allergy for a solution of allergenic material used in testing or for treatment.

EXTRINSIC: An allergen or antigen that originates outside the body, such as pollen or house dust. A synonym is *exogenous.*

FALSE-NEGATIVE REACTION: An erroneous or misleading negative skin test reaction.

FALSE-POSITIVE REACTION: A positive skin test reaction for allergy which cannot be verified by clinical trial. False-positive reactions are more common with skin tests for foods which are ingested and undergo chemical changes in the process of digestion than they are for inhaled substances such as pollen and dusts.

FOCUS OF INFECTION: A place or organ in the body where bacteria are harbored without producing any outward symptoms or signs of infection. The tonsils have long been considered to be a possible focus of infection. Abcessed teeth are another site in which germs may exist without being recognized. There are others.

FUNGUS: A parasitic vegetable which feeds on organic material, lacks chlorophyl as compared to other plants, and reproduces by spores. Fungi include molds, mildews, mushrooms, toadstools, rusts, and smuts. In allergy, this group is important because some filaments of these plants can enter the atmosphere and produce allergy symptoms. The term *mold* is often used as a synonym although it is only one part of the fungus.

GASTROINTESTINAL ALLERGY: Symptoms due to allergy, originating in the stomach or intestines. The symptoms may vary from mild indigestion to severe diarrhea. Gastrointestinal allergy must be distinguished from *food allergy,* which refers to food as a cause of allergy symptoms not necessarily limited to the stomach or intestinal tract.

HORROR AUTOXICUS: An old axiom in medicine stating that the body has a fear (or horror) of injuring or poisoning itself and therefore prevents one from being allergic to one's own tissue cells. This concept has been modified by the recognition of autoimmune diseases.

HYPERSENSITIVITY: Literally this term means an excessive or abnormal reaction to certain substances as judged by an adequate control group. It has been used synonymously with allergy: sensitivity, usually increased, based on a specific physiological and immunological mechanism. The adjective is *hypersensitive.* The opposite, a decreased reactivity, is *hyposensitivity* and the adjective form is *hyposensitive.*

HYPERSENSITIVITY VASCULITIS: An inflammation of the small blood vessels or organs due, it is believed, to an allergy. This is often confused with *collagen disease* in which a similar pathological entity occurs. Collagen disease and hypersensitivity angiitis or vasculitis frequently overlap.

HYPODERMIC: Under the skin. Usually applied to an injection of a medicine which is placed just under the layers of the skin. When the injection is not as deep and is placed within the layers of the skin it is called *intracutaneous* or *intradermal;* when it is given within the muscle it is *intramuscular.* A synonym for hypodermic is *subcutaneous.*

HYPOSENSITIVITY: Reduced ability to react to a given exposure. This is the aim of desensitization therapy. *Hyposensitization* is the name for the procedure and is preferred by some allergists to desensitization.

"ID": A type of allergy reaction to a bacteria or a fungus that appears on the body at a site distant from the locale of the original infection. For example, ringworm of the toes (athlete's foot) can produce an "id," *trichophytid,* a rash on the hands or elsewhere. Usually an "id" appears long after the original infection has taken place.

IDIOBLAPTIC ALLERGY: This is a term coined by the late Dr. A. F. Coca to indicate a type of allergy which is familial and in which one cannot demonstrate the antibodies (reagins). For that reason, he also called it *familial non-reaginic allergy* and recommended diagnosing the cause, usually foods, by counting the pulse after eating a suspected food. A rise in pulse rate is presumed to indict that particular food.

IDIOSYNCRASY: A term once used to indicate an unusual reaction and often used synonymously with allergy. At the present time it is reserved for drug reactions which are not necessarily produced by allergy as strictly defined.

IMMEDIATE REACTION: A positive allergic reaction that occurs within minutes after contact with the allergen. When intracutaneous or scratch allergy tests are performed, the immediate reaction is apparent in ten to thirty minutes. This is in contrast to the delayed reaction of bacterial allergy and patch tests which do not appear until twenty-four, forty-eight, and sometimes as long as seventy-two hours after the tests are applied.

IMMUNE: Being secure or protected from infections. In allergy it is applied to protection from symptoms resulting from contact with allergens. It is rarely absolute. The state of being immune is termed *immunity*. The science which studies the mechanisms involved in immunity is called *immunology*. The antigen-antibody reaction is the basic mechanism in the production of immunity.

IMMUNOLOGY: The science that deals with immunity and its various manifestations, involving the antigen-antibody reaction.

IMMUNOSUPPRESSIVE: That which suppresses the immune mechanism (allergic reaction). In the process of transplanting organs from one person to another, in order to prevent their rejection as foreign to the body, immunosuppressive drugs are used. These are frequently the same drugs used to kill cancer cells. The corticosteroids (cortisone and its derivatives) so often used for allergic disease are also employed for this purpose.

INFECTANT: An infective agent, usually a microbe.

INFESTANT: An agent, such as a worm or other parasite, that can infest the body and cause allergy symptoms.

INHALANT: An airborne substance, such as pollen or dusts, which can be the cause of allergy symptoms when breathed into the respiratory tract.

INJECTANT: A substance which when injected can cause allergy symptoms. The most common are serums, drugs, and the venom of insects transmitted through their bites or stings.

INOCULATE: To introduce into the body (by injection) vaccines or other antigenic material (allergenic extracts) for preventive, curative, or experimental purposes. There are other meanings of this term, such as communication of a disease by the transfer of its virus. In allergy, the term is most often used to describe the desensitization (hyposensitization) treatments to inhalant substances.

INTRACUTANEOUS OR INTRADERMAL: Within the layers of the skin. It usually refers to an injection of an antigen within the layers of the skin for treatment or testing.

INTRINSIC: From within. This usually refers to allergy to a substance which is present within the person's body, such as the bacteria of an existing infection. *Extrinsic* refers to allergens that originate outside the person's body, such as inhalants.

IRREVERSIBLE: Permanent. Most allergy reactions are reversible—that is, they are not permanent. In other diseases the damage done very often cannot be remedied; it is *irreversible*.

LEUCOPENIC INDEX: A change in the normal white blood count which has been considered by some to indicate the presence of allergy. For example, if after eating a certain food the white blood count is decreased, some allergists believe that this change indicates a specific allergy to the food that has been eaten. It is a test that is not universally accepted and is infrequently used.

LOCAL REACTION: A reaction that may consist of swelling, itching, and inflammation at the site of the injection of an allergen. This must be differentiated from a *constitutional reaction* which is a generalized reaction, not limited to the site of the injection.

MOLD: The part of a fungus that gets into the air and produces allergy symptoms. The term is often used synonymously with fungus. A more common term is *mildew*.

MUCOSA (MUCOUS MEMBRANE): The lining tissues of the body. They are found in the eye, nose, throat, sinuses, gastrointestinal tract, bladder, and practically every hollow organ. Mucous membrane allergy tests are done in the eye, nose, and bronchi.

MUCUS: A viscid and slippery secretion produced by glands in the mucous membranes which it moistens and protects.

NEURODERMATITIS: This is an old French term frequently shortened and pronounced "neurodermeet" to indicate *allergic eczema* or *atopic eczema,* an inflammatory reaction of the skin marked by itching. It has numerous synonyms. Some of these are Prurigo Besnier, Disseminated Neurodermatitis, Infantile Eczema, Eczematoid Dermatitis, Flexural Eczema. The characteristic locations of the skin inflammation are in the bends of the elbows, the backs of the knees, and on the neck and face. The skin is usually thick and scaly, with evidence of scratching promoted by the accompanying itching.

NON-ALLERGIC: Not due or related to allergy.

NON-SPECIFIC THERAPY: Any treatment not related to the one for the allergy symptoms. It may be a medicine or a protein substance.

OFFENDER: Any material, physical, or psychological agent that is able to produce an allergy reaction. It is used as a loose term for allergen.

PASSIVE TRANSFER: A method of demonstrating the presence of the skin-sensitizing antibody. The technique was first described by Doctors Prausnitz and Küstner and has become known as the *Prausnitz-Küstner test* or reaction. It consists of injecting intradermally (within the layers of the skin) into a non-allergic person at a number of different sites a small amount of the liquid portion of the blood serum of an allergic person. Since this serum contains the allergic antibodies (reagins or skin-sensitizing antibodies), the local area where the subject has been injected becomes allergic to whatever substance the donor is allergic to. If the site is tested with a specific allergen and the test is positive, there will be a characteristic reaction—a hive—at the site. A control test is done with the specific antigen on a site not inoculated with the donor's serum. This test is employed when for any reason it is impractical to do direct skin testing.

PATCH TEST: A type of allergy skin test that is used to determine the cause of *contact dermatitis.* The suspected substance, in proper dilution, is placed on the skin, covered with a cotton or plastic strip, and allowed to remain in place for twenty-four to forty-eight hours. A positive reaction is indicated by redness and itching, at times reproducing in miniature the original rash which is being investigated. Usually several patch tests can be performed at one time.

PHOTOSENSITIVITY: A reaction of the skin to the rays of the sun that occurs only when a person takes certain drugs and medicines. There is a suggested allergic cause which in many instances can be demonstrated.

PHYSICAL ALLERGY: Allergy symptoms due to physical causes such as heat, light, cold, pressure, and even effort. It is believed that the mechanism producing the symptoms is identical with that produced by inhalants, foods, and other allergens, but the antibody is difficult to demonstrate.

POLLEN: The male reproductive agent in plants. When the pollen is wind-borne from one plant to another the atmosphere withholds a considerable amount, and persons who are allergic to pollen will develop symptoms. It is a fine dust and can be seen only under the microscope. The term is also used as an adjective to indicate the cause of symptoms. Examples are *pollen asthma* and *pollen rhinitis. Pollinosis* refers to symptoms due to pollen and is usually applied to nasal symptoms. The term is used often by doctors as a synonym for hay fever.

POLYP: A pendulous projection of the mucous membrane (lining) caused by an excess accumulation of fluid. Nasal polyps are not uncommonly due to allergy. They obstruct breathing and are usually irreversible. However, if produced by allergy to inhalant substances and adequately treated, they often disappear.

POST-NASAL DRIP: A drip of mucus from the back of the nose into and down the throat. This is a common symptom of nasal disturbances where the nasal membrane is so swollen that it does not allow the mucus to be blown out of the nose. In hay fever, where the membrane of the nose is inclined to be water-logged, this is a prominent complaint.

PRAUSNITZ-KÜSTNER TEST: Another name for a Passive transfer test.

PRE-SEASONAL: Before the season, usually referring to allergy injection treatment given before the pollinating season occurs.

PROPEPTAN: A partially digested food extract treated with body enzymes recommended by some as a diagnostic aid and symptomatic treatment for food allergy.

PROTEIN EXTRACT: An extract of the protein portion of the allergen which is used for testing and treating in allergy. The extract is prepared in the same way that an extract of tea or coffee is made, except that there is no boiling or any form of heat used.

PROVOCATIVE TEST: The deliberate use of a suspected allergen in order to reproduce symptoms. When used with foods it is a relatively safe procedure and can be used in conjunction with the elimination or trial diet. (See Elimination Diet and Trial Diet). The use of dry pollen delivered to the nose in order to reproduce symptoms of nasal allergy, or inhaled into the lungs to reproduce asthma, are examples of provocative tests which require more care since the symptoms they produce may be very disturbing. They are not routine procedures, but at times may be necessary.

PSYCHOSOMATIC: Derived from the Greek words for mind and body. The term is used to describe an organic disease of the body (soma) which is influenced or produced by the mind (psyche).

PUNCTURE TEST: A modification of the allergy scratch skin test.

REAGIN: The term given to the allergic antibody found in some people. It is different from the ordinary antibodies, which all people have and which protect them from disease. The reagin is able to sensitize a normal person's skin. When it travels through the blood-stream to a "shock tissue" and joins with its respective antigen, it causes the release of certain chemicals which produce allergy symptoms, instead of protecting the individual by eliminating or reducing symptoms.

REVERSIBLE: Capable of changing from an abnormal state to a normal condition. This is true of many of the allergy diseases when the cause has been removed and treatment instituted; the tissues return to their normal state. It is particularly evident in nasal polyps due to allergy. When they are fully developed they can occlude the entire nasal passageway. If caused by allergy and the cause is determined (e.g., house dust), desensitization with a house dust antigen often reduces the size of the polyps, and the lining of the nose returns to normal.

RHINITIS: Literally, inflammation of the nose, or more exactly, inflammation of the lining of the nose (the nasal membrane or mucosa). A simple "cold" can be considered a rhinitis. In allergy, rhinitis is characterized by watery discharge with itching at the tip of the nose. The nasal membrane is pale and swollen. The various terms used to describe the allergic inflammation are *allergic rhinitis, allergic coryza, hay fever,* and *pollinosis.* Allergic rhinitis is *seasonal* if it occurs only during certain seasons and *perennial* if it occurs throughout the year. *Vasomotor rhinitis,* a purely physiological term that fits all types of rhinitis, is used by some to indicate a rhinitis that has all the symptoms of allergy but in which there is no demonstrable allergy present. Thus, it has the connotation of being due to an emotional disturbance. This is not necessarily true. Strictly speaking, "vasomotor" refers to the state of the blood vessels, either constriction or dilation. Since "allergic" refers to the cause, the term "allergic rhinitis" and "vasomotor rhinitis" are not synonymous.

SCRATCH TEST: One of the methods of testing for the cause of allergy in a suspected sufferer. The allergen is placed on an area of the surface of the skin which has previously been scratched or scarified. A positive reaction is the appearance of a wheal and a surrounding area of redness in ten to thirty minutes. The scratch test is also called the *scarification test;* a variation is known as the *puncture test.*

SECONDARY EFFECTS: Used in connection with adverse drug reactions. An example is the diarrhea that may occur following the excessive use of antibiotics in some persons. This reaction is not due to allergy.

SENSITIZATION: The act of acquiring allergy. It involves primary contact with an antigen after which the specific antibody is produced. At this point the person is sensitized and is ready for the antigen-antibody reaction on subsequent exposure to the same antigen with its attendant symptoms.

SERUM: The liquid portion of the blood from which the clotting element is absent.

SERUM SICKNESS: A type of allergic reaction that may follow the use of a serum, such as tetanus or diphtheria antitoxin and snake antivenoms. The reaction does not appear immediately but may develop ten days to two weeks later. The symptoms are generalized and consist of hives, angioedema, fever, joint pains, and swollen glands. The term *serum sickness type* of allergic reaction is used to describe one that does not have all the characteristics of a true allergic reaction and results from penicillin or other drugs. The symptoms are more severe than those usually encountered in allergy.

SHOCK TISSUE: The type of allergic symptoms that may appear is determined by the location of the antigen-antibody union in the body. The site is called the *shock tissue.* In bronchial asthma, the shock tissue is the wall of the muscles of the small bronchial tubes; in hay fever, the lining of the nose is the shock tissue; in cases of dermatitis or skin allergy, the shock tissue is the skin. Practically any tissue or any organ can be the shock tissue and the allergic individual may have practically any symptom depending on the site.

SIDE EFFECTS: A term usually employed in reference to an adverse reaction to a medicine. The effect is not the one for which the drug was given. It does not necessarily mean that the unwonted effect is caused by allergy.

SINUS: An air cavity within a bone. In the head there are four pairs of sinuses: the frontals in the forehead above the eyes, the maxillaries in the cheekbones on either side of the nose, the sphenoids in the base of the skull, and the ethmoids in the upper part of the head between the top of the nasal cavity and the skull. Any of these sinuses may be involved in allergy, which produces thickened lining membranes and the formation of fluid in the cavities.

SKIN TEST: A method used to demonstrate the presence of allergy and to determine which allergen is at fault. The suspected allergen is introduced into the skin by scarification (scratch or puncture) or by intradermal (intracutaneous) injection. A positive reaction is characterized by a wheal (typical hive) surrounded by a zone of redness (erythema). The severity of the response is measured by the size of the wheal, the presence of pseudopods (irregular protrusions from the wheal), and the amount of erythema surrounding it. Usually the scale used to denote severity is one to four plus (+ to + + + +), a large wheal with several pseudopods indicating the stronger reaction (three to four plus), and a small wheal with little erythema indicating a milder reaction (one to two plus). The *passive transfer* or Prausnitz-Küstner test is another form of skin test used on occasion (see Passive Transfer). The *patch test* is still another in which the suspected allergen is placed in direct contact with the skin for variable length of time (see Patch Test).

SOMATIC: Pertaining to the body (in contrast to *psychic,* which relates to the mind). These two terms, psychic and somatic, are often put together to form *psychosomatic,* a term used by psychologists to indicate the influence of the mind on the body. *Somatopsychic* indicates the effect of bodily illness on the mind.

STATUS ASTHMATICUS: A condition in which the person has severe, persistent bronchial asthma which resists the ordinary methods of treatment. In extreme cases there are changes in the ratio of oxygen and carbon dioxide in the blood. Aggressive treatment must be administered to correct this and to prevent permanent bodily changes.

STOCK VACCINE: A suspension of bacteria obtained from sources other than the cells or secretions of the person who is to receive it. Most stock vaccines are made up of several different kinds of common organisms. A frequently used stock vaccine in allergy is a *respiratory* vaccine, prepared from organisms frequently encountered in respiratory infections.

SUBCUTANEOUS: Under the skin. (*Subdermal* is a synonym.) Subcutaneous injections are the usual form employed in allergy desensitization (hyposensitization) therapy, and must be differentiated from those which are *intradermal* (within the layers of the skin), *intramuscular* (into the muscle), and *intravenous* (into the vein).

SYSTEMIC REACTION: Synonymous with *constitutional reaction,* indicating a series of generalized symptoms resulting from the administration of an allergen.

THERAPY: Treatment.

THERAPEUTIC TEST: The use of a given drug or form of treatment to verify the diagnosis. An example in allergy is the use of an injection of epinephrine to relieve an asthmatic attack. If relief is obtained the diagnosis is verified. Non-allergy examples are the use of quinine for certain types of malaria, and colchicine for gout. Another is relief of a runny nose or hives by antihistamines. Sometimes a therapeutic test is used to differentiate one disease from another (differential diagnosis). For example, if asthma is relieved by the use of a medicine which aids the function of the heart muscle, a diagnosis of *cardiac asthma* rather than *bronchial asthma* is made.

TISSUE FLUID: The fluid that bathes all the cells of the body. It acts as an intermediary between the cells and the blood in the very small blood vessels.

TOXICITY: This is a term used in connection with adverse reactions to drugs. Literally it means "a state or degree of being poisonous," but since practically all medicines used may be poisonous if given in large enough doses, toxicity does not indicate a true poison in the common meaning of the word. Usually allergy is not involved in adverse (toxic) reactions.

TOXIN: Any poisonous substance of microbic, vegetable, or animal origin. When injected into the animal or human body, it stimulates the production of the antitoxin which is its antibody.

TOXOID: A toxin which has been deprived of its poisonous quality but is still able to stimulate the production of antitoxin. This form is almost universally used today as immunization injections against tetanus and diphtheria. It is sometimes used in other diseases as well.

TRIAL DIET: The use of a diet excluding foods that are suspected as the cause of the person's allergy symptoms. If symptoms are relieved on the trial diet, it can be assumed that one or more of the foods which have been excluded is the cause. (See Elimination Diet.)

TUBERCULIN TEST: An allergy skin test to indicate the susceptibility of an individual to tuberculosis. The test is done in exactly the same manner as the allergy intradermal test, using as the testing material or allergen an extract of killed tuberculosis bacteria, properly diluted. The delayed reaction does not become positive until twenty-four to forty-eight hours after the injection. In addition, the reaction is not just a wheal and flare reaction like the reaction to direct allergy tests, but is a deeper involvement of the skin, with swelling and inflammation. There are alternatives to the intradermal tuberculin test for tuberculosis: one is the scarification test; another is the patch test.

URTICARIA: Hives or nettlerash. The origin of the term is the plant *urticatus,* which produces a characteristic hive on contact—even in people who are not allergic. The lesion is a raised white wheal (hive) surrounded by a zone of redness (erythema). The hives may range in size from the head of a pin to a silver dollar or larger. There may be just one hive but usually there are many scattered all over the body. Some may run into each other to form several immense wheals with large irregular outlines. When the deeper structures are involved in the process the urticaria is called *giant hives, angioedema,* or *angioneurotic edema.*

VACCINE: An extract prepared from live or dead bacteria or viruses. Although a vaccine may be used for testing and for treatment, it is primarily employed to provide immunization from disease. *Poliomyelitis vaccine* and *smallpox vaccine* are examples. Sometimes allergy protein extracts or other allergy extracts used for diagnosis and treatment are termed vaccines. This is an erroneous use of the word.

VERNAL CONJUNCTIVITIS: An inflammation of the mucous membrane which lines the eyelids and is reflected into the eyeball (conjunctiva). The term "vernal" would appear to signify that this condition is most prevalent in the spring but this is not precisely so since it may occur at any time of the year, and very commonly occurs in the fall or all year around. Vernal conjunctivitis is usually considered an allergy disease, but the detection of the cause and response to allergy treatment are not as satisfactory as in other allergy diseases. For that reason some feel that it is not always or entirely due to allergy and that there are other factors, as yet unknown, that can produce it.

WHEAL: The raised white lesion that is characteristic of a hive and of the positive allergy skin test. It is usually surrounded by a zone of redness (erythema), and is actually a localized swelling of the skin.

Index

Abalone as mollusks, 107
ACTH (adrenal hormone), 128
Agranulocytosis, 246
Air conditioners, 154, 158, 171, 230
Allergens, definition of, 10
Allergic coryza, *see* Allergic rhinitis
Allergic rhinitis (hay fever), 27, 28, 95, 96, 217,
    243, 246, 247, 259, 309
  bronchial asthma and, 24
  cause of, 2-3, 6, 7, 9, 11, 12, 21-22, 139, 141,
    152-53, 160, 275, 277, 279, 285, 289,
    302, 308, 335
  diagnosis of, 104, 150, 155-56, 307
  drug reaction and, 90-91
  eczema and, 213, 216, 223
  headaches and, 234, 257-58, 336-37
  history of, 24, 29
  occupational allergies and, 268, 275, 277, 279
  as perennial, 61, 149, 152, 153, 170
  as seasonal, 149-51, 170
  treatment for, 85-87, 156-57, 171, 327
  See also Pollen; Ragweed
Allergy
  definition of, 5-6, 8-10, 17
  diagnosis of, 309
  explanation of, 14-15
  treatment of, 310-11, 322-40
  See also specific allergy
Almonds, 105
Amino acids, use of, 338
Aminopyrine, 128-29
Anemias, 129, 246, 287, 295, 296
Anaphylaxis, definition of, 5, 12
Anergex treatment, 325, 339
Anesthetics, reactions to, 127, 133-34, 138
Angina pectoris, 243-44, 258
Angioedema, *see* Hives
Angora hair, *see* Goat hair allergy
Animals, allergy to, 22, 28
  hairs of, 9, 15, 21, 23, 35, 62-69, 76, 88, 93,
    150, 154, 182, 213, 216, 274-75, 282,
    283, 286, 302, 317, 318, 326
  See also specific animal
Ant bites, reaction to, 139, 148
Anthrax, 261
Antibiotics, reaction to, 22, 126, 128, 129, 138,
    265

Antibodies
  definition of, 10-11
  formation of, 15-17
  theory of blocking, 81, 91
Antigen-antibody reaction, definition of, 10-11,
    13-14
Antigens, definition of, 10, 11
Antihistamines, reactions to, 121, 133, 138
Antitoxins, *see specific antitoxin*
Anus, itching of, 250, 253-54, 260
Aphids, allergy to, 76, 79
Aphthous stomatitis, 250-51, 259
Apiarist's asthma, 275
Aplastic anemia, 129
Argyrol for nasal allergy, 328, 339
Arsenic, reaction to, 128, 129, 134, 332, 340
Arteritis, *see* Collagen diseases
Arthropods, 107, 119
Asparagus, 105
Aspirin, drug allergy and, 123, 124, 132, 138,
    176, 210
Asthma, 95, 261, 301, 308
  allergic rhinitis and, 170
  bronchial asthma and, 202-4
  causes of, 11, 21, 68-69, 74, 132-33, 302-6,
    309, 316
  definition of, 173, 175-76
  diet diary and, 99
  drug reaction and, 125, 137, 138
  eczema and, 213, 216, 223
  exercise and, 23
  insect bites and, 139, 141
  physical allergies and, 226
  tests for, 104
  treatments for, 7, 135, 310, 322-23, 325-27,
    329-32, 334-35, 337-39
  See also Bronchial asthma
Asthma powders, 323
Athlete's foot, 221, 224
Atomic explosions, anemia and, 129
Atopic dermatitis, *see* Eczema
Atopy, definition of, 12
Autohemotherapy, 210, 324-25
Autoimmune disease, 242, 245, 249, 252, 285-
    87, 292, 295, 297, 298

361

Bacon allergy, 107
Bacteria, dust and, 62, 67, 70, 71, 76
Bagassosis, 273
Baker's asthma, 273-74, 283
Banana allergy, 102
Barbituates, reaction to, 124, 127, 230
Bathrooms, allergies and, 316-17
Baths for eczema, 214-15
Bean allergy, 35, 275, 282, 283
Bedbug allergy, 76, 79, 139, 148
Bedrooms, allergies and, 313-16
Bed wetting, 256, 260
Bee allergy, 6, 45, 125, 139, 41, 143-45, 147,
    148, 275, 327
Beef allergy, 107, 108
    See also Meats
Beetle allergy, 76, 79
Berylliosis, cause of, 277
Bird feathers, see Feather allergy
Blood
    abnormalities of, 128, 137
    injection of, 210, 324-25
    sample of, 326, 339
Bone granulomas, 296, 298
Botanical relationships, 105-7, 119
Box elder bugs, 139
Breast-fed baby, allergies and, 22
Breathing, 174-75
    exercises for, 197-201, 206
    oxygen for, 201-2
Bronchial asthma, 217, 225, 243, 244, 285
    allergic rhinitis and, 24, 150
    asthma and, 202-4
    causes of, 11, 24, 125, 176, 203-5, 267-69,
        274-77, 279, 309
    complications from, 179-81
    definition of, 173, 177-79, 204
    treatment for, 39, 178, 181-202, 205-6, 328,
        334, 335
    See also Asthma
Bronchial inhalation tests, 39, 42
Bronchitis, 24, 76, 170, 180, 205, 269, 278
Buckwheat allergy, 102
Buerger's disease, 245
Butterfly allergy, 76, 79, 153

Calcium treatment, 335-36, 340
Camel hair allergy, 69
Canker sores, 250-51, 259
Cardiovascular system, allergy of, 242-46, 258
Castor bean allergy, 73, 74, 79, 275, 282, 283
Cat hair allergy, 9, 21, 23, 63-64, 76-77, 309
Cataracts, allergy and, 249

Cathartics, rash from, 22, 209, 210
Cattle hair allergy, 70, 77
Celery allergy, 102
Cellulose, 62, 76
Central nervous system, allergies of, 233-45
Cereal allergy, 75, 102, 105, 118, 213, 273, 283
Chemicals, reactions to, 94, 127, 167, 220, 224,
    265-68, 275, 279, 283
    See also Medicines; Plastics; specific chemical
Chicken allergy, 22, 102, 107
    feathers and, 10, 69, 78, 133, 315
Chihuahua dog as asthma cure, 325-26, 339
Children, homes for asthmatic, 197, 331, 340
Chloral hydrate for asthma, 192
Chocolate allergy, 102, 208, 239
Chrome dermatitis, 264, 267, 283
Cigarettes for asthma, 323-24
    See also Tobacco smoke
Clams as mollusks, 107, 119
Cleaning, allergies and, 314-15
Climatic treatment, 330-31, 340
Clonal selection theory, 15-18
Closets, allergies and, 318
Cluster headache, 234
Coal tar allergy, 262
Cocaine for asthma, 192-93
Cockroaches, bites of, 140
Cocoa butter allergy, 254
Codeine, 168, 197
Coffee allergy, 73-75, 79, 275, 283
Cold, allergy to, 225, 227-28, 232, 244
Colic, 253, 260
Colitis, 251-52, 259, 287
Collagen diseases, 130, 137, 285, 287, 291-98
Conjunctiva, 37-38, 41-42, 65, 247-48, 260
Contact dermatitis, 207, 217-24, 246-47, 262-
    68, 279, 319
    See also Eczema; Hives; Rash; Skin
Corn allergy, 102, 108, 273, 318
Cornea, inflammation of, 248
Coronary insufficiency, 244
Cortisone
    gland production of, 179, 301
    side effects of, 194-96, 205
Cosmetics, reactions to, 39, 72, 220, 224, 246-
    47, 259, 264-65, 317
Cotton allergy, 150, 274, 315
Cottonseed allergy, 35, 61, 67, 70, 78, 102, 108,
    315
Crab allergy, 6, 107, 119
Crayfish as arthropods, 107
Crohn's disease, 252
Cutaneous tests, see Scratch tests
Cystic fibrosis, 202-3
Cystourethritis, 256, 260

Decongestants, 209
Dehumidifiers, 333, 340
Dermatitis, *see* Contact dermatitis; Eczema; Hives; Skin eruptions
Dermatomyositis, 291, 292
Desensitization, 80-93, 145-46, 148, 159-67, 169, 171, 182, 205, 216, 225-28, 231, 233, 235, 237, 240, 255-56, 258, 281-82, 284, 302
Desert air lamp, 333
Detergents, 153, 214, 218, 266-67, 283, 317
Devil's darning needle, bite of, 142
Diabetes, steroid usage and, 194, 195, 205
Diagnostic food ingestion test, 96, 103-4, 119
Diets, 96, 99-104, 119, 235-36, 311-12, 320, 329-30, 339
Diptera, bite of, 141
Diptheria antitoxin, 4, 6, 7, 13, 22, 90, 245
Disseminated lupus, 287, 291, 298
Dog hair allergy, 23, 62-63, 76-77, 88
Dragonfly, bites of, 142
Drugs, *see* Medicines
Duck feather allergy, 10, 69, 78, 315
Dusts, 23, 28, 182
  in house, 9, 10, 15, 39, 61-62, 67, 74, 76, 88, 93, 150, 153, 154, 167, 170, 235, 257
  in occupational allergies, 266, 269, 273, 274, 276, 283
  to prevent, 156-59, 171, 315-16, 318, 326
  See also Molds; Pollen
Dyes, reaction to, 134, 138, 230, 264, 267, 278-79, 283, 319, 321

Ear, allergies of, 254-56, 260
Eczema, 207, 212-16, 222, 223, 249, 254, 259, 260, 263, 285, 307, 308
  cause of, 9, 11, 127, 141, 234, 309
  drug reaction and, 125-27, 137
  history of, 36-37
  tests for, 36-37
  treatment of, 310-11
Effort, allergy to, 225, 232
Eggs, allergy to, 2, 7, 15, 95, 102, 107-10, 118, 133, 181, 213, 239
Elm tree allergy, 47, 59
Emotional factors in allergy, 25-26, 29, 155-56, 195, 205, 211, 214, 223, 235, 236, 241, 253, 299-306
Emphysema, 179-80, 197-202, 204-6
Endocarditis, 245, 259
Endophthalmitis phacoanphlactica, 249, 287
Enuresis, allergies and, 256, 260
Environmental factors, 22-23, 28, 29
Enzymes, reactions to, 133

Eosinophiles, definition of, 27
Ephedrine, 184, 205, 226, 269, 277, 282
Epilepsy, 128, 129, 241-42, 258
Epinephrine, 182-83, 210, 269, 277, 282
Ergot, 242
Erythromycin, reactions to, 132
Ether for asthma, 192
Excipients, reactions to, 134
Expectorants for asthma, 185
Eye, allergies of, 166, 246-53, 260, 286

Farmer's lung, 273
Feather allergy, 61, 62, 67, 69-70, 76, 78, 88, 93, 108, 150, 182, 213, 216, 274, 311, 315
Fertilizers, food allergies and, 94
Filters, 156-59, 171, 181
Fireplace, allergies and, 316, 321
Fish allergy, 4-5, 7, 35, 102, 107, 119, 208, 239
Flaxseed allergy, 22-23, 35, 71-72, 78-79, 274, 316
Fleas, reactions to, 23, 76, 79, 139, 142, 148, 211-12, 223
Flour, inhaling of, 73, 79, 274, 275
Fly allergy, 76, 79, 139, 141, 148, 153, 274
Food allergy, 9, 10, 22, 35, 41, 42, 82, 91-92, 94-119, 130, 153, 154, 173, 181, 208, 209, 213, 222, 234-36, 239, 241, 243, 244, 248, 250, 252, 254, 256-57, 259, 260, 286, 301, 311, 317, 320, 326
  See also Diets; *specific food*
Frankfurters, ingredients of, 112
Fruit allergy, 97, 119, 208, 213
  See also specific fruit
Fume allergy, 40
Fungus spores, 170
  See also Molds
Fur allergy, 65, 68-69, 78, 275, 283, 318
Furnaces, filters for, 157-58, 171

Gallbladder disease, 252-53, 261
Garlic, 105
Gases, allergies and, 40, 269
Gastrointestinal tract, 28, 29, 94, 95, 250-54, 260
Gay treatment for asthma, 332, 340
Genitourinary tract, allergies of, 257-58, 261
Glandular treatment, 329-30, 339
Glomectomy, 202, 206
Glue, inhaling of, 73, 79, 274
Gnat bites, 139
Goat hair allergy, 65, 66, 77, 316, 318

Gold for asthma, 327, 339
Gold salts, reactions to, 124, 128, 129
Goose feathers, 10, 69, 78, 315
Grains, inhalation of, 272-74, 283
  See also specific grain
Granulomas, 296, 298
Grass, *see* Pollen; *specific grass*
Gums, inhaling of, 73, 79

Hair, human, 68, 153
  See also Animals
Halogens, reaction to, 278
Ham allergy, 107
Hapamine treatment, 333, 340
Haptens, definition of, 11
Hashimoto's goitre, 287
Hashimoto's thyroiditis, 286
Hay fever, *see* Allergic rhinitis
Headaches, 28, 233-40, 257, 258
Heart, allergies and, 195, 205, 243-45, 259
Heat, allergy to, 225-30, 232, 244
Heat lamps, 168, 333-34
Heleidae insects, 142
Hematopoietic disturbances, 246
Hemolytic anemia, 295, 296
Hemp, inhaling of, 73, 74, 79
Heredity of allergies, 9, 12, 16-17, 18, 25
  See also History of patients
Herpes simplex, 248
Histamine
  desensitization with, 228, 240-41, 258
  reaction of, 255-56
  release of, 11, 14, 225, 231, 232, 333
Histamine cephalalgia, 234, 240-41, 258
History of patients, 19-29, 96-98, 119, 209-10,
  237, 250, 258, 279-80, 284, 308, 320, 321
Hives, 4-5, 7, 9, 11, 23, 31, 33, 35, 48, 95, 104,
  125, 126, 132, 135-38, 142, 207-13, 217,
  222, 226-32, 282, 285, 295, 307, 310, 324-
  25, 336
Hog hair allergy, 68, 317
Homograft, 285, 288-91, 297
Honey
  for allergies, 326-27, 339
  as allergy, 102
Hormones, reactions to, 127, 128
Hornets, 1, 7, 139-41, 144, 145, 148
Horse hair allergy, 64-65, 76, 77
Horse serum, 64-65, 208-9
Hydroarthrosis, intermittent, 257, 260
Hydrochloric acid, 337
Hypersensitivity, definition of, 12

Hypersensitivity vasculitis, *see* Collagen diseases
Hypertension, allergy and, 244, 258
Hyposensitization, *see* Desensitization

"Id" reactions, 130-31, 207, 221-22, 224
Idiopathic thrombocytopenic purpura, 291, 296
Idiosyncratic reaction, 13, 17, 122, 123, 136
Ileitis, 252
Immunizations, reaction to, 22
  See also Vaccines; *specific immunization*
Infrared lamp, use of, 333
Ingestion, food allergies and provocative, 96,
  103-4, 119
Inhalants, *see specific inhalant*
Inhalation tests, 280-81, 284
Injection, giving of, 88-89, 91, 93
  See also Desensitization; *specific injection*
Insecticide allergy, 71, 94, 182
Insects, contact with, 1, 6, 7, 67, 75-76, 79, 139-
  53, 209, 211, 223, 274
  See also specific insect
Insulin reaction, 133, 138
Intestinal tract allergies, 251-52
Intractable asthma, 178, 204
Intradermal (intracutaneous) tests, 34-36, 41,
  98, 171, 280
Iodides, reaction to, 124, 128, 129, 134
Ionizing devices, 332-33, 340
Iontophoresis tests, 41, 42
Isoproterenol, 183-84
Italian ryegrass, 3, 7

Jaundice, 129, 130, 135, 137
Joints, allergies of, 257, 260
June grass allergy, 49
Jute, inhaling of, 73, 74, 79

Kapok allergy, 35, 62, 71, 76, 78, 182, 274, 302,
  315
Keratitis, 248, 259
Keratoconus, definition of, 249
Kissing bugs, 139, 142
Kitchens, allergies and, 317-18, 321

Lamb allergy, 49
Lard allergy, 107
Latex fixation test, 294

Lens cataracts, 249
Lermoyez' syndrome, 255, 296
Leucocytes, extract of, 337
Lice bites, 139
Lichen simplex chronicus, 216, 223
Lids (eye), rash on, 246-47
Light, allergy to, 225, 228-30, 232
Linseed allergy, 71-72, 78-79, 316-18
Liver allergy, 102, 107
Liver disease, 129, 130, 137, 252, 260, 269
Living rooms, allergies and, 316
Lobster, 95, 107, 119, 209
Loeffler's syndrome, 274
Lupus erythematosus, 287, 291-94, 298

Maple bark disease, 275
Maple tree allergy, 59
Marihuana allergy, 74
Measles antitoxin, 90, 91
Meats, allergy relationship of, 107, 119
Medicines, reactions to, 11, 13, 17, 21-22, 120-
    41, 173, 176, 178, 182-96, 205, 209, 210,
    222, 249, 250, 252, 254, 259, 265-66, 283,
    292, 295, 301, 310, 320
    See also specific medicine
Melon allergy, 102
Mendelian law, 6, 18
Meniere's disease, 255, 260
Meperidine for asthma, 192
Mercury drugs, reactions to, 124, 129, 133, 134
Metal allergy, 254, 267, 276-78, 282-84, 319,
    321
Migraine headaches, 1, 2, 234, 235, 237-40,
    258, 302
Milk
    allergy to, 1, 2, 24, 95, 108-9, 134, 213, 236,
        242, 253, 254
    foods containing, 110-11
    penicillin reaction and, 126, 130, 210
    as treatment, 327-28, 338, 340
Miller's asthma, 273-74
Mineral waters, 330-32
Miner's asthma, 273
Mites, bites of, 140
Molds (mildew), 10, 22, 62, 67, 70, 71, 74-76,
    79, 88, 93, 153-54, 158, 248, 259, 273
Mollusks, 107, 119
Monkey allergy, 68, 78
Morphine for asthma, 192, 193
Mosquito bites, 6, 139, 140, 148, 209
Mosquito hawk, 142
Moth allergy, 76, 79, 318
Mouth, allergies of, 250-51

Mucus thinners, 184-85, 205
Multiple sclerosis, 242, 258
Mustard allergy, 35
Myocarditis, 245, 259

Nasal allergy, 24, 328, 339
Nasal inhalation ("sniff") tests, 38-39, 42
Nasal manipulation, 336, 340
Negative ions, 332-33
Nettle rash, see Hives
Nettlefish allergy, 4-5
Neurodermatitis, see Eczema
Nosaki for allergy, 337
Nose, filters for, 158
Nose drops, 159-60, 167, 171, 183, 236, 237,
    258, 330, 339-40
Novocain, reactions to, 133
Nut allergy, 35, 97, 102, 105, 208, 239, 251

Oak tree allergy, 59
Oat allergy, 102, 273
Occupational allergies, 261-84
Ocelot allergy, 64
Onion, 105
Ophthalmia, sympathetic, 249, 286
Optic nerve edema, 249-50, 262
Orchard grass allergy, 49
Organ transplants, see Homograft
Organic compounds, reaction to, 278-79
Oriental rug allergy, 63, 68
Orris root allergy, 39, 72, 79, 317
Osteoporosis, cortisone usage and, 194, 195
Oxygen for asthma, 201-2
Oysters as mollusks, 107, 119

Papular urticaria, 211-12, 223
    See also Hives
Passive transfer tests, 36-37, 41, 229
Patch tests, 39-40, 217, 224, 266-67, 277, 280,
    284, 319
Pea allergy, 102, 105, 239
Peach allergy, 105
Peanut allergy, 239
Penicillin, reactions to, 124, 126-31, 133, 136-
    38, 209, 210, 222, 243, 257, 265, 292, 295,
    308
    identification card for, 134
Periarteritis nodosa, 291-92, 298
Perfumes, allergy to, 72, 79, 154, 167, 317

Pericarditis, 245, 259, 287
Pertussis, *see* Whooping cough
Petroleum product allergy, 262
Pets *see* Animals; *specific animal*
Phenacetin, reactions to, 128
Phenobarbital for asthma, 192
Phenolphthalein, rash from, 22
Phenothiazine medicines, 129
Photosensitivity reaction, 128, 229, 230
Physical allergies, 225-32, 244
Physical examination for allergy, 27, 29
Pigweed allergy, 49
Piromen, 337, 340
Plants, allergy to, 268, 283
    See also Pollen; *specific plant*
Plastics, reactions to, 220-21, 262, 269-72, 283
Pleurisy, 287
Pneumoconiosis, dust and, 273
Poison ivy, 8, 12, 127, 137, 217, 221, 223, 262, 268, 283, 308, 319, 321, 337
Poison oak, 8, 127, 137, 217, 221, 223, 268, 283, 319, 321, 339
    extract from, 325
Poison sumac, 8, 127, 137, 217, 224, 268, 283, 319, 321
Polio vaccines, 25, 90, 91, 130
Pollen, 3, 6, 7, 10, 15, 22, 43-60, 86-87, 92-93, 156-59, 173, 205, 248, 262, 312, 320, 323, 326, 331
    See also Allergic rhinitis; Ragweed allergy
Polyarteritis, 291-92, 298
Polyps, 167, 169, 171, 334
Poplar tree allergy, 59
Pork allergy, 102, 107, 208, 239
Porphyria, 230
Post-myocardial infarction syndrome, 287
Potassium iodide, 123, 337, 340
Potato allergy, 102
Prausnitz-Küstner tests, 36-37, 41, 229
Pregnancy
    bronchial asthma and, 181
    endocarditis in, 245
    migraine headaches and, 239
Pressure, allergy to, 225, 231-32
Prick (puncture) tests, 34, 41
Primrose, reaction to, 268
Printer's allergies, 268, 276, 283
Procaine treatment, 328-29, 339
Propeptans, 96, 104, 118, 119
Protein hydrolysates, 338
Prunes, 105
Pruritis ani, 250, 253-54, 260
Pruritis vulvae, 256-57, 260
Psoriasis, 216-17
Psychological relationship, *see* Emotional factors

Pulmonary eosinophilia, transient, 274
Pulmonary fibrosis, 270
Pulse-counting technique, 96, 104, 119
Puncture (prick) tests, 34, 41
Punkies, bites of, 142
Purpura, definition of, 128, 137, 246, 291, 295-96
Pyrethrum, allergy to, 71, 78

Quinine allergy, 124, 127, 129

Rabbit hair allergy, 65-66, 76, 77
Rabies, 25
Ragweed allergy, 3, 7, 9, 44, 47, 49, 59, 91, 96, 160, 289, 327, 331
    See also Allergic rhinitis; Pollen
Rash, 11, 20, 22, 29, 123, 132-34, 137, 138, 229, 261, 309, 310, 319, 321
    See also Contact dermatitis; Eczema; Hives; Skin eruptions; *specific rash*
Reagins, 13, 15, 80-81, 139
    See also Antibodies
Rectum, allergies of, 253-54
Redtop grass allergy, 59
Regional enteritis, 252
Resins, inhaling of, 73, 79
Respiratory diseases, occupational allergies and, 268-79
Respiratory vaccine therapy, 334, 340
Retinal detachment, 250, 259
Rheumatic fever, 291, 294-95, 298
Rheumatoid arthritis, 258, 287, 291, 294
Ringworms, reaction to, 221, 224
Rose fever, *see* Allergic rhinitis
Russian thistle allergy, 49
Rusts, *see* Molds
Rye allergy, 49, 273, 274, 318

Sagebrush allergy, 49
Salicylates, reactions to, 124
Sand fly, 142, 153
Sausage allergy, 107
Sawdust allergy, 73, 75, 79
Scallops, 107, 119
Schönlein-Henoch purpura, 295, 296
Sclera, 249, 259
Scleroderma, 291-93
Scorpion bites, 139
Scratch tests, 31-35, 41, 98, 153, 171, 280
Seborrheic dermatitis, 216

Secretory otitis, 170
"Self-allergy," see Autoimmune disease
Sensitization, definition of, 12
Serum sickness, 125-26, 130, 137, 295
Shellfish allergy, 35, 102, 107, 119, 208
Shock tissue, definition of, 11-12
Shrimps, 107, 119
Side effects of drugs, 121-23, 136
    See also Medicines
Silk allergy, 35, 73, 79, 316
Sinusitis, 167-69, 171, 236, 237, 326, 334
Sisal, inhaling of, 73, 74, 79
Sjögren's syndrome, 286-87
Skin, allergies of, 126-28, 136, 207-24
    See also Contact dermatitis; Eczema; Hives;
       Rash
Skin tests, 3, 7, 15, 30-37, 39-42, 48, 65, 71, 83-
    84, 94, 98-99, 118, 119, 125, 131, 136,
    150, 171, 210, 217, 222, 224, 225, 235,
    237, 239, 250, 253, 257, 266-67, 277, 279-
    81, 308, 309, 319, 320
Sleeping pills, reactions to, 21-22
Smallpox vaccine, 4, 25, 90, 91, 214, 223
Smoke inhalation, 197, 205, 316
    See also Tobacco smoke
Smuts, see Molds
Snails as mollusks, 119
"Sniff" tests, 38-39, 42
Soybean allergy, 73, 79, 275, 283
Spas, 330-31, 340
Spice allergy, 208
Spider bites, 139
Spleen, extract of, 337
Sprays, nasal, 159-60, 167, 171, 183, 236, 237,
    258
Squirrel hair, 69
Staphylococcus bacteriophage, 334, 340
Status asthmaticus, 178-79, 193, 201-2, 204
Steam inhalation, 168, 185, 205
Steroids, see Cortisone
Stomach, allergies of, 251
Strawberry allergy, 6, 9
Streptomycin, reactions to, 127
Sublingual tests, 41, 42, 104, 119
Sulfa drugs, reaction to, 124, 127-29, 131-32,
    138, 229, 230, 292
Sweets, allergy to, 97
Sympathetic ophthalmia, 249, 286
Symptoms, systematic review of, 26-27, 29
Syphilis, "id" reaction to, 221

Template theory, 15-18
Testing solutions, strength of, 35

Tests, diagnostic, 30-42, 309
    See also specific test
Tetanus antitoxin, 4, 7, 25, 65, 91, 125, 245,
    250
Tetracyclines, reactions to, 132, 138
Textile allergy, 263-65, 282, 283
Thalidomide, 123
Theophylline for asthma, 184
Thouricil, reaction to, 129
Thromboangiitis obliterans, 245, 258
Tick bites, 140
Timothy grass allergy, 49
Tobacco leaf allergy, 267-68, 283
Tobacco smoke, 72, 79, 93, 167, 235, 243-45,
    258
Tomato allergy, 102
Toxic reactions, 122
Tranquilizers, 129, 191-92
Transplant, see Homograft
Trees, pollination of, 49, 59, 152, 153
    See also specific tree
Tuberculosis, 40, 195, 221, 278
Turkey feathers, allergy to, 78
Typhoid vaccine, 211, 334-35
Tyral for allergy, 337

Ulcerative colitis, 287
Ulcers, 194-95, 205, 251-52
Undecylinic acid, use of, 337-38
Urine injections for allergies, 324, 339
Urticaria, see Hives
Uveal tract, allergy of, 249

Vaccines, 107-8, 133, 138, 166, 169, 334-35,
    340
    See also specific vaccine
Vasomotor rhinitis, see Allergic rhinitis
Veal allergy, 107
Vegetable oils, 108
Velvet grass allergy, 49
Vitamins
    for allergies, 335, 340
    elimination diets and, 103
    reaction to, 22, 209, 210

Walnut tree allergy, 47, 59
Wasps
    description of, 141
    desensitization to, 145
    eradication of, 143, 144
    reactions to, 139, 140, 148, 152

Weather, allergies and, 154, 197, 205, 209
Weeds, 49, 152, 153, 182
    See also Pollen; *specific weed*
Weevils, inhaled allergy to, 76, 79
Wheals, *see* Hives
Wheat, allergy to, 95, 96, 102, 109, 111-12,
    213, 239, 273, 318
Whooping cough, 40
    immunization for, 25
Wood allergy, 266, 274-76, 283, 316, 321
Wool allergy, 61, 62, 66-67, 76, 77, 88, 93, 150,
    181, 182, 209, 263, 315, 316
    See also Textile allergy

X rays, aplastic anemia and, 129

Yellow jackets
    description of, 141
    desensitization to, 145
    eradication of, 143-44
    reaction to, 139, 140, 148

Date Due